Fish, Omega-3 and Human Health

Fish, Omega-3 and Human Health

Second Edition

William E.M. Lands

AOCS PRESS

Champaign, Illinois

AOCS Mission Statement
To be the global forum for professionals interested in lipids and related materials through the exchange of ideas, information, science, and technology.

The paper used in this book is acid-free and falls within the guidelines established to ensure permanence and durability.

Library of Congress Cataloging-in-Publication Data
Lands, William E. M., 1930–
Fish, Omega-3 and human health / by William E.M. Lands.-- 2nd ed.
p. cm.
Includes bibliographical references and index.
ISBN 1-893997-81-2 (alk. paper)
1. Fish as food. 2. Heart--Diseases--Nutritional aspects. 3. Essential fatty acids in human nutrition. I. Title.

QP144.F56L36 2005
616.1'20654--dc22

2005002993

CIP

Printed in the United States of America.
16 15 14 13 12 5 4 3 2

A full, balanced life
Has many events
Known and unsensed
Transient and enduring.

We treat and prevent
With mineral and nutrient
From seas and lands
Of fish and man.

Contents

Foreword ix
Preface xi
Introduction xiii

Part 1. Relating Diet to Disease
1 Epidemiology and Curiosity 3
2 Foods, Drugs, and Disease Mechanisms 13
3 Essential Fatty Acids 21
4 Common Factors in Heart Disease, Heart Attacks, and Strokes 31
5 Heart Disease: Atherosclerosis and Serum Lipids 33
6 Heart Attack: Coronary Thrombosis 47
7 Vasospasm: Cardiac Output and Coronary Flow 63
8 Strokes 71
9 Hypertension 75
10 Immune Responses 83
11 Cell Proliferation and Cancer 105

Part 2. Metabolic Differences Among Polyunsaturated Fatty Acids
12 Maps and the Unknown 115
13 Acyl-CoA Pathways 120
14 Pathways to Prostaglandins 139
15 Prostaglandin Formation Following Changes in Diet 152
16 Pathways to Leukotrienes 155

Part 3. Choosing Diets
17 Polyunsaturated Acids in Tissues and Foods 163
18 Overall Supply of n-3 Fatty Acids 171
19 Alternative Diets 186

Glossary 201
About the Author 213
Index 215

Foreword

I am pleased to recommend *Fish, Omega-3 and Human Health* to all readers interested in the basis of disease and nutritional strategies that can be used to support better health. Valuable insights can be gained on many diverse topics. What is amazing is that everyone, from the layman interested in good nutrition to research scientists who specialize in essential fatty acids, can gain valuable insights from this book. Graduate students will find many directives for important thesis projects for many years to come. Bill Lands unfolds his story in a most readable manner, starting from the beginning and gaining technical force as he finishes chapters with technical sections. He has a passion for the prevention of eicosanoid-mediated disease; disease that he convincingly shows can be prevented or diminished by more careful selection of the foods that we eat. His thesis is that we must better balance n-3 and n-6 fatty acid intake to moderate an over active eicosanoid system that is leading to the development of many of the chronic inflammatory diseases that plague the present day industrialized world. Chapters 13 and 14 were especially delightful for me, his insightful analysis of fatty acid and lipid metabolism and eicosanoid formation and regulation. His perspective and broad scope is one gained from the brilliant research career of a pioneer in these areas.

Norm Salem, 2004
2002 AOCS/Supelco Research Awardee

Preface to the Second Edition

This second edition of *Fish, Omega-3 and Human Health* reaffirms that essential fatty acids in the foods we eat form hormones that have powerful effects on human life. Many find it hard to believe that a simple change of diet can affect so many things in their lives. This second edition adds information to help readers sense the slow shift in attitudes about the relationship between foods and disease.

Since the first edition in 1986, the names for n-3 and n-6 structures became known as omega-3 and omega-6. However, understanding of how food choices affect so many serious aspects of life was delayed by two general attitudes. One attitude had faulty logic in interpreting some associated markers as causal mediators of disease and death, and the other attitude was a bias for curative/treatment interventions that neglected preventing initial dietary causes of disease and death. This edition expands the glossary of words and concepts to help readers recognize how specific nutrient imbalances in our normal diets can contribute to disease and death.

I thank the various editors who have invited me to reflect on my absorbing and enjoyable career of discovery, especially Mary Lane who assured me that I could update this book and Howard Knapp and Jodey Schonfeld who helped me be diplomatic. I also thank the AOCS which awarded me the 1997 Supelco/Nicholas Pelick-AOCS Research Award.

Above all, I thank the friends who shared my curiosity and helped me find words to speak of my own slow step-by-step growth in understanding: Norberta Schoene, Etienne Lamoreaux, Pat Springer, Bill Smith, Lenny Rome, Martin Hemler and Rich Kulmacz. Also, I thank the many colleagues who published the hundreds of interesting research reports that make *Fish, Omega-3 and Human Health* a rich field of discovery.

I hope that the new information will help people build a positive attitude toward changing harmful food habits and building a better quality of life. Preventing children from developing nutritional imbalances before the problems become severe is likely every parent's goal. My parents have died, and another generation has arrived since the first edition. I hope that some of what we now know will help my four great-grandchildren have a long healthy life. May this small book help all who read it enjoy a long, healthy life with their families filled with understanding and love.

William E. M. Lands

Preface to the First Edition

Curiosity is the beginning of understanding, and a steady pursuit of our questions seems to always lead us into new adventures and new understandings. When I was a young child, my mother and father explained to me why eating undercooked pork was often not safe. In doing so, they created for me a new understanding of how the custom of forsaking this form of food had health benefits for the tribes who followed it. My parents also told me of some benefits of that "daily spoon" of fish liver oil that we took before the days of coated vitamin pills. Over the years, they somehow convinced me to think about what would be a moderate, balanced daily diet. The more I think about our "normal" diets and our "normal" ways of life, the more curious I am about what is normal.

Now I can no longer turn to my parents for advice because in the "normal" course of events my father died (as did his father) of a heart attack before the age of 65 and my mother is paralyzed and without speech as a result of a cerebral stroke many years ago. Stories that they can no longer tell me are steadily filling new books on the shelves of our libraries, and in them I can find new ways of following the questions "What if?" and "How come?"

This book is dedicated to all those who sought answers and shared their understanding with the rest of us who want to know. I share their stories with you and my children and my grandchildren.

William E. M. Lands

Introduction

Eicosanoids

Many disorders of human health are linked to an imbalanced overproduction of hormone-like materials derived from the polyunsaturated fatty acid, arachidonate. This twenty-carbon fatty acid is converted in our bodies to hormone-like materials called eicosanoids (Fig. I-1). An overproduction of eicosanoids occurs in many health disorders such as thrombosis or asthma. Medications can slow down the overproduction of eicosanoids, decreasing the severity of the disorders and some unpleasant symptoms. Our food intake also can affect that undesired overproduction. This book examines some dietary ways to regulate eicosanoid production and action to give us some of the benefits associated with certain medical treatments.

The quickest and most dramatic relief from the effects of eicosanoid overproduction is usually obtained with specialized medicines that inhibit the enzymes that produce eicosanoids. With this inhibition, the medicines rapidly establish a new balance among the hormone-like materials in our tissues. This effect is important in treating an acute health crisis when we want immediate relief. Also, some of the synthetic drugs may be used either on a short-term or long-term basis when arranging for the prophylactic (preventive) treatment of people who are at risk of disorders related to an undesirable overproduction of the eicosanoids.

Preventing Diet-based Disease

This book focuses on a long-term approach to prophylactic treatment. Because eicosanoids are derived only from dietary fatty acids, a long-term preventive approach is proposed that involves considering the type of fat consumed in daily diets. Proper nutrition and food selection can be important in programs for preventive medicine or health maintenance. There are many ways in which careful planning of the daily balance in our various foods can improve our health. With what is now known about eicosanoids, new programs that recognize the dietary origins of the arachidonate in our tissues can be designed to change the balance of formation

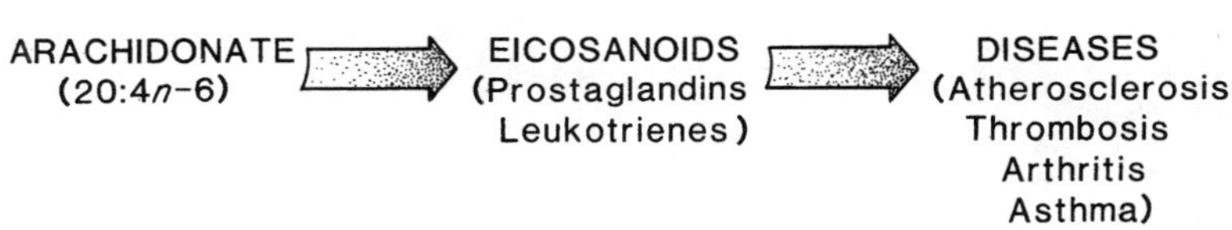

Fig. I-1. Eicosanoids from arachidonate.

among eicosanoids in our bodies over a long period without the use of drugs. Some people achieve this type of health maintenance program when following their traditional cultural food habits.

Arachidonate is an essential fatty acid that we cannot make on our own and can obtain only through the foods we eat. Often, arachidonate (20:4n-6)* is derived from a shorter acid of the (n-6) type of polyunsaturated fatty acid, linoleate (18:2n-6),* that animals and humans obtain from plants (Fig. I-2). (*The number notation 20:4n-6 indicates the size of the fatty acid, 20 carbons; the number of double bonds, 4; the location of the last double bond, n-6. With linoleate there are 18 carbons, 2 double bonds, and the last double bond is at the n-6 position. [Illustrations of these structures are in the Glossary.])

Competition by n-3 and n-6 Acids

Our tissues can convert dietary linoleate (n-6) into a variety of polyunsaturated fatty acids, all of the n-6 type. A closely related group of fatty acids, the linolenate (n-3) type, also comes to us through diet. An important part of the story discussed in this book relates to the balance between these two kinds of polyunsaturated fatty acids, the n-6 and n-3 types. Both types come into our food chain from plant origins, and they compete with each other for our enzyme systems. Understanding the competitions leads us to consider four dietary approaches to antagonize or decrease imbalanced formation of n-6 eicosanoids from arachidonate. They are mentioned only briefly here, and the basis for their health effects is discussed in detail later in this book.

One early suggestion for shifting the balance of eicosanoids was to eat large amounts of vegetable oils containing linoleate (18:2n-6) as in reports of Dayton et al (1966) and Galli et al (1981). This approach was based initially on an interest in lowering high blood cholesterol levels and on very preliminary evidence that megadoses or supraoptimal amounts of linoleate (11-15% of the daily energy intake) might antagonize eicosanoid formation. The proposed antagonism (represented in Fig. I-3 by the line marked "1") raised hopes for "megadose" linoleate treatments, but it now seems unlikely. In contrast, drugs and eicosapentaenoate (20:5n-3) do block this conversion.

Since the amount of the essential fatty acid, linoleate (18:2n-6) adequate for the needed eicosanoid formation seems to be less than 1% of daily energy intake (1 en%), a second approach could be to reduce the average daily intake of linoleate from current high amounts to a level near 1 en%. The lower intake might keep the

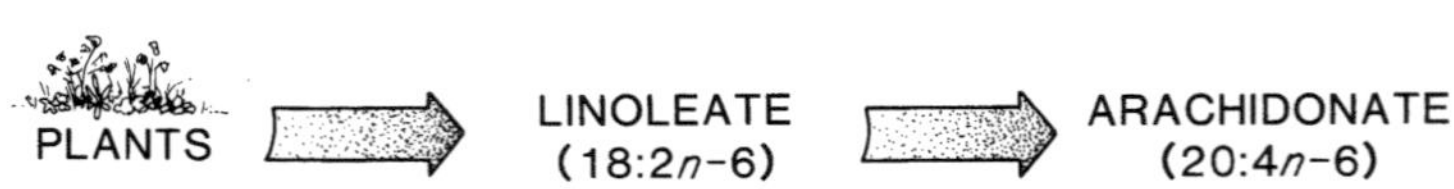

Fig. I-2. Arachidonate from linoleate.

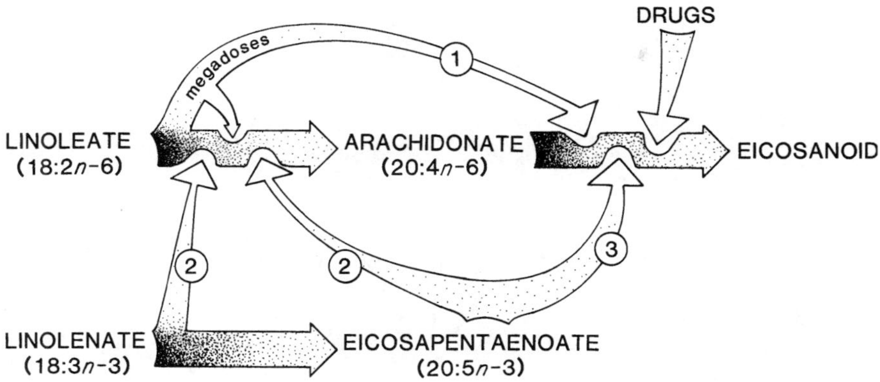

Fig. I-3. Competition between n-3 and n-6 types of polyunsaturated fatty acids and drug action can both diminish n-6 eicosanoid formation and action.

proportion of n-6 acids in tissue membranes at moderate values and cut the likelihood of overproducing eicosanoids from arachidonate. A third approach is to consume vegetable oils that contain as much linolenate (18:3n-3) as linoleate (18:2n-6). It is based on well-established results indicating that competitive antagonism by the n-3 fatty acids decreases the conversion of dietary linoleate (18:2n-6) to tissue arachidonate (20:4n-6) as well as increasing eicosapentaenoate that antagonizes oxidative conversion of 20:4n-6 to eicosanoids (noted by lines marked 2 and 3, respectively, in Fig. I-3).

The fourth approach is to eat fish or fish oils. It is based on competitive concepts similar to the third approach, but has an additional strength due to the greater competitive effectiveness of the longer, more unsaturated analogs of n-3 fatty acids (20:5n-3 and 22:6n-3) that occur in maritime foods, such as fish, shrimp, and seaweed. From this last alternative comes the title of this book.

PUFA and Human Health

This book introduces readers to the natural origins of polyunsaturated fatty acids in dietary fat and offers some basic insights into three general processes by which their competitive interactions affect human health: membrane structures, eicosanoid actions and gene expression (Fig. I-4).

1. Tissue EFA form specific lipid-protein membrane complexes needed for cellular structures at specific stages of tissue development and differentiation. In particular, adequate supplies of EFA are vital during brain and retina development. A growing realization of the importance of EFA transfer from mothers to infants is now alerting the health community to possible nutritional deficits of n-3 EFA

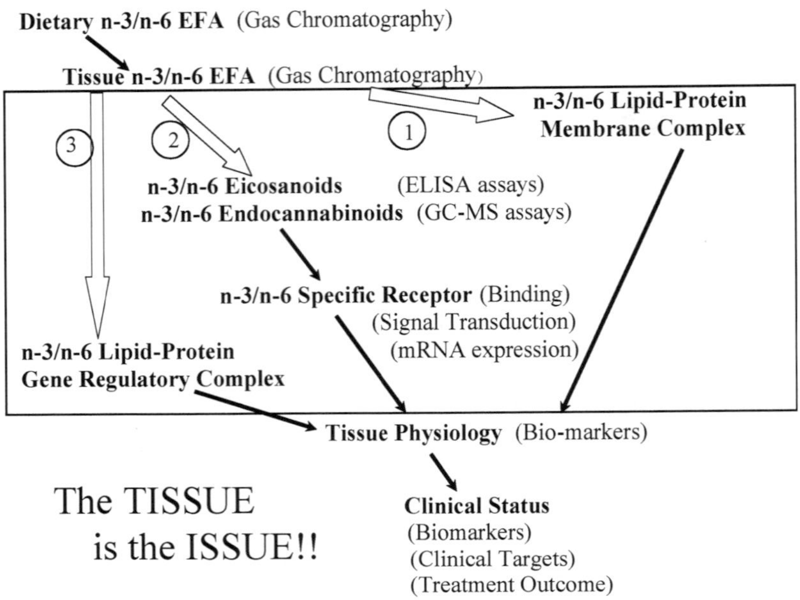

Fig. I-4. Three general processes for EFA action in tissues and how the actions are monitored. In health and disease, the tissue is the issue.

causing postpartum depression in mothers and behavior disorders in children. Chapters 3 and 7 include vital new insights into EFA actions in human growth and in the development of cognition. A supply of n-3 EFA from seafoods may have made possible the large brain expansion during the long evolution of hominids to Homo sapiens. New dimensions of EFA requirements are now emerging with provocative new evidence associating low seafood intakes with a greater incidence of major depression, aggression, suicide, and homicide (Chapter 3).

2. Tissue EFA form hormone-like self-healing autacoids (auto=self; akos=healing) that signal important fine-tuning adjustments of healthy tissue responses to stimuli. The n-3 and n-6 acids compete during metabolism converting dietary EFA to the 20- and 22-carbon highly unsaturated fatty acids (HUFA) in tissues. As a result, their relative abundance in the diet affects the relative proportions of autacoid likely to be formed and the relative intensity of response by the tissue. Eicosanoids are often monitored by enzyme-linked immunoassay (ELISA), and endocannabinoids by mass spectroscopic monitoring of gas chromatographic separations (GC-MS analyses). The different actions of n-3 and n-6 eicosanoids through specific receptors (Chapter 14) remain a principal reason for this book. In addition, the earlier awareness of transient inter-cellular signaling by

eicosanoid autacoids is now expanded with a newly recognized class of autacoid, the endocannabinoids (Chapter 2). These autacoids are likely to gain in physiological importance as we learn more about their specific receptor-mediated signaling processes. In addition, the major EFA-based autacoids cited in the 1982 Nobel Award, prostaglandins and leukotrienes (Chapters 14 and 16), are now accompanied by many other related and newly recognized products (hydroxyeicosatetraenoates, lipoxins, lipoxylins, isoprostanes, and neuroprostanes) whose actions are still not fully characterized. All of these products may have different actions depending on their n-3 or n-6 structure.

3. Tissue EFA form specific lipid-protein regulators of gene expression that control the cellular formation of enzymes that catalyze important metabolic processes and of proteins that mediate intercellular interactions. Current evidence in this area of molecular regulation of cellular processes points to selective actions of the HUFA, but has not yet shown appreciable differences in actions between the n-3 and n-6 types of EFA. As a result, the effect that a dietary change will have remains uncertain. Chapter 13 includes some new advances in knowledge about the potentially important ways that EFA affect gene expression.

Arrangement of Information

Biochemical and cellular interactions that mediate the influence of eicosanoids in certain diseases are in Chapters 2-11 and the fundamental biochemical processes in nutrition and metabolism that regulate that influence are in Chapters 12-16. Chapters 17-19 examine how to choose new food combinations to maintain whatever balance is needed to fit a personal level of risk aversion.

The information in many chapters is divided into a general description followed by a more detailed technical part. I hope that this arrangement will help each reader find the amount of detail needed. Each reader must examine the evidence and then choose the balance of polyunsaturated fatty acids that he/she wishes to use in his/her diet. Those who are developing programs in preventive medicine or health maintenance, will need complete nutritional, biochemical and physiological interpretations that are beyond the scope of this book; however, I've listed additional sources of information for the detailed data they will need.

The first edition of this book was published in 1986. Since then, more evidence about the cause of heart attacks is available (see chapters 4 to 8), making it even more certain that eating fish and seafood benefit human health. The benefit is now evident in recommendations by the American Heart Association for primary (Krauss et al, 2000) and secondary (Kris-Etherton et al, 2002) prevention of cardiovascular disease.

The metabolic discrimination during conversion of n-3 and n-6 dietary EFA into tissue EFA and into eicosanoid actions is now described in more detail in Chapters 13 and 14. Also, quantitative diet-tissue relationships were developed and added to Chapter 17 to guide specific personal food choice planning for a healthy balance among tissue eicosanoid precursors and modulators. That empirical metabolic relationship also helps evaluate epidemiological evidence on health benefits of eating the essential fatty acids in seafood, and it helps design and interpret future controlled clinical intervention studies. When used with the nutrient information in Chapter 18, it informs people of specific food combinations that help prevent excessive n-6 eicosanoid-mediated diseases. Specific examples of daily menu plans are in Chapter 19.

This second edition adds new insights and viewpoints on how health is affected by the vitamin-like EFA in food. Expanded and updated discussion of the concepts is often followed by more technical details and reference lists. The National Library of Medicine website (http://www.ncbi.nlm.nih.gov/entrez/query.fcgi) contains the latest biomedical details for any term(s) of interest. I've included examples of PubMed search results at the end of each chapter.

References

Dayton S, Hashimoto S, Dixon W, et al. Composition of lipids, in human serum and adipose tissue during prolonged feeding of a diet high in unsaturated fat. *J Lipid Res* 7:103-111, 1966.

Galli C, Agradi E, Petroni A, et al. Differential effects of dietary fatty acids on the accumulation of arachidonic acid and its metabolic conversion through the cyclooxygenase and lipoxygenase in platelets and vascular tissue. *Lipids* 16:165-172, 1981.

Krauss RM, Eckel RH, Howard B, et al. AHA Dietary Guidelines: revision 2000: A statement for healthcare professionals from the Nutrition Committee of the American Heart Association. *Circulation* 102:2284–2299, 2000.

Kris-Etherton PM, Harris WS, Appel LJ, for the Nutrition Committee. Fish consumption, fish oil, omega-3 fatty acids, and cardiovascular disease. *Circulation* 106: 2747-2757, 2002.

Part 1—Relating Diet to Disease

Calmly
fish
teach us
life.

1—Epidemiology and Curiosity

Two thirds of the earth is covered by oceans, and to the present day they provide us with routes to new adventures and new explorations. One is the significance of ocean-generated polyunsaturated fatty acids in human health, which led to my irresistible urge to explore the idea of "What is a normal way of life at home?" compared with "What is 'normal' in faraway places?" This book details that exploration; please notice how the smell of the sea drifts in and out around the dry facts of this story. The facts serve as safe harbors in which we can anchor our imagination, after each trip in this story takes us beyond our customary land. My adventure is recorded here. Please join me and then explore beyond where I could not go. Tell me what you see.

Sea vs. Land-Based Diets

For many the roots of our daily customs go deep into the soil, and our normal folk custom is to shun the perils of the open sea. My friends and I learned long ago that land is home while the seas are a place of homeless wandering. The sea was a place of fearful monsters, and it may still be. I wonder if the sea (when we turn to face it squarely) should really be all that frightening. Even though some may continue to avoid traveling on the sea or living on the sea or eating foods from the sea, we still can learn something more about our own life and death if we take a closer look at the products of the sea.

The first part of this book is about people who live near the sea and feed their families food gathered from the sea. These people have lives rich in tradition, which are slowly "modernizing". Their treatment of families and friends resembles ours; yet in some way they have very different patterns of sickness and causes of death. We can begin to learn about ourselves as we study them. Why are diseases that are average and normal for families that live near the sea not normal for those who live far from the sea?

One of the most frequently noted differences in health between fishing villagers of Japan or Greenland and workers in Western industrialized nations is the low incidence of heart attacks. Somehow maritime people have much less risk of heart disease than others. Medical scientists have identified a large number of activities and conditions or *risk factors* that correlate with the probability of suffering a heart attack. Several of these risk factors for heart attacks are lower for the fishing villagers than for people in Western industrialized nations. There are still other patterns in the frequency of other major diseases. Not only do the fishing villagers have a low incidence of heart attacks, but they also appear to have less frequent occurrences of bronchial asthma, psoriasis, diabetes, and autoimmune diseases although stroke rates are high in Japan. Since eicosanoids derived from our diet are important in producing some of the symptoms recognized in these diseases, a new possibility arose. Could the differences in disease frequency reflect differences in eicosanoid formation? This is an idea worth considering. It can lead to some interesting questions about the relationships between diet and disease. Could the severity and frequency of many of the diseases commonly occurring in our lives be due to a hyperresponsive state that results from the way that we use polyunsaturated fatty acids in our daily food? Fig 1-1 simplifies some of the data on incidences of illness or death among the populations listed in more detail in Tables 1-1 and 1-2. See tables 1 and 2 in the Technical Details section (page 11) for more info.

Studies of the villagers in the Upernavik district of Greenland reported that the two most prevalent types of disease among Eskimos were hemorrhagic stroke (apoplexy) and cancers (Kromann and Green, 1980), and that acute myocardial infarctions were extremely rare among these people (Fig. 1-1). These results contrast considerably with the corresponding frequencies of these disorders for Danes of similar age and weight. These findings also resemble the disease pattern reported for Alaskan natives for whom the major causes of death were infections and cancer (Arthaud, 1970). Among those people also, the rupture of aneurisms and hemorrhage were more prevalent forms of vascular disease than myocardial infarction, which was extremely rare. There is a similar relationship between a maritime diet and low rates of thrombotic events in residents of Japanese fishing villages. Knowing some of these relationships, scientists have searched for decades for an understanding of how to interpret the effect of the ocean-generated diet on human health. We will follow some of their searches to learn how diet and health can be related. The story began with epidemiology of ocean-based diets.

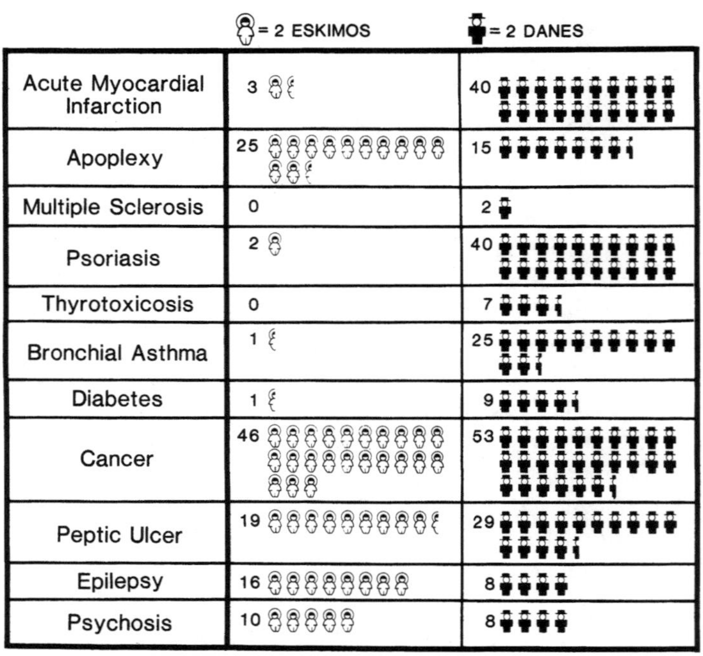

Fig. 1-1. Morbidity and mortality among arctic maritime populations.

Eicosanoids in Disease

It will be necessary to understand more about how diseases occur and how *eicosanoids* function in the diseases. If fishing villagers have fewer heart attacks, we may learn as much about ourselves as we do about them by asking "Why do we have more?" rather than "Why do they have less?" We study each disease that occurred at different rates to learn which could be related to diet and lifestyles.

Scientists discovered a more detailed understanding of the biochemistry of many disease processes in the past decade. This new information gives a fresh interpretation of the different patterns of disease observed in fishing villages compared with those in urban centers. Many disease mechanisms can involve processes that include the conversion of n-6 polyunsaturated essential fatty acids to the powerful physiologic agents—*prostaglandins, thromboxane*, and *leukotrienes*—that we call eicosanoids (Chapter 2).

Diet and Coronary Disease

An international cooperative study showed reliable data on the customary diets of people from different countries and how they relate to the incidence of coronary heart disease and serum cholesterol levels (Keys, 1970). The 1970 report correlated the number of coronary infarcts per 100 citizens and the average percentage of calories in the diet that were in saturated fats as well as the average level of cholesterol in the serum and the average percentage of calories in the diet from saturated fat. Since serum cholesterol and death from coronary infarcts both positively correlated to the same dietary feature, they also showed a close correlation with one another. How can we use that information to get an idea of the underlying cause of coronary infarcts? In which events are the correlations merely parallel effects of diet? Is cholesterol or fat the cause of death?

Understanding the full significance of cholesterol in plasma developed slowly, even as the mechanisms of heart disease and thrombosis became evident (Chapters 4–6). In the 1980s, the mediating roles for eicosanoids began to be assimilated into medical practice. Clues to the involvement of such factors were available in earlier epidemiologic data (Wilber and Levine, 1950), as they also are in the recent results shown later in Figure 1-2. At that time, medical scientists were unable to interpret the results; the role of eicosanoids in thrombosis came 25 years later. In 1950 Wilber and Levine stated: "*In the literature there are repeated references to an alleged causal relation between development of atherosclerosis and dietary cholesterol intake. It is postulated that a low blood cholesterol will delay arterial deposition, of the lipid. In the Alaskan Eskimos, however, there is a consistently high serum cholesterol, on one hand; repeated clinical surveys, on the other, indicate an almost total absence of cardiovascular-renal diseases in the population. These results taken in connection with the conclusion of Keys ['Neither in the younger (18–25 years) nor older (45–55 years) men is there any relation between blood cholesterol and habitual intake of cholesterol'] show the causative role of serum cholesterol in development of atherosclerosis to be somewhat dubious.*"

When considering the epidemiologic vs. autopsy data, there were too many uncontrolled variables to reach a conclusion about the way that diet influenced mortality. Epidemiologists can help us learn what is correlated and what might fit a hypothesis, but associative data do not prove the causes and the mechanisms. Some useful answers come from knowing the disease mechanisms described in the following chapters. If we knew more about the cause of a disease, we could make better decisions on how to minimize our risk.

Significance of Diet

An important idea at this stage is to check in more detail for evidence that difference in diet can be a cause. We can modify our food intakes more easily than our genes. People in industrial nations might tend to have more heart attacks just because of their genes. After all, there are genetic differences among people! Maybe Eskimos in Greenland and Alaska are genetically similar to the Japanese fishermen. Of course this idea may be helpful to us, but other data establish that the pattern of disease cannot be attributed simply to genetic differences between the two groups. For example, Bang and Dyerberg (1981), reflecting on the decreased incidence of ischemic heart disease in Norway during World War II, noted that it paralleled the increased consumption of fish and fish products. This decrease in ischemic heart disease was accompanied by observations of a decreased frequency of postoperative thrombosis and embolism in a large surgical department. We need to understand how the decreased consumption of meat and eggs and total calories, and the increased consumption of fish products can relate to such a decrease in thrombotic tendencies.

The wartime experience was helpful in indicating that nutritional factors may play an important role in the frequency of heart attacks. Related to this decreased morbidity is the greater bleeding tendency among Greenland Eskimos, summarized by Bang and Dyerberg (1980). The longer bleeding times, for which records extend back 500 years, are common among Greenlanders living on typical Eskimo food, and the bleeding times may be decreasing with recent changes in dietary habits and increasing urbanization. Since heart disease is a major problem in the United States, I focused on that problem. However, as I studied Fig. 1-1, I became intrigued by the other diseases that were also relatively low among the Eskimos. What if they were also related to diet? By this time I was aware that the correlations could not prove any causal role of diet (and they could not even indicate which part of the diet was related), but they aroused my curiosity. Could these diseases have common factors derived from diet? Can polyunsaturated fatty acids influence diseases such as bronchial asthma, thyrotoxicosis, multiple sclerosis, psoriasis, and atherosclerosis? All of these, like acute myocardial infarction, occur at exceedingly low rates among the Eskimo population, and we should study the role of diet in these diseases.

Fat Composition and Disease

This book examines some disease mechanisms to illustrate ways in which differences in dietary fat composition might be related to a disorder. Later chapters show

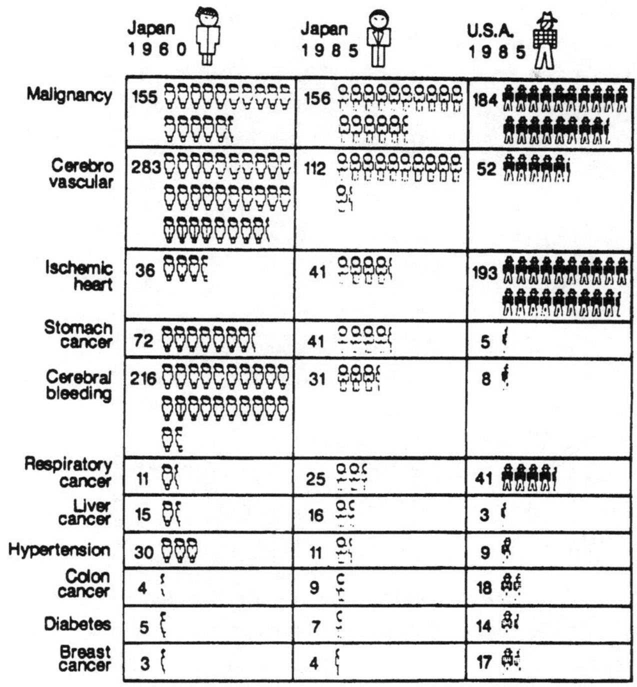

Fig 1-2. Death rates from specific diseases are quite different in different populations. Results were gathered by the US–Japan Malnutrition Panel of the US–Japan Cooperative Medical Science Program. (Reprinted from Lands et al, 1990 with permission of the senior author.)

how (without intending to at the beginning) I began to learn more about immune inflammatory diseases. These diseases involve eicosanoids with blood cells, but each has very different consequences. We still need to know more precisely how diets influence their behavior.

Curiosity has been a joy for me. Gaining knowledge from exploring seems to me almost as needed for human health as breathing air, drinking water, or eating food. I once thought that just helping people see new information about health risks from their food choices would stimulate them to change their lives to decrease the risk, but I failed to see how often we humans do not act in accord with logic. The classic book *The Structure of Scientific Revolutions* (Kuhn, 1962) evaluates how and when groups of people will convert information into belief and action. Kuhn called the broad change in attitude a *paradigm shift.* It involves complex sociological factors and attitudes that intrude into logic whenever people discuss evidence. For example, many social factors blocked acceptance of the published astronomical interpretations of Copernicus and Galileo. Eventually, a paradigm shift away from an earth-centered solar system to a sun-centered system occurred as modern science came into being with the help of Newton. The lengthy delay in moving past the narrow cholesterol-centered view of cardiovascular disease led me to add here some comments about often ignored limits in interpreting epidemiological risk factors. Readers who recognize those limits can develop more useful views linking diets to disease and participate in a new paradigm shift. Remember, not all associated markers are causal mediators.

Risk Factors and Disease

Hundreds of diseases are defined by clinical signs agreed upon by appointed experts who create the International Classification of Disease. Each disease name has an associated cluster of clinical signs useful for recognizing or "determining" its presence. Such signs are *determinants*, but not necessarily causes of the disease. Similarly, a factor closely associated with a disease is a risk factor that predicts likelihood of developing disease, and it may also be a clinical sign characterizing the disease. However, a close association alone does not prove a causal role in the mechanism for disease and death. The following several criteria help assign a causal role to a risk factor, and each criterion has limitations.

1. The risk factor appears before the clinical signs of disease (and death), although another unidentified factor might cause both the risk factor and the clinical signs.
2. The risk factor should have higher levels with higher incidence of disease (and death), although another unidentified factor might cause both the risk factor and the clinical signs.
3. The risk factor and clinical signs (and death) are lowered by controlled clinical interventions, although intervention may lower another unidentified factor that causes both the risk factor and the clinical signs.
4. The risk factor should have a plausible mechanism of how it contributes to disease pathogenesis (and death), although controlled evidence for mechanisms needs different conditions, interventions, and measurements than are customary in clinical trials and epidemiological studies.

The fourth criterion, involving difficult-to-measure transient signaling actions, is often neglected in clinical and epidemiological studies as investigators prefer stable biomarkers able to endure shipping, storage, and cheap assays of the hundreds or thousands of clinical samples that are used to overcome statistical problems. The first edition of this book noted plausible mechanisms by which a dietary imbalance of n-6 and n-3 essential fatty acids (EFA) can imbalance the EFA stored in tissues and contribute to cardiovascular disease and death (and to other diseases also). The mechanisms involve normal, transient, reversible actions of self-healing *autacoid* (auto = self; akos = healing) hormones that sometimes become excessive and produce irreversible harm. This edition confirms those mechanisms (especially platelet thrombosis, Chapter 6) and adds new information on inflammatory (Chapters 5 and 10) and arrhythmic (Chapter 7) processes obtained in the past 15 years.

Thirty years after the discovery that the n-6 autacoid, *thromboxane* is a major mediator of thrombotic ischemic death, many practitioners advocate administration of low-dose aspirin to stop platelet formation of n-6 thromboxane and decrease the risk of heart attacks. However, the underlying nutritional imbalance in dietary n-3 and n-6 EFA that enhances excessive n-6 thromboxane formation and sudden death also should be considered. This book addresses how nutrient imbalance can result when people do not consume a healthy diet; and describes ways to prevent the imbalance and its consequences.

Diversity in Food Choices

Diverse voluntary food choices made worldwide provide diverse EFA intakes that produce widely diverse tissue EFA compositions and eicosanoid response intensities. Comparison of disease incidence rates continues to stimulate curiosity as did comparisons between Greenlanders and Danes in Fig 1-1. This was later extended to Japanese and Americans (Fig. 1-1; Lands et al, 1990) in discussing the dietary habits that are steadily changing in Japan (Lands, 2003). Similar comparisons also spark interest in Mediterranean diets, and a figure for that population resembling Figs. 1-1 and 1-2 will likely appear soon. The effect of specific food choices on the pattern of tissue EFA linked to diseases is examined further in Chapters 18 and 19.

Ethnic Differences

Although cross-country comparisons include many sociological variables, an observed close fit of coronary heart disease (CHD) mortality rates with tissue EFA compositions also occurs for different ethnic groups within the same province (Quebec) of the same country (see Fig. 1-3). The association between mortality and tissue EFA composition has plausible mechanisms: conversion of dietary EFA to tissue EFA and the conversion of the tissue EFA to eicosanoids and their actions.

The strong correlation coefficient (>0.95) in Figure 1-3 confirms important EFA actions in "normal" living and dying. Now, more than 50 years past the advice of Wilbur and Levine (1950) that results "show the causative role of serum cholesterol in development of atherosclerosis to be somewhat dubious," public attention is slowly turning to known inflammatory, thrombotic and arrhythmic actions of n-6 autacoids. Since publication of the first edition of this book in1986, we continue to discover more harmful health consequences from neglecting a common imbalance in tissue EFA. Some people correct this by eating seafood. Imbalance in n-3 and n-6 nutrients is seen in analyses of unbalanced highly unsaturated fatty acids (HUFA) in blood plasma; this comes from imbalanced dietary EFA (Lands, 1993, 2003). Fig. 1-3 shows how this tissue biomarker of dietary EFA balance relates to CHD mortality. Clearly, people's food choices affect the risk of this disease. Hopefully, something will soon trigger a "paradigm shift" toward broader awareness of the widespread influence of n-3 and n-6 EFA actions in human health. Much needs to be done in applying specific diet-disease knowledge to improve primary prevention programs that move people from the upper right corner of Figure 1-3 toward the lower left.

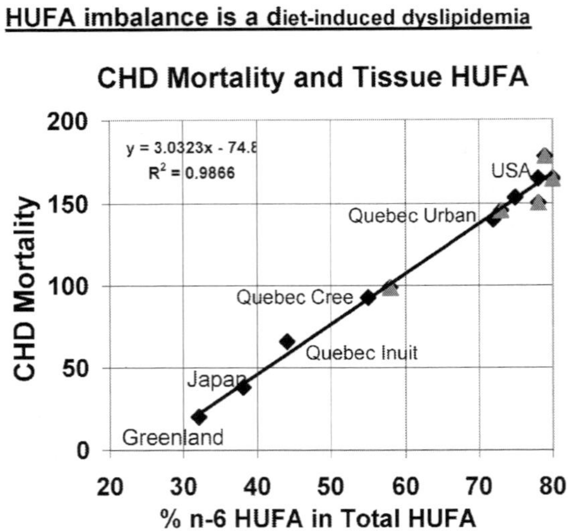

Fig 1-3. CHD Mortality Rates and Tissue HUFA. The values for the proportion of n-6 highly unsaturated fatty acids (HUFA) in total plasma phospholipid HUFA on the horizontal axis were calculated by gas chromatographic analyses. Results from USA, Japan, and Greenland were discussed earlier (Lands 1992; Lands et al., 1992) as were those from Quebec Inuits (Dewailly et al, 2002a), Quebec Cree (Dewailly et al, 2002b), and Quebec overall (Dewailly et al, 2001). The CHD mortality deaths per 100,000 = 3 x (% n-6 in HUFA) – 75 with a correlation coefficient of 0.99. (Reprinted from Lands, 2003a with permission of the author).

Technical Details

The data in Table. 1-1 were condensed from the report of Kromann and Green (1980), which described the frequency of several diseases in the Upernavik district of northwest Greenland. The population of about 1800 villagers represented one of the remaining whaling and sealing populations of Greenland. From 1950 to 1974, they represented approximately 30- 40% of the people of Greenland. The report was derived from the files of Upernavik Hospital listing all cases of the diseases indicated for 1950- 1962 and 1963-1974. Age-specific incidence rates expected for a corresponding European (mainly Danish) group of men and women were provided for comparison (see Table 1-1).

A study of Alaskan natives (Arthaud, 1970) gave further information on the nature of diseases among Eskimos by describing the cause of 339 deaths confirmed by autopsy. This information is extended by the more recent data shown in Fig. 1-3. The overall results were similar to those in an earlier report of 103 cases (Study 1, Gottmann, 1960). Eskimos constituted about 52% of the Alaskan natives in the 1960 U.S. Census; 34% were Indians and 14%, Aleuts. The specific diseases listed in Table 1-2 occurred at different frequencies among the three groups, but the number of cases

TABLE 1-1
Incidence of Chronic Diseases in Greenland (1950–1974)

Disease recorded	1950–1962 Men	1950–1962 Women	1963–1974 Men	1963–1974 Women	Observed total	Expected (for Danes)
Cancer	4	11	13	18	46	53
Apoplexy	6	5	8	6	25	15
Epilepsy	5	5	2	4	16	
Peptic ulcer	4	2	10	3	19	29
Rheumatic	5	1	2	3	11	NR
Polyarthritis	3	5	0	1	9	NR
Glomerulonephritis	0	2	2	0	4	NR
Pyelonephritis	0	1	0	1	2	NR
Psychosis	2	0	3	5	10	8
Myocardial infarction	0	1	1	1	3	40
Psoriasis	0	1	1	0	2	40
Bronchial asthma	1	0	0	0	1	25
Diabetes mellitus	0	0	1	0	1	9
Thyrotoxicosis	0	0	0	0	0	7
Multiple sclerosis	0	0	0	0	0	2

[a]Results from Kromann and Green (1980).
[b]NR indicates that a value was not reported.

TABLE 1-2
Primary Causes of Death of Alaskan Natives

	Study 1 (1956–1958) percentage (cases)		Study 2 (1959–1968) percentage (cases)	
Infections	24.3	(25)	24.8	(84)
Tuberculosis	9.7	(10)	4.7	(16)
Malignancies	26.2	(27)	21.2	(72)
Cardiovascular	5.8	(6)	10.3	(35)
Congenital	7.8	(8)	10.9	(37)
Prematurity	13.6	(14)	7.4	(25)
Trauma	—	5.9	(20)	
Others	12.6	(13)	14.8	(50)

seems too small to make a generalization here. The overall results summarized in Table 1-2 indicate much higher rates of death due to infection than occur in most Western societies. The general pattern—infection > malignancy> cardiovascular—tends to be the opposite of that found among the Western industrialized nations. This may reflect a lower level of anti-infective therapy available to these people. Chapter 10 briefly examines possible effects of dietary fatty acids on immune responses.

References

Arthaud B. Cause of death in 339 Alaskan natives as determined by autopsy. *Arch Pathol* 90:433-438, 1970.

Bang, H0, Dyerberg J. The bleeding tendency in Eskimos. *Dan Me Bull* 27:202-205, 1980.
Bang, H0, Dyerberg J. Personal reflections on the incidence of ischaemic heart disease in Oslo during the Second World War. *Acta Med Scand* 210:245-248, 1981.
Dolecek TA, Granditis G. Dietary polyunsaturated fatty acids and mortality in the Multiple Risk Factor Intervention Trial (MRFIT). *World Rev Nutr Diet* 66: 205-216, 1991.
Dewailly E, Blanchet C, Gingras S, et al. Cardiovascular disease risk factors and n-3 fatty acid status in the adult population of James Bay Cree. *Am J Clin Nutr* 76(1): 85-92 (2002a).
Dewailly E, Blanchet C, Gingras S, et al. Relations between n-3 fatty acid status and cardiovascular disease risk factors among Quebecers. *Am J Clin Nutr* 74(5):603-611(2001).
Dewailly E, Blanchet C, Lemieux S, et al. n-3 Fatty acids and cardiovascular disease risk factors among the Inuit of Nunavik. *Am J Clin Nutr* 76(1):85-92, 2002b.
Gottmann AW. A report of 103 autopsies on Alaskan natives. *Arch Pathol* 70:117-124, 1960.
Keys, A. Coronary heart disease in seven countries. *Circulation* 41: (Suppl. 1) 1:162-179, 1970.
Kromann N, Green A. Epidemiological studies in the Upernavik district, Greenland. *Acta Med Scand* 208:401-406, 1980.
Kuhn T. *The Structure of Scientific Revolutions,* 3rd ed. Chicago: University of Chicago Press, 1996.
Lands WEM. Biochemistry and physiology of n-3 fatty acids. *FASEB Journal* 6:2530-2536, 1992.
Lands WEM. (1993) Eicosanoids and health. In Lee KT, Oike Y, Kanazawa T (eds.). *The Third International Conference on Nutrition in Cardio-Cerebrovascular Diseases*). New York: New York Academy of Sciences, 1993, pp 46-59.
Lands WEM. Functional foods in primary prevention or nutraceuticals in secondary prevention? *Current Topics in Nutraceutical Research* 1(2):113-120, 2003a.
Lands WEM. Primary prevention in cardiovascular disease: Moving out of the shadows of the truth about death. *Nutrition, Metabolism and Cardiovascular Diseases* 13:154-164, 2003b.
Lands WEM, Hamazaki T, Yamazaki K, et al. Changing dietary patterns. *Am J Clin Nutr* 51:991-993, 1990.
Lands WEM, Libelt B, Morris A, et al. Maintenance of lower proportions of n-6 eicosanoid precursors in phospholipids of human plasma in response to added dietary n-3 fatty acids. *Biochim Biophys Acta* 1180:147-162, 1992.
Wilber CG, Levine VE. Fat metabolism in Alaskan Eskimos. *Exp Med Surg* 8:422-425, 1950.

2005 National Library of Medicine Search Results:

(http://www.ncbi.nlm.nih.gov/entrez/query.fcgi)
cardiovascular = 838,673; cardiovascular fish = 3,703; cardiovascular omega-3 = 1,226
CHD = 7,781; CHD fish = 112; CHD omega-3 = 84; CHD Inuit = 6
diabetes = 229,463; diabetes fish = 510; diabetes omega-3 = 338

2—Foods, Drugs, and Disease Mechanisms

Descriptions of the metabolic and chemical differences among the different fatty acids in our tissues appear later in this book. They describe how the n-3 type of fatty acids present in fish oil can antagonize the conversion of *arachidonate* into potent hormone-like materials and affect human health. Since the early 1970s, results of medical research have indicated ways in which these hormone-like derivatives of arachidonate can be important in diseases. However, clinical scientists still cannot classify which of the different hormone-like actions is good or bad. Although they know that these derivatives are important; they do not yet know precisely how important each derivative is in a particular disease mechanism.

Mechanism of Disease

Because we all have so little understanding of disease mechanisms, many pharmaceutical corporations customarily invest a high percentage of their assets in exploring disease mechanisms at the same time that they are testing new therapeutic agents. Often, by studying the way in which a new agent is effective in decreasing some undesired symptom, medical investigators can better understand the disease process itself.

This pattern of discovery and application of new drug information was evident following John Vane's 1971 recognition that aspirin had its beneficial analgesic and anti-inflammatory effect, principally by inhibiting the enzymatic conversion of arachidonate to prostaglandins (Fig. 2-1). Although aspirin was used as a pain reliever for many decades, medical scientists did not know much about how it worked. When Vane and his colleagues reported that aspirin, and a number of other aspirin-related drugs, work at the specific metabolic step converting arachidonate to prostaglandins, researchers recognized that the aches and pains may have been caused by that metabolic step.

Extrapolating from this, others successfully applied medicines of this type to a wide range of experimental disease models. They obtained new evidence that the prostaglandins derived from arachidonate were actually participating in the different disorders (see Fig. 2-2). That led to increasing new agents to treat these different dis-

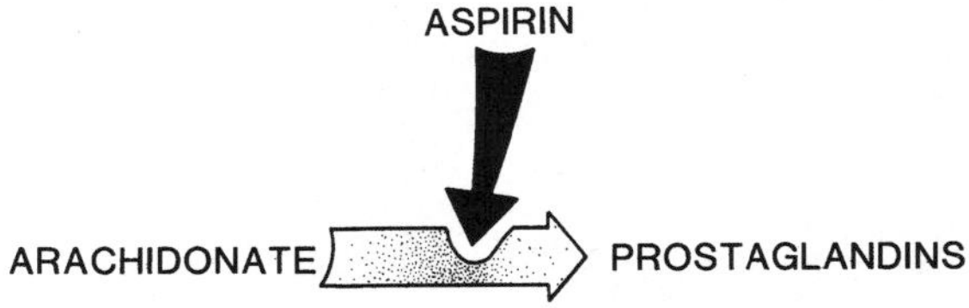

Fig. 2-1. Aspirin action.

orders. This cycle of discovery and application benefits us all as we progress from treating symptoms to understanding the mechanism of a disease.

Although there are some similarities in the symptoms of allergic responses and inflammatory disorders, clinical investigators found that drugs such as aspirin (that were effective against inflammation) were ineffective against asthma and some inflammatory disorders. Thus, blocking prostaglandin formation with aspirin-like drugs was not enough in those cases. Further research then led Bengt Samuelsson and his colleagues (1980) to the recognition of another type of arachidonate derivative, the *leukotrienes*. These compounds play a major role in the allergic or immune responses that are so important in asthma. In only five years, from 1974 to 1979,

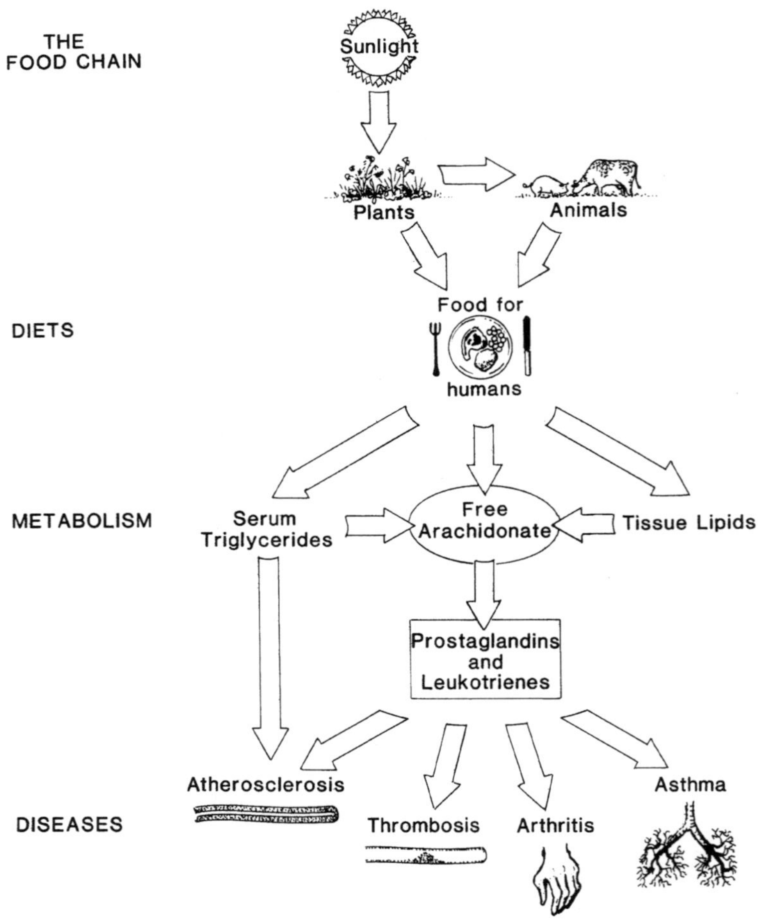

Fig. 2-2. Relationships of polyunsaturated fatty acids in the food chain with human diseases.

medical research produced *thromboxane* (Chapter 6), *prostacyclin* (Chapter 14), and *leukotrienes* (Chapter 16). Then new interpretations of disease mechanisms were possible. We can now reexamine our earlier knowledge with newer understanding. Chapters 4 to11 indicate some ways in which eicosanoids participate in disease processes.

Data from the epidemiological studies noted in Chapter 1 gave medical investigators further clues to the possible involvement of arachidonate derivatives in several diseases. Perhaps the average diet of the fishing villagers might shift the balance among the different eicosanoids in ways causing very different frequencies of disease. If that idea is correct, we may later apply that insight to the design of new nutritional studies and therapeutic approaches. This could lead to a new cycle of discovery on the application of diets that modify eicosanoid formation. From better understanding comes the ability to ask better questions and make better observations and then still better understanding. The evidence from the fishing villagers now takes on a new significance when we consider that changing the dietary polyunsaturated fatty acids could give health benefits that were not previously recognized.

We now need to look at each disease more carefully to see how eicosanoid actions can be involved and how diet influences those actions. The process of sifting through the mass of information on health and disease and converting it into a useful plan for action seems slow and uncertain. Even after we learn about the benefits of wisely selected therapeutic approaches to polyunsaturated fatty acid nutrition, progress is uncertain. We may all share ideas about foods, but the actual day-to-day diet decisions will be made by individuals who act by free choice. Individuals need a chance to know more of what to expect from the polyunsaturated fatty acids in their daily foods.

Effects of Changing PUFA Intake

An altered dietary intake of polyunsaturated fats might be more effective for long-term preventive or prophylactic approaches rather than for immediate, therapeutic treatments such as are generally used with common pharmaceutical agents such as aspirin. The dramatic effects obtainable with many pharmaceutical agents often give more convincing evidence for the desirability of the use of such agents to gain FDA approval. The slower effects that we may obtain by adjusting dietary polyunsaturated acids may be harder to prove, but they are based on removing primary causes rather than treating symptoms.

It is difficult to document the effectiveness of any protective agent administered over a long term. Conclusive proof of health benefits requires that many volunteers be studied for a long time before enough statistically reliable evidence is accumulated. The cost of such extensive human clinical research is significant in time, energy, and funds.

Financial risks with the heavy investment in time and skill associated with new drug development are frequently combined with a strong desire for the financial security provided by a substance patent. In this way, the costs of developing and testing a drug can be recovered. At this time, no U.S. patent security is available to corporations considering administration of natural foods in the long-term to contribute to the general health maintenance of a population.

It will be hard for a food producer to prove without doubt that a food or combination of foods can relieve a chronic disease or disorder. Though this was achieved in the early part of the 20th century for vitamins, once the essential material and its source was identified, the basic and clinical research on how it actually worked to relieve deficiency disorders proceeded at a slow rate.

We know that vitamins are needed, and average minimal amounts are recommended. However to-date, researchers cannot explain the causal mechanisms for the symptoms observed during deficiencies or overdoses of well-known vitamins. More than 70 years ago, the n-3 and n-6 fatty acids that form the eicosanoids were recognized to be essential (vitamin-like) materials. However, as with the vitamins, we have limited answers on the mechanisms by which those essential acids actually help our health or what is the minimum daily requirement of arachidonate or whether we are overdosing on n-6 nutrients.

Because of the lack of information on the physiological effects of foods, rationales for future approaches to nutritional therapy may come more rapidly from applying detailed research findings of the pharmaceutical industry. Scientists in that industry have gained much evidence for the role of the n-6 eicosanoids in disease mechanisms. Thereby they have sharpened the focus for others to consider health consequences of essential fatty acids. This information may be used to plan new drug-free ways to balance the apparent overproduction of eicosanoids from arachidonate and decrease our dependency on the drugs that have been developed for that purpose. The following chapter examines how essential fatty acid actions were recognized and found to be linked to eicosanoid actions.

Note that the essential n-3 nutrients abundant in seafoods compete with n-6 nutrients for storage in body tissues and for formation of potent hormone-like eicosanoids that act with different intensities. Knowing the balance between the n-3 and n-6 types of nutrient-based processes is the key to understanding how diet can have so many different profound effects on health.

Significance of Autacoids

Herein, to emphasize important signaling mediators in disease mechanisms, we use the 100-year-old name and concept of *autacoids* (auto=self, akos=healing), self-healing agents that the body produces while fine-tuning important cellular signaling processes. Healthy self-healing responses are transient and reversible, allowing tissues to adapt to environmental changes and then return to normal function. The self-healing actions are the way that certain nutrients from foods behave as hormones. Tissues form autacoids from essential vitamin-like nutrients that come only from the diet. Important autacoids (and their essential nutrient precursors) are *histamine* (histidine), *serotonin* (tryptophan), *nitric oxide* (arginine), and *eicosanoids* (n-6 and n-3 essential fatty acids).

Autacoids usually act intermittently and transiently through tissue receptors as they amplify low-intensity signals and produce adaptive tissue responses. The transient fine tuning of amplifying and suppressing signals gives successful self-healing actions that eventually terminate the signals and restore the tissue to a quiet normal state.

However, chronic excessive amplification by autacoids gives over-reactions that go beyond the limits of time and intensity for normal responses and cause loss of normal tissue function with serious impairment of people's quality of life. Such chronic excesses are particularly evident in inflammatory immune over-responses. Drug stores have hundreds of drugs that give relief by decreasing excessive formation of autacoids and their amplifying actions at specific receptors. Because our tissues store the EFA that make balanced eicosanoid responses possible, the success achieved by some populations in preventing diet-based chronic over-amplified actions of n-6 eicosanoids sets the stage for this book.

Health benefits come from preventing excessive n-6 eicosanoid signaling. Proof of this principle continues to come from the extensive worldwide marketing of aspirin and related nonsteroidal anti-inflammatory drugs (NSAIDs) that prevent excessive n-6 eicosanoid signaling (see Chapter 14). We know that excessive n-6 eicosanoid actions occur in thrombosis and arrhythmia of heart attacks, inflammatory immune events in atherosclerosis, arthritis and asthma, and in headaches, menstrual cramps and tumor proliferation. Unfortunately, current therapies seem to focus on suppressing *clinical signs* of a disease with patented pharmaceuticals; many treatments do not address preventing the *primary causes* of the diet-driven disease.

The "business" of medical treatment sometimes tends to emphasize reimbursable treatment plus investments in expensive, high tech procedures and equipment instead of preventing people from developing health problems in the first place. The emphasis on treating only people with clear signs and risk factors can shift medical resources to the highest risk individuals in higher education and income brackets. Often population-based nutritional initiatives that would benefit poor and ill-informed people are overlooked (Morgan, 2000).

The focus on treating clinical signs can neglect the underlying causal mechanisms of the disease process that remain as chronic underlying imbalances while the clinical signs are suppressed and removed from sight. This type of bias for treatment/curative activity that ignores early prevention can require that patients are maintained on lifelong medications.

If viewed as a marketing strategy, this means that we all must experience disease before receiving treatment. Ironically, many health economists calculate cost effectiveness of various treatment regimens (usually favoring one pharmaceutical product over another); but little or no attention goes to calculating the overall value of preventing the early causes of the disorder in a population. Removal of clinical signs by a drug does not correct the nutritional imbalance that remains an underlying cause.

Careful study of tissues from the PDAY study (see Chapter 5) of more than 3,000 young Americans (15 to 34 years old) who died of external causes between 1987 and 1994 (Zieske, 2002) indicates a steady progressive accumulation of inflammatory arterial atherosclerotic plaques long before clinical signs appear. This evidence indicates that it would be sound to begin primary prevention of atherosclerosis in childhood or early adolescence, before serious vascular damage occurs.

This book notes much about imbalances in n-3 and n-6 nutrition that contribute to the disease. Unfortunately, a whole generation of biomedical specialists was taught that arteriosclerosis was just a process of depositing lipid from cholesterol-rich blood (Taubes, 2002). After much delay, attention is shifting finally to studying the vascular immune inflammatory signaling that drives development of atherosclerosis and type-2 diabetes, serious risk factors that predict early mortality from a heart attack. Ironically, now that inflammation is finally becoming an "acceptable" concept in heart disease, many scientists are finding that the statin class of drugs that was developed to slow the formation of cholesterol may give health benefits more from an anti-inflammatory action than from lowering plasma cholesterol levels.

The biomedical community may now be in the midst of a paradigm shift, as old information on cardiovascular disease is viewed from a new perspective of immune inflammatory processes and autacoid signaling. This is an important advance in understanding and a valuable change in attitude. Hopefully, the dietary imbalances in n-6 and n-3 fats that aggravate inflammatory, thrombotic and arrhythmic conditions in humans will soon gain more attention. The need for primary prevention with nutrition education is clear.

The earlier edition of this book noted briefly that the public can get information about expensive large clinical trials that show evidence of efficacy of a drug (see below) but may not learn about the significance of nutritional imbalance of n-3 and n-6 EFA that results from the foods eaten. Since 1986 I've realized that simply indicating a public health problem with a plausible mechanism of nutritional imbalance may not be a sufficient stimulus for the people who sell foods to generate the needed solutions. Providing more information for the public may bring about a change in attitudes. Some of the quantitative metabolic relationships by which dietary EFA maintain EFA in body tissues are now included in Chapters 13 and 17.

This quantitative diet-tissue relationship is now combined with extensive nutrient data from the U.S. Department of Agriculture in a personalized interactive computer food choice program (that can be downloaded free from http://ods.od.nih.gov/eicosanoids/ or http://efaeducation.nih.gov/) to help people prepare daily menu plans that have dietary n-3 and n-6 EFA in specific amounts that give whatever balance in tissue EFA they desire. Examples of such menu plans are now included in Chapter 19.

Recent research developed information about a new set of EFA-based autacoids (self-healing agents) and their receptors: the endocannabinoids (Hillard, 2000; Porter and Felder, 2001; Schmid et al, 2002). These self-healing agents are formed in tissues from EFA, and they act through specific receptors in brain, blood vessels and leukocytes to affect neural and immune signaling systems. At this early stage, attention has focused on two endocannabinoid autacoids formed with n-6 arachidonic acid; arachidonoyl glycerol and arachidonoylamido ethanol.

We need more information about the actions of n-3 analogs at cannabinoid receptors before we'll know whether different food choices and tissue EFA compositions will influence signaling intensities in the endocannabinoid autacoid system. The naturally occurring receptors for endocannabinoids also bind compounds introduced from the environment (like tetrahydrocannabinol, the active component in marijuana) and give signals that are based on events other than normal tissue autacoid adaptation. Caution with these agents is prudent because chronic excessive signaling through autacoid receptors frequently generates pathology. We need to learn the safe balance for activating the cannabinoid signaling system and whether different dietary EFA supplies affect that balance. Responses by the cannabinoid system seem likely to be altered by the EFA balance in diets and tissues. Will more dietary n-3 EFA make the system less active or more active?

The first edition noted difficulty in finding financial support for the long-term primary prevention interventions needed to show that dietary EFA balance affects tissue EFA balance and health. That problem remains today.

The biomedical community can be slow to use the epidemiological evidence of strong effects of diet (see Chapter 1, Fig. 1-3) as evidence to recommend diet changes for primary prevention. There may be bias toward the format of "randomized, placebo-controlled clinical trials" in secondary prevention with people already impaired by long-term chronic imbalances. Many seem more oriented to ***treating*** problems with a pill rather than ***preventing*** them by sound nutrition advice.

Chapter 5 details the tragic progression of diet-induced inflammatory vascular damage that begins in childhood and occurs for decades until older people are finally accepted as patients and regarded as candidates for drug treatments. Belated advice to "watch their diets" is too unfocused and too late. I hope that broader awareness of EFA actions with the specific new information in Chapters 17 and 19 will help young people alter their voluntary food choices to prevent a lifetime of excessive n-6 eicosanoid responses in their tissues.

References

Hillard CJ. Endocannabinoids and vascular function. *J Pharmacol Exp Ther* 294(1):27-32, 2000.

Morgan S, Barer M, Evans R. Health economists meet the fourth tempter: drug dependency and scientific discourse. *Health Economics* 9:659-667, 2000.

Porter AC, Felder CC. The endocannabinoid nervous system: unique opportunities for therapeutic intervention. *Pharmacol Ther* 90(1):45-60, 2001.

Samuelsson B, Borgeat P, Hammarstrom S, et al. Leukotrienes: A new group of biologically active compounds. In Samuelsson B, Ramwell PW, Paoletti R (eds.) *Advances in Prostaglandin and Thromboxane Research,* vol. 6. New York: Raven Press, 1980, pp1-18.

Schmid HH, Schmid PC, Berdyshev EV. Cell signaling by endocannabinoids and their congeners: Questions of selectivity and other challenges. *Chem Phys Lipids* 121(1-2):111-134, 2002.

Sparrow CP, Burton CA, Hernandez M. Simvastatin has anti-inflammatory and antiatherosclerotic activities independent of plasma cholesterol lowering. *Arterioscler Thromb Vasc Biol* 21(1):115-121, 2001.

Taubes G. Does inflammation cut to the heart of the matter? *Science* 296:242-245, 2002.

Vane JR. Inhibition of prostaglandin synthesis as a mechanism of action for aspirin-like drugs. *Nat New Biol* 231(25):232-235, 1971.

Zieske AW, Malcom GT, Strong JP. Natural history and risk factors of atherosclerosis in children and youth: The PDAY study. *Pediatr Pathol Mol Med* 21(2):213-237, 2002.

2005 National Library of Medicine Search Results:

(http://www.ncbi.nlm.nih.gov/entrez/query.fcgi)
NSAID = 124,961; NSAID thrombosis = 3,310; NSAID ulcer = 5,397; NSAID fish = 404
clinical trials = 509,292; clinical trials NSAID = 17,887; clinical trials platelet = 10,554; clinical trials eicosanoids = 6,059; clinical trials arthritis = 9,587; clinical trials fish = 1,387

3—Essential Fatty Acids

In the early 1900s scientists discovered many vitamins by observing symptoms that occurred after certain substances were removed from the diet and studying which could be relieved when one of these substances was then added to the diet. Such studies led to the understanding that vitamins and certain essential amino acids were necessary for normal health and that they could not be made by animals or humans.

In 1930, scientists discovered essential fatty acids that could somehow help us maintain normal health, but they did not know then how these acids acted. They only knew that the n-6 type of fatty acid was needed for the growth and health of laboratory animals. Now, medical researchers know that eicosanoids are formed in our bodies from these essential fatty acids, and the new data on these compounds (Fig. 3-1) help explain some of the nutritional effects that were noted so long ago.

In summarizing the evidence for essential fatty acids, Holman (1958) suggested a narrow definition:

"Properly, the term essential fatty acids should include only those substances which are active both for growth and for maintenance of dermal (skin) integrity, limiting the term to linoleic and arachidonic acids and to such other acids as may be derived metabolically from them."

Now, we can consider that the n-6 fatty acids may have essential fatty acid activity only insofar as they can be converted via arachidonate to the important physiologically active eicosanoids (e.g.,Table 14-4 in Chapter 14). Acids that did not form prostaglandins were not potent in the biological assay for essentiality. However, our concept of "essentiality" will need to become still further sophisticated and recognize added roles for n-3 EFA. There may not be a single minimal daily requirement, but rather a flexible daily requirement that depends on interactions with other nutrients that each individual consumes. Finally, different physiologic events may have different EFA requirements. At one time, the U.S. Food and Nutrition Board suggested 1 en% as the minimum allowance of dietary essential fatty acids for humans. Advice for linoleate was repeated in many subsequent reports (Crawford et al., 1978), but arachidonate still has not been adequately studied. The fact that arachidonate was at least three times more effective than its precursor (Turpeinen 1938) is further evi-

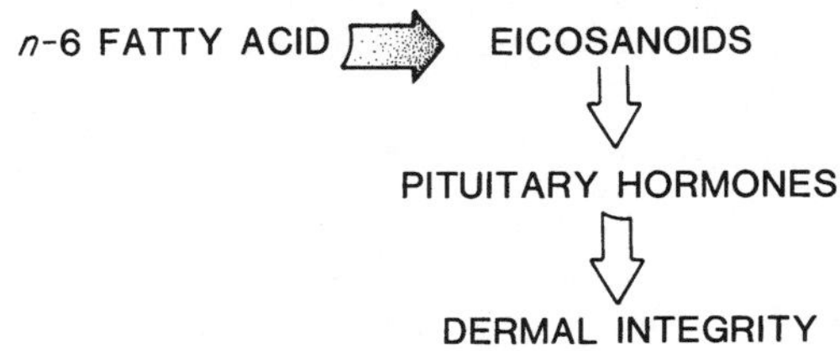

Fig. 3-1. Essential fatty acids.

dence for its role in "essentiality" and for greater effects of 20-carbon HUFA compared to 18-carbon EFA.

Essential n-6 Fatty Acid: How Much?

Once minimal EFA needs are met and we are sure that our diet has no deficiency, we need to consider nutritional strategies that can alter the balance between stimulation and inhibition of eicosanoid synthesis. We need to approach the question of whether it is sensible to ingest a high caloric diet containing much linoleate (18:2n-6) if the diet is also rich in meat with pre-formed arachidonate (20:4n-6) without planning for some suppression of eicosanoid formation of the sort that can be achieved by ingesting aspirin or competing n-3 EFA. Does the meat-rich diet of industrial nations increase the need for anti-eicosanoid pharmaceuticals and dietary n-3 HUFA?

Eating large amounts (11 en%) of the essential fatty acid, linoleic acid, might even cause a paradoxical apparent increase in the "minimum requirement" for that essential fatty acid in the diet (Galli et al., 1981). Possibly, higher amounts of dietary n-3 fatty acids can decrease the conversion of linoleate to arachidonate or diminish the conversion of linoleate to arachidonate and to active eicosanoids as suggested in Fig. I-3. This might require a higher than minimal intake of 18:2n-6 to compensate for the antagonism by the n-3 acids. Further quantitative nutrition research directed toward this end seems needed to clarify this possibility.

Nutritional Strategies

As we incorporate new knowledge of prostaglandin and leukotriene behavior into our definitions and rationales of normal health, an important consideration will be how much of the essential n-6 fatty acid is necessary for a balanced existence and how much n-6 intake might constitute an undesirable "overload." The topic of overload of the vitamin-like essential n-6 fatty acids has not been adequately addressed in scientific circles, although an overload phenomenon is clearly recognized for the fat-soluble vitamins A and D.

Early researchers established the desirability of including linoleate in the diet, but no one has carefully assessed the impact of eating 10 or 13% of daily calories as linoleate. Only after scientists learned about prostaglandins and leukotrienes did they begin to recognize the human need to diminish the over-mobilization of arachidonate that accompanies many pathophysiologic conditions (e.g., see Chapter 2). The information generated since the 1970s invites a reexamination of the interpretations of linoleate requirements.

The current edition of this book recognizes that progress in understanding the impact of essential fatty acid (EFA) nutrition on human health was impaired by continued denial or neglect of two simple concepts: the current intake of n-6 EFA in the United States (mostly from vegetable oils, see Chapter 18) is very much above that supporting adequate health, and the current U.S median intake of long-chain (20- and 22-carbon) n-3 EFA (mostly from seafoods) is below that supporting adequate health. This edition corrects those oversights. Much evidence accumulated in the past 20 years reaffirms the powerful impact of EFA imbalances in American diets. In addition, completely new measures of "essential function" are now being defined (see below and Chapter 7).

Quantitative metabolic studies of growth of laboratory rats (Mohrhauer and Holman, 1963) showed a strong competitive hyperbolic relationship between the intake of n-3 and n-6 EFA and the resultant tissue proportions of their highly unsaturated fatty acid (HUFA) derivatives. Those competitive metabolic results were known, but not widely discussed in detail (and they still are not!). Fig. 3-2 shows graphically how 0.3 en% linoleate or linolenate was adequate for growth of healthy normal animals, and the dietary EFA compete for storage as tissue HUFA. Importantly, the hyperbolic form of those 1963 results suggests that half-adequate amounts of dietary EFA for HUFA formation and growth might be near 0.1 en%. This quantitative information sets a useful baseline to interpret other information about EFA adequacy and to evaluate the likely impact of daily eating 100 times that amount.

The n-9 HUFA accumulated in the absence of dietary EFA is competitively displaced in acyl-CoA pathways (see Chapter 13) as n-3 or n-6 HUFA accumulate in tissues. Maximal growth of laboratory rats occurred near 1 en% EFA when the n-9 HUFA was still about 20% of tissue HUFA. The predicted curves are from a simple saturable hyperbolic relationship with half-saturation at 0.1 en% or 0.08 en% dietary EFA.

As we began quantitative measurements of diet-tissue relationships in laboratory animals in 1986, we were surprised that the competitive hyperbolic pattern for diet-tissue composition had a half-adequate nutrient level around or below 0.1 en% dietary linoleate (represented by the constant PC_6 described in Chapter 17). Of course, we were re-discovering the low values of the earlier reports of Mohrhauer and Holman (1963) graphed in Fig. 3-2.

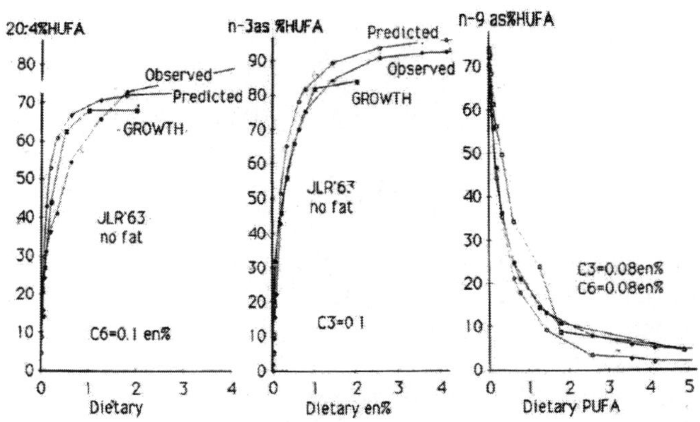

Fig. 3-2. Tissue HUFA Patterns and Diet

To correct my previous presentations, I've showed Fig. 3-2 repeatedly in talks during the past 19 years. Sometimes a picture is truly worth a thousand words! The low dietary level for adequacy was further supported by showing that adding more dietary n-6 acids to the standard chow diet gave little increase in tissue n-6 HUFA (Prasad et al, 1987), whereas adding dietary n-3 acids competitively lowered the accumulated tissue n-6 HUFA. Tissues of chow-fed animals were already at the high plateau (near 80%) in the range of n-6 proportions in tissue HUFA (Fig. 3-3). The standard laboratory chow diet gives a strong n-6 bias to all existing studies of "normal" tissue eicosanoid responses by research animals. It skews attitudes about what a "normal" physiological response actually is.

Hyperbolic Competition Makes HUFA in Humans

The next surprise we had was in seeing that the competitive hyperbolic diet-tissue relationship in rats with half-adequate nutrient level (around 0.1 en%) also closely fitted data for humans in Chicago (Lands et al, 1992). This confirmed the well-known observation that metabolic selectivities of many enzymes in humans and rodents are very similar. Apparently, the standard laboratory rat (that is given no choice of its food) matched adult Americans who were voluntarily eating high amounts of linoleate that kept n-6 proportions in tissue HUFA near the upper extreme of the possible metabolic range.

In contrast, voluntary food choices of humans worldwide give proportions of n-6 HUFA in plasma HUFA ranging from 15% to 90% (see Fig. 1-3). Americans, who are mostly at the upper end of this range, should consider whether the likely intensities of their current typical ("normal"?) eicosanoid responses are at a desired level. If not, they can be lowered readily by increasing n-3 and decreasing n-6 in the diet.

The apparent "half-adequate" level near 0.1 en% for rats and Chicagoans (PC_6 = 0.044; PC_3 = 0.055; see Chapter 17) caused us to look more carefully at earlier published results with human infants. Babies fed 0.07 en% linoleate had half of the clinical signs of EFA deficiency as those fed with 0.04 en% (Wiese et al, 1958; Hansen et al, 1963). Such unique evidence of adequacy for low levels of the n-6 acid in preventing deficiency can no longer be gathered in humans in an ethical manner, and the experiment is not likely to be repeated. However, the result quantitatively fits the animal results of Mohrhauer and Holman (1963) and supports Cuthbertson's conclusion (1976) that 0.5 en% linoleate is more than adequate to meet human needs for essential fatty acid with an ample margin of safety. Such results make the current median USA adult intake above 6 en% linoleate (see Chapter 18) seem far in excess of what is needed. Our results in Chicago gave the empirical diet-tissue relationship in Chapter 17 that helped us realize that the first edition of this book had overlooked the important evidence that an adequate intake of n-6 linoleate was below 1 en% for humans.

Attempts to correct my oversight (Lands, 1992; 1993; 1995; 1999; 2001) and alert people to the current unbalanced intakes of n-6 relative to n-3 EFA in the

United States had limited success. Recently, the U.S. Food and Nutrition Board of the Institute of Medicine of the National Academies gave no clear use of the above evidence (National Academies, 2002; reviewed in Lands, 2002). Contrary to the evidence cited in their report, board members surprisingly recommended eating *at least* 5 en% linoleate and eating very much less n-3 HUFA. Conditions still seem not ready for a paradigm shift away from using megadoses of dietary n-6 linoleate, a practice already viewed with concern in the 1986 edition of this book. More time and education still seem needed for people to recognize important facts that were published many decades ago.

New Dimensions of Essentiality

For some unexplained reason, the inclination of many nutrition experts to advise high intakes of n-6 EFA is not paralleled by similar advice for n-3 EFA. The neglected roles of the n-3 type of essential nutrient became particularly poignant in the 1990s as reports increasingly described health costs of failing to provide sufficient 20- and 22-carbon n-3 HUFA to pregnant mothers for adequate transfer to the developing child (Neuringer and Connor, *NutrRev* 44:285-294, 1986; Birch et al, 1992; Uauy et al, 1990 and 1992; Crawford, 1993; Makrides et al, 1993; meta-analysis by Anderson et al, 1999).

Awareness of the need for n-3 essential fatty acid nutrients to build important cellular structures in retina and brain (e.g., Kodas et al, 2002) began to supersede the unconvincing evidence that n-3 nutrient is only required to prevent dermal problems (reviewed by Anderson and Connor, 1989). The biomedical community has slowly come to realize that the high contents of n-3 EFA (particularly 22:6n-3, docosahexaenoic acid, DHA) in developing human brain and retina place demands upon pregnant and nursing mothers who may become progressively depleted if not supplemented with dietary n-3 HUFA (Crawford et al, 1978; Hibbeln, 2002).

Deficits of n-3 EFA are now seen associated with a higher incidence and severity of postpartum depression (Fig. 3-3) as well as with subsequent conduct disorder in the children from deficient mothers (Hibbeln, 2002). Studies relating human behavior to n-3/n-6 imbalances in inflammatory cytokine signaling (Smith RS, 1991) proposed fish oil (n-3 fats) as a prophylaxis against depression whereas n-6 fats promote the disease. Correlations of clinical symptoms of depression with a low supply of dietary n-3 HUFA relative to n-6 linoleate (Hibbeln and Salem, 1995)) were extended further (Hibbeln, 1998; Adams and Sinclair, 1996) and confirmed with a highly successful small intervention trial (Stoll, 1999). This concept is now rapidly developing and expanding to include the hypothesis of Hibbeln and Salem (1995) that increased consumption of linoleate-rich vegetable oils after 1950 may have caused recent rises in depression and neurologic disorders in Americans. Shifts in food handling and marketing over the past century in the USA have increased dietary n-6 EFA intakes and neglected n-3 EFA in ways that may be creating many more widespread societal risks than were previously recognized. Behavioral research will con-

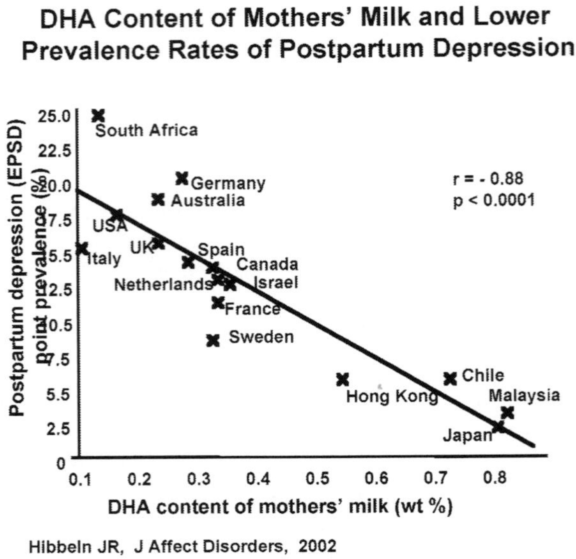

Fig. 3-3. Postpartum depression relates to dietary supply of n-3 HUFA.

tinue to identify new health dimensions by which we will define essential needs of humans for n-3 EFA nutrition.

Observational associations that show greater rates of aggression, homicide (Hibbeln, 2001) and depression (Tanskanen, 2001) among populations eating less seafood are stimulating powerful new research questions about how the n-3 EFA in seafood may be essential in human health and culture. The phenomenon likely relates to an association between low levels of n-3 EFA in plasma and low efficacy of serotonin (Hibbeln et al, 1998). The close epidemiological association between depression and cardiovascular mortality, identified by the World Health Organization as the two most common diseases worldwide, may involve common mediators related to n-3 and n-6 autacoids controlling autonomic tone and heart rate variability (Chapter 7). This area of neuroscience seems certain to excite curiosity about new essential functions of EFA in human life.

Omega-3 HUFA in Brain Development

The clearly evident need of the developing human brain for sufficient supplies of n-3 EFA (particularly 22:6n-3, DHA) may have been an important nutritional factor facilitating the expanding volume and complexity of brains during evolution of thinking hominids, *Homo sapiens*. Humans appear to have adapted to coastal marine environments in Africa by 125,000 years ago and expanded and dispersed out of Africa along coastal and riparian regions where n-3 HUFA are abundant in seafood and fish (Walter, 2000; Crawford, 2002). The rich traditions of people who live near the sea noted in Chapter 1 include diets that now link food from the sea with human culture and health in many more detailed ways than is commonly discussed. The following chapters note some of the links between fish and human health that affect the cardiovascular system (Chapters 4-9), autonomic nervous system (Chapter 7) and immune inflammatory system (Chapters 5 and 10). Over recent centuries, increases in n-6 EFA and decreases in n-3 EFA in typical foods led to more and more people having greater proportions of n-6 HUFA in their tissues. We should consider what that change in "normal" foods may have done to human health and behavior.

In the context of evolution and the supply of n-3 and n-6 EFA, a useful story comes from feeding and raising rainbow trout. These fish share with all vertebrates the need to eat a balanced supply of n-3 and n-6 fats to maintain their health. However, their evolution over millions of years was in an environment rich in n-3 fats with low supplies of n-6 fats. By now, the normal autacoid signaling in this species is balanced in such a way that trout fed high supplies of dietary n-6 fats suffer seizures and sudden death when disturbed (Castell et al, 1972). Clearly, farmers must avoid feeding excessive amounts of n-6 fats if they wish to prevent losing their livelihood. This interesting phenomenon may have parallels in psychiatric, cardiovascular and immune disorders of humans. The nutrient balance that maintains healthy autonomic and immune system responses may differ somewhat among different vertebrate species, but it cannot be ignored. Humans need to know what constitutes a healthy balance of n-3 and n-6 HUFA in their tissues to avoid accidentally creating a balance that is harmful.

Technical Details

The abnormally high skin permeability to water that occurs during a deficiency of essential fatty acids (EPA) (e.g., Hansen, 1982) reflects a variety of dermal symptoms that are not fully relieved by supplementation with the n-3 polyunsaturated fatty acids from tuna oil (Privett et al., 1959). This ineffectiveness coupled with the inability of linolenate (18:3n 3) to prevent the problems in reproduction for EFA-deficient rats (Quackenbush et al 1942) is part of the reason why linolenate and its related members of the n-3 family of fatty acids were omitted from a list of EFA (DeJongh and Thomasson, 1956; Thomasson, 1962). A later study showed no evidence for any requirement for n-3 fatty acids (Tinoco et al 1971) when animals had sufficient dietary n-6 fats. The corresponding protocol of examining the physiology of animals with sufficient dietary n-3 fats remains poorly studied.

The apparent need for EFA of the n-6 type to maintain the integrity of the pituitary gland (Greenberg and Ershoff 1951 Panos et al 1959) represents an important endocrinologic aspect to the dietary intake of n-6 fatty acids and their n-3 analogs that may be partial antagonists. Clearly, the lack of both n-6 and n-3 acids that occurs in EFA deficiency has a strong, harmful impact on hormonal regulation. The mechanism whereby EFA deficiency impairs pituitary function merits much more careful study.

The mechanism of this impairment seems even more important in light of the fact that removal of the pituitary gland (hypophysectomy) leads to dermal symptoms resembling those in EFA deficiency (Haeffner and Privett, 1973). Pituitary hormones may be needed to prevent the dermal symptoms, and n-6 eicosanoids are needed to facilitate release of those hormone(s). Loss of either the dietary n-6 acids or the pituitary could lead to the same symptoms (see Tan and Privett, 1973).

Although prostaglandins may have an important modulatory role in the release of pituitary hormones, no harmful antagonism by either aspirin-like drugs or n-3 fatty acids has yet been described. Can n-3 fatty acids support normal pituitary function? The question still has not yet been carefully explored. Excellent reviews on the topic of "essentiality" (Aaes-Jorgensen, 1961, 1982; Holman, 1968) provide an important base of knowledge to reexamine and reinterpret the biological effects of the n-3 and n-6 polyunsaturated fatty acids.

References

Aaes-Jorgensen E. Essential fatty acids. *Phvsiol Rev* 41:1-51, 1961.

Adams PB, Lawson S, Sanigorski A, et al. Arachidonic acid to eicosapentaenoic acid ratio in blood correlates positively with clinical symptoms of depression. *Lipids* 31(suppl):S-157-S-161, 1996.

Anderson GJ, Connor WE. On the demonstration of omega-3 essential-fatty-acid deficiency. *Am J Clin Nutr* 49:585-587, 1989.

Anderson JW, Johnstone BM, Remley DT. Breast-feeding and cognitive development: A meta-analysis. *Am J Clin Nutr* 70:525-535, 1999.

Birch DG, Birch EE, Hoffman DR, et al. Retinal development in very-low-birth-weight infants fed diets differing in omega-3 fatty acids. *Invest Opthamol Vis Sci* 33:2365-2376, 1992.

Castell JD, Lee DJ, Sinnhuber RO. Essential fatty acids in the diet of rainbow trout (Salmo gairdneri): lipid metabolism and fatty acid composition. *J Nutr* 102(1):93-99, 1972.

Castell JD, Sinnhuber RO, Lee DJ, et al. Essential fatty acids in the diet of rainbow trout (Salmo gairdneri): physiological symptoms of EFA deficiency. *J Nutr* 102(1):87-92, 1972.

Castell JD, Sinnhuber RO, Wales JH, et al. Essential fatty acids in the diet of rainbow trout (Salmo gairdneri): growth, feed conversion and some gross deficiency symptoms. *J Nutr* 102(1):77-85, 1972.

Crawford MA. The role for essential fatty acids in neural development: implications for perinatal nutrition. *Am J Clin Nutr* 57(suppl):703S-710S, 1993.

Crawford MA, Hassam AG, Rivers, JPW. Essential fatty acid requirements in infancy. *Am J Clin Nutr* 31:2181-2185, 1978.

DeJongh HL, Thomasson HL. Essential fatty acid activity of docosapolyenoic acids from brain glycerophosphatides. *Nature* 178:1051, 1956.

Galli C, Agradi E, Petroni A, et al. Differential effects of dietary fatty acids on the accumulation of arachidonic acid and its metabolic conversion through the cyclooxygenase and lipoxygenase in platelets and vascular tissue. *Lipids* 16:165-172, 1981.

Greenberg SM, Ershoff BH. Effects of chorionic gonadotropin on sex organs of male rats deficient in essential fatty acids. *Proc Soc Exp Biol Med* 28:552, 1951.

Haeffner EW,Privett OS. Development of dermal symptoms resembling those of an essential fatty acid deficiency in immature hypophysectomized rats. *J Nutr* 103:74-79, 1973.

Hansen, H. S. (1982). Essential fatty acid-supplemental diet decreases renal excretion of immunoreactive arginine-vasopressin in essential fatty acid-deficient rats. *Lipids* 17:321, 1982.

Hansen AE, Wiese HF, Boelsche AN, et al. Role of linoleic acid in infant nutrition. Clinical and chemical study of 428 infants fed on milk mixtures varying in kind and amount of fat. *Pediatrics* 31:171-192, 1963.

Hibbeln JR. Seafood consumption, the DHA content of mothers' milk and prevalence rates of postpartum depression: a cross-national, ecological analysis. *J Affect Disord* 69(1-3):15-29, 2002.

Hibbeln JR. Seafood consumption and homicide mortality. A cross-national ecological analysis. *World Rev Nutr Diet* 88:41-46, 2001.

Hibbeln JR. Fish consumption and major depression. *Lancet* 18:351(9110): 1213, 1998.

Hibbeln JR, Salem Jr N. Dietary polyunsaturated fats and depression: When cholesterol alone doesn't satisfy. *Am J Clin Nutr* 62:1-9, 1995.

Hibbeln JR, Umhau JC, Linnoila M, et al. A replication study of violent and non-violent subjects: cerebrospinal fluid metabolites of serotonin and dopamine are predicted by plasma essential fatty acids. *Biol Psychiatry* 44:243-249, 1998.

Holman RT. Essential fatty acids. *Nutr Rev* 16, 33, 1958.

Holman RT. Essential fatty acid deficiency. *Prog Chem Fats Other Lipids* 9:275, 1968.

Kodas E, Vancassel S, Lejeune B, et al. Reversibility of n-3 fatty acid deficiency-induced changes in dopaminergic neurotransmission in rats: critical role of developmental stage. *J Lipid Res* 43:1209-1219, 2002.

Lands WEM. Biochemistry and physiology of n-3 fatty acids. *FASEB Journal* 6:2530-2536, 1992.

Lands WEM. Eicosanoids and health. In KT Lee, Y Oike, T Kanazawa (eds.). *The Third International Conference on Nutrition in Cardio-Cerebrovascular Diseases*. The New York Academy of Sciences, pp. 46-59, 1993.

Lands WEM. Long-term fat intake and biomarkers. *Am J Clin Nutr* 61(suppl):721-725S, 1995.

Lands WEM. Balancing fatty acids. *Food Technology* 53: 120, 1999

Lands WEM. Impact of daily food choices on health promotion and disease prevention. In OR Kochli (ed.). *Fatty Acids and Lipids – New Findings*. World Rev. Nutrition and Diet. Karger, vol.88, pp 1-5, 2001.

Lands WEM. Please don't tell me to die faster. *Inform* 13: 896-897, 2002.

Makrides M, Neumann MA, Byard RW, et al. Fatty acid composition of brain, retina, and erythrocytes in breast- and formula-fed infants. *Am J Clin Nutr* 60:189-194, 2002.

Mohrhauer H, Holman RT. The effect of dose level of essential fatty acids upon fatty acid composition of the rat liver, *J Lipid Res* 4:151-159, 1963.

Neuringer M, Connor WE. Omega-3 fatty acids in the brain and retina: Evidence for their essentiality. *NutrRev* 44:285-294, 1986.

National Academies (2002) report on Macronutrients (http://www.nap.edu/books/0309085373/html/)

Panos TC, Klein GF, Finerty JC. Effects of fat deficiency on pituitary gonad relationships *J Nutr* 68:509-540, 1959.

Prasad MR, Culp B, Lands WEM. Alteration of the acyl chain composition of free fatty acids, acyl-CoA and other lipids by dietary polyunsaturated fatty acids. J *Biosciences* 11:443-453, 1987.

Privett OS, Aaes-Jorgensen E, Holman RT, et al. The effect of concentrates of polyunsaturated acids from tuna oil upon essential fatty acid deficiency. *J Nutr* 67:423, 1959.

Quackenbush FW, Kummerow FA, Steenbock H. The effectiveness of linoleic, arachidonic, and linolenic acids in reproduction and lactation. *J Nutr* 24:213-224, 1942.

Smith RS. The macrophage theory of depression. *Med Hypoth* 35:298-306, 1991.

Stoll AL, Severus WE, Freeman MP, et al. Omega-3 fatty acids in bipolar disorder: A preliminary double-blind, placebo-controlled trial. *Arch Gen Psychiatry* 56(5):407-412, 1999.

Tan WC, Privett O. Studies on the synthesis of prostaglandins in the vesicular, glands of essential fatty acid-deficient and hypophysectomized rats. *Biochem Biophys Acta* 296:586-592, 1973.

Tanskanen A, Hibbeln JR, Hintikka J, et al. Fish consumption, depression, and suicidality in a general population. *Arch Gen Psychiatry* 58(5): 512-513, 2001.

Tanskanen A, Hibbeln JR, Tuomilehto J, et al. Fish consumption and depressive symptoms in the general population in Finland. *Psychiatr Serv* 52(4):529-531, 2001.

Thomasson HJ. Essential fatty acids. *Nature* 194:173, 1962.

Tinoco J, Williams MA, Hincenbergs I, et al. Evidence for nonessentiality of linolenic acid in the diet of the rat. *J. Nutr* 101:937-946, 1971.

Turpeinen O. Further studies on the unsaturated fatty acids essential in nutrition. *J Nutr* 15:351-366, 1938.

Uauy RD, Birch DG, Birch EE, et al. Visual and brain function measurements in studies of n-3 fatty acid requirements of infants. *J Pediatr* 120:S168-180, 1992.

Uauy RD, Birch DG, Birch EE, et al. Effect of dietary omega-3 fatty acids on retinal function of very-low-birth-weight neonates. *Pediat Res* 28:485-492, 1990.

Walter RC, Buffler RT, Henrich Bruggemann J, et al. Early human occupation of the Red Sea coast of Eritrea during the last interglacial. *Nature* 405:65-69, 2000.

Wiese HF, Hansen AE, Adam DJD. Essential fatty acids in infant nutrition. *J Nutr* 66:345-360, 1958.

2005 National Library of Medicine Search Results:

(http://www.ncbi.nlm.nih.gov/entrez/query.fcgi)

essential fatty acid = 31,391; essential fatty acid brain = 2,515; essential fatty acid fish = 972; essential fatty acid omega-3 = 2,276; essential fatty acid depression = 419; essential fatty acid development = 2,028

4—Common Factors in Heart Disease, Heart Attacks, and Strokes

Understanding the events associated with heart attacks and strokes requires that we understand a bit about blood flow and about three separate phenomena that can cause a decrease in blood flow: *atherosclerosis*, *thrombosis*, and *vascular spasm*. All three of these phenomena may play some role in the ischemic incidents that are fatal to so many people in Western industrialized nations.

Atherosclerosis results from a slow, chronic process of deposition of lipids (fat and cholesterol that accompanies a thickening of the blood vessel walls, and thereby is associated with a narrowing of the "pipe" that carries the vital blood supply to the tissue.

Thrombosis represents a more acute event in which a clump of aggregated platelets and associated materials that we call a thrombus blocks the blood vessel and causes the ischemia (prevents blood from flowing) that leads to an infarction (tissue that has irreversibly lost its function).

Vascular spasm of the muscle around the blood vessel is another acute event which can rapidly constrict the diameter of the vessel and thus cause ischemia with its subsequent damage to the tissue. The ischemic lack of sufficient oxygen that occurs with either of the two acute events may cause the steady rhythm of the heart muscle to falter (arrhythmia) in ways that then impair further blood flow to the heart. This can lead to sudden death.

The long-term chronic process causing atherosclerosis is the basis for what we call vascular disease or "heart disease." On the other hand, abrupt, short-term events of thrombosis and arrhythmia cause "heart attacks." These short-term events are much more likely to occur closely associated with the chronic atherosclerotic "diseased" condition that decreases the effectiveness of the blood vessels and predisposes the individual to a greater risk of sudden death. The following three chapters demonstrate how dietary polyunsaturated fatty acids modulate these processes and thereby have an important impact on the frequency and severity of heart attacks.

Readers should wonder why the medical literature has accumulated more than one-half million published reports about heart disease (see National Library of Medicine search results at the end of the chapter). Why have we not prevented it more successfully? The first edition of this book noted that cardiovascular death involves imbalanced autacoid self-healing signals that amplify each other during inflammatory, atherosclerotic, thrombotic, and arrhythmic processes. Signaling by n-6 eicosanoids is a healthy process that can go out of control when pushed by imbalances in tissue HUFA that come from imbalances in dietary supply. Excessive eicosanoid signaling is a common factor in heart attacks (and many other disease processes). The years since 1986 have added much more insight into how dietary n-3 and n-6 EFA imbalances (rather than plasma cholesterol levels) cause normal self-healing signaling to go from healthy reversible events to irreversible pathology during signaling of immune inflammatory vascular atherogenesis (Chapter 5 and 10), platelet thrombosis (Chapter 6), and vasospasm or cardiac arrhythmia (Chapter 7).

Much new information exists on arrhythmic effects of n-6 eicosanoids and anti-arrhythmic effects of n-3 EFA. The unsteady rhythm of an ischemic heart is partially corrected by "free" fatty acids released from the energy-deprived ischemic heart muscle (Chapter 7). However, arrhythmia still occurs when the released acids include high proportions of the n-6 eicosanoid precursor, arachidonate. Unfortunately, current typical American food choices make arachidonate the most abundant HUFA in most body tissues. Fortunately, voluntary food choices can be altered to give proportions of n-6 HUFA in tissue HUFA ranging from 15% to 90% (Chapter 19).

The American Heart Association recommended at least two meals of fatty fish per week as a way to improve primary prevention of cardiovascular death (Krauss et al, 2000). It recently extended that advice to 1g/day of n-3 HUFA for secondary prevention in people with known cardiovascular problems (Kris-Etherton et al, 2002). A question of ethics remains in deliberately withholding dietary advice from people who do not yet "qualify" as heart patients but would likely benefit from similar diet advice as a part of effective community-wide primary prevention. With millions waiting for further dietary guidance, it seems useful to remember that "There has never been a cardiologic treatment that worked as a secondary prevention that didn't also work as primary prevention" (Harris, 2003).

References:

Krauss RM, Eckel RH, Howard B, et al. (2000) AHA Dietary Guidelines: Revision 2000: A statement for healthcare professionals from the Nutrition Committee of the American Heart Association. *Circulation.*102: 2284–2299.

Kris-Etherton PM, Harris WS, Appel LJ, for the Nutrition Committee. Fish consumption, fish oil, omega-3 fatty acids, and cardiovascular disease. *Circulation* 106:2747-2757, 2002.

Harris WS. Quoted in omega-3 oil: Fish or pills? *Consumer Reports*, July 2003, pp. 30-32.

2005 National Library of Medicine Search Results:

(http://www.ncbi.nlm.nih.gov/entrez/query.fcgi)
heart disease = 568,977; heart disease eicosanoid = 3,494; heart disease omega-3 = 763
coronary heart disease = 149,005; coronary heart disease eicosanoid = 1,452
heart attack = 101,524; heart attack eicosanoid = 617; heart attack omega-3 = 126
stroke = 90,152; stroke eicosanoid = 520; stroke omega-3 = 96

5—Heart Disease: Atherosclerosis and Serum Lipids

For decades an association of serum cholesterol and fats with atherosclerosis and coronary or cerebral artery disease has been noted. The emphasis on the type and amount of serum lipids and on their deposition in arteries occurred because of the very visible evidence of unusually large deposits of lipid in the arteries nourishing the brain and the heart. It seems particularly sad that these arteries, of all those in our body, should be so vulnerable to this disorder. The heart and brain seem too valuable to be permitted such a weakness. When epidemiologists succeeded in correlating the incidence of coronary and cerebral artery disease with the serum levels of cholesterol (and also with the level of serum triglycerides), a clear linkage of vascular disease to hypercaloric, fat-rich diets was developed. This knowledge led to a major effort to modify some aspects of diet. We have still more to do.

From the very beginning, a paradox seemed to exist from the studies of Alaskan Eskimos in whom a consistently fat-rich diet and high average levels of serum cholesterol were associated with an almost total absence of clinically recognizable signs of cardiovascular or renal diseases (Wilber and Levine 1950; Feldman et al. 1972). At that time such data illustrated that the causative role of high serum cholesterol in developing atherosclerosis was not established. Other factors were certainly also important in causing the disease. If only we knew then how to use information on diets and eicosanoids more effectively. As the Quebec data (Dewailly et al, 2001; 2002) show in Chapter 1, Fig. 1-3, the relationship between diet and disease remains.

Lowering of Serum Lipids

Long ago, Ahrens et al. (1959) and Kingsbury et al. (1961) demonstrated that diets that replaced saturated fats with polyunsaturated fats could lower the levels of plasma cholesterol and decrease the total serum triglycerides, irrespective of the content of the n-6 essential fatty acids in the oil. Fish oils that had little n-6 acid were very effective in decreasing the levels of serum lipid. Although eating fish (rather than just the oil) had similar effects, Peifer et al. (1962) demonstrated that the component in fish that was most responsible for the beneficial lowering of serum lipids was in the oils of the fish rather than in the protein or carbohydrate. Thus, most research attention is now directed to the effects of the polyunsaturated fatty acids in the oils. The manner in which these fatty acids affect the activity of the enzymes that form fat in our tissues and blood stream is important.

The way that public attention to foods turned away from the sea and sought the polyunsaturated acids from the land is still hard to explain or justify. Scientists had clear evidence that the n-3 polyunsaturated acids from fish were beneficial, but n-6 polyunsaturated fats from seeds and grains were more convenient to obtain, and they were vigorously marketed. During the two decades between 1950 and 1970, while evidence was accumulating on how dietary polyunsaturated oils including fish oil could cause a reduction in serum lipids, an unusual pioneering study was conducted by A. M Nelson and reported in 1972. This study of 80 patients on diet therapy extended over 16 to19 yr, during which the amount of cholesterol and the ratio of phospholipid/cholesterol in blood were monitored. Significant amounts of fish were included in the diet in the later years of the study to test in humans the applicability of the beneficial results that were reported by Peifer et al (1962) and Peifer (1966) for rats. Although many difficulties were encountered in the design and execution of such a long-term extended diet therapy regimen, the observed decreased amounts of blood cholesterol and increased ratio of phospholipid/cholesterol were interpreted by Nelson as vast changes of great significance.

Further effects of including n-3 fatty acids in the diet were indicated by the serum lipid analyses for Eskimos and for people from Japanese fishing villages both populations had lower values for serum triglycerides relative to other populations, and they had a very low incidence of coronary atherosclerosis. The hypolipidemic effect of eating fish was further described by Bang et al. (1971). They compared plasma lipid patterns of Eskimos in Umanak with a group of Eskimos who were living in Denmark. The level of pre-beta-lipoproteins and serum triglycerides was much lower in the Greenland Eskimos than in the Danish controls, and this finding was confirmed and extended in a later report (Bang and Dyerberg, 1972; Dyerberg et al., 1975; see also the review by Goodnight et al., 1982).

Cellular Interactions Involved

While research on the effects of high serum triglycerides was undergoing continued reinforcement, concepts began to evolve about the tissue changes involved in developing atherosclerosis (atherogenesis). The concepts came from attempts to describe the cellular interactions that occur in the blood vessels during the formation of atherosclerotic plaques (Ross and Glomset, 1976a, b). A significantly different aspect in this approach was the assignment of different roles for endothelial cells, smooth muscle cells, monocytes, platelets and neutrophils (See Fig. 5-1). A series of events was proposed to lead to this type of artery disease. In essence, the endothelial cell, smooth muscle cells, platelets, neutrophils, and monocytes interact in what resembles a defensive, inflammatory "wound-healing" or self-healing response. The eicosanoids are part of the signals used by these cells when "talking" to each other. A combination of normal self-healing responses at local sites within blood vessels then amplifies any slight stimulus by releasing chemotactic and growth-promoting agents, which then enhance the migration and proliferation of smooth muscle cells and monocytes at the surface of the vascular lumen.

Once these cells arrive at the surface, they may be exposed to elevated serum lipoprotein concentrations. Whenever such conditions occur (especially following

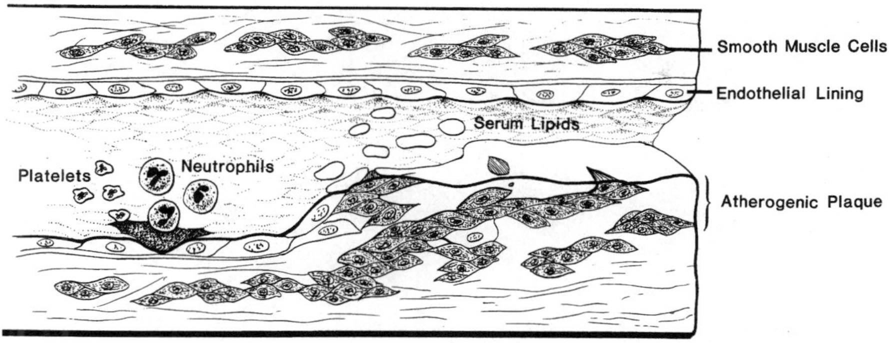

Fig. 5-1. Atherogenesis is a chronic inflammatory condition of vascular walls involving many different cells.

fat-rich hypercaloric meals), the smooth muscle cells may accumulate fat and develop the fatty streaks which gradually evolve into atherosclerotic plaques. In this hypothesis of the process for heart disease, the chain of events leading to plaque formation might be diminished either by impairing the release of factors from platelets or neutrophils or by decreasing the levels of serum lipoproteins released from the liver in response to food intake.

The important role of platelet and/or neutrophil responses in atherogenesis has inevitably brought attention to the dietary polyunsaturated acids that mediate these cellular responses by forming the eicosanoids prostaglandins and leukotrienes Fish oils contain much of the n-3 fatty acids that can antagonize the conversion of n-6 acids to eicosanoids. Recognition of the important mediating role of the eicosanoid modulators of these cells therefore puts a completely new orientation on the role of fish oils in diminishing cardiovascular disease (Lands et al., 1980). These oils not only decrease the level of serum lipids (see also Bronsgeest-Schoute et al., 1981), they also decrease the cellular interactions that cause the disease. Those cellular interactions are described further in Chapter 6.

CHD Risk Development from Childhood

Slow progressive inflammatory damage of the endothelium that lines vascular walls starts early in life for people who eat like Americans. The inflammatory disease develops for decades before clinical signs and symptoms of vascular disease make older people seek a doctor's advice and become a patient who needs treatment (Fig. 5-2). This book was written because vascular damage and cardiovascular death is less among people who eat food from the sea. Comprehensive autopsy measurements by the Pathobiological Determinants of Atherosclerosis in Youth (PDAY) researchers showed fatty streaks in the abdominal aortas of approximately 20% of 15- to 19-year-old Americans, and this percentage was approximately 40% for 30- to 34-year-olds (McGill et al, 2000). Raised fatty streaks were present in the right coro-

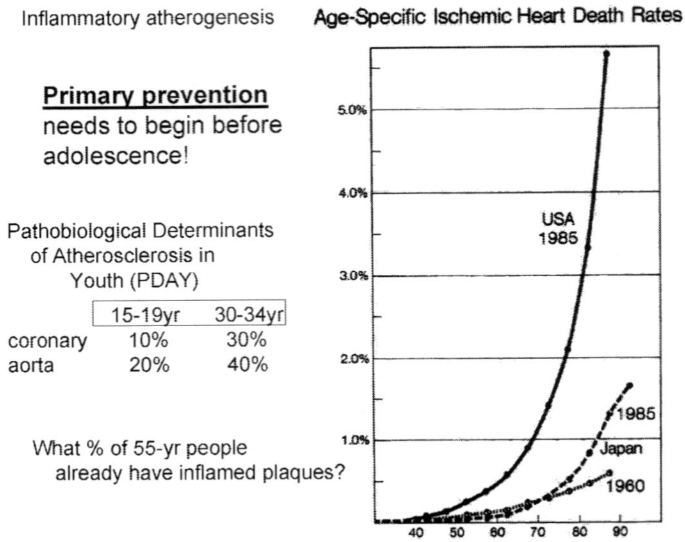

Fig. 5-2. Accelerated Risk of Death with Age. Age-specific cardiovascular death rates on the vertical axis fit the age-cohorts noted on the horizontal axis. Vascular damage may be in 30-40% of 30-35 year olds who still have death rates near 0.1%. (Modified from Lands, 1993.)

nary arteries of approximately 10% of 15- to 19-year-old people, and this percentage was approximately 30% for 30- to 34-year-olds (McGill et al, 2000), confirming earlier reports of vascular pathology in young soldiers killed in Korea (Enos, 1953). Fifty years of knowledge have still not brought an effective program of primary prevention for young Americans who are likely to continue the tragic epidemic trend.

The inflammatory damage begins with two nutritional imbalances: a relatively greater intake to expenditure of energy and a relatively greater n-6 to n-3 essential fatty acids. The past decade brought much public attention to healthy energy balance, and now national attention to the problem is strong. However, much more attention is needed to the balance of essential fatty acids in our foods and our tissues. The age-specific rate of cardiovascular death dramatically accelerates with age (see Fig. 5-2), but it is less among people with more n-3 fats in their diet. The diet-disease link prompts efforts to understand the life-long chain of events that drifts from preventable and reversible conditions in the young to those that become inevitable and irreversible in the elderly. Because the existing number of disease segments in arteries is a strong predictor of future progression of coronary disease, preventive nutrition efforts need to begin early—with children and adolescents who now are eating greatly imbalanced proportions of n-3 and n-6 EFA.

Although almost one in three 20-40 year-old adults have inflammatory vascular damage (PDAY group, 1990; McGill et al, 2000), few have visible external clinical signs of disease and few express concern about the explosive rise of diet-induced

CHD death rates that their age group will experience later in life. Unfortunately, current treatment of older patients with severely advanced disease tends to ignore the diet-based tissue imbalances that should have been corrected many years earlier by primary prevention and nutrition education. By the time that significant clinical symptoms cause 50- and 60-year old people to seek a doctor's help, a majority of their age group already have a seriously impaired arterial system—a condition that could have been prevented by earlier action.

Inflammation and Oxidative Stress After Meals

Large meals elevate blood levels of glucose and non-esterified fatty acids, which create transient oxidative/inflammatory responses (Bae et al, 2001; Hsieh et al, 2002) with leukocyte adhesion, stress-related responses and impaired endothelial function (Griendling et al, 2000). If the transient post-prandial inflammatory events were 99.9% reversible, three meals per day would give over 1,000 events per year with only one event (0.1%) remaining as an unresolved inflammatory focus. This may seem harmless at first, but when the 0.1% accumulates year by year, 30 or 40 years of accumulated inflammatory plaques (McGill et al, 2000) eventually give arteries with greater calcium deposits and intimal-medial thickness characteristic of elderly Americans. Because inflammatory plaques are less in people eating more n-3 EFA, the progressive inflammatory arterial disease is likely due to chronically imbalanced EFA and is not a "normal" aging process (Rumberger et al, 1996).

The 1986 edition noted "new concepts" of Ross and Glomset, (1976a,b) regarding the progressive cellular interactions in atherogenesis as an inflammatory disease. Ross continued until his death to affirm the inflammatory nature of the cellular interactions in this vascular disease (Ross, 1999). Unfortunately, general neglect of inflammatory immune intercellular signaling was extensive after the Consensus Conference and its National Cholesterol Education Program diverted attention and resources almost exclusively toward lowering the amount of cholesterol circulating in blood (Consensus Conference, 1985). Now that the "cholesterol-lowering" medications are shown to have anti-inflammatory actions, the biomedical community will likely re-examine the long-standing evidence of dietary imbalances that interfere with the ability of n-3 fats to lower serum triglycerides and to moderate excessive n-6 eicosanoid inflammatory actions. Hopefully, the re-examination will go beyond treatment tactics and inform people how to prevent the two causal risk factors noted in the upper left corner of Figure 5-3.

The anti-inflammatory enzymes, paraoxonase and PAF acetylhydrolase, in high density lipoprotein complexes (HDL) likely affect signaling events and vascular health more than the widely-publicized cholesterol molecules that are carried on the HDL complexes. Similarly, very low density lipoproteins (VLDL) secreted by liver release large amounts of non-esterified fatty acids in the plasma as they form low density lipoproteins (LDL). The released acids promote oxidant stress and impair endothelial integrity more than the cholesterol molecules carried on the resulting

LDL complexes. The large flow of fatty acids after a meal and their resulting oxidant conditions create signals that affect vascular health by forming highly active oxidized phospholipids (that mimic PAF). Cholesterol molecules decorating HDL lipoprotein complexes accompany beneficial actions linked to HDL and are loosely described as "good" cholesterol. In contrast, cholesterol decorating LDL lipoprotein complexes accompany harmful actions linked to LDL and are loosely described as "bad" cholesterol. An important point here is that "good" and "bad" labels are for actions of lipoprotein complexes and not for cholesterol itself. The amount of cholesterol in blood can be a marker of nutritional imbalances and a predictor of risk of death as noted in Fig. 5-3, but its role in actually causing death remains uncertain after many years and billions of dollars of marketing.

Antioxidants

Because oxidants are involved in amplifying inflammatory events, many people have attempted to reduce injury by eating antioxidant supplements to stop amplified oxidant chain reactions. Success depends on the intensity of the amplified responses and whether the antioxidant reacts rapidly enough with the different mediating oxidants and their diverse targets. Some of the enzyme-catalyzed reactions which produce hydroperoxide signaling agents (HOOH and ROOH) are poorly inhibited by general non-specific radical trapping agents (see cyclooxygenase in Chapter 14 and lipoxygenase in Chapter 16) even though added antioxidants may "re-direct" the resulting

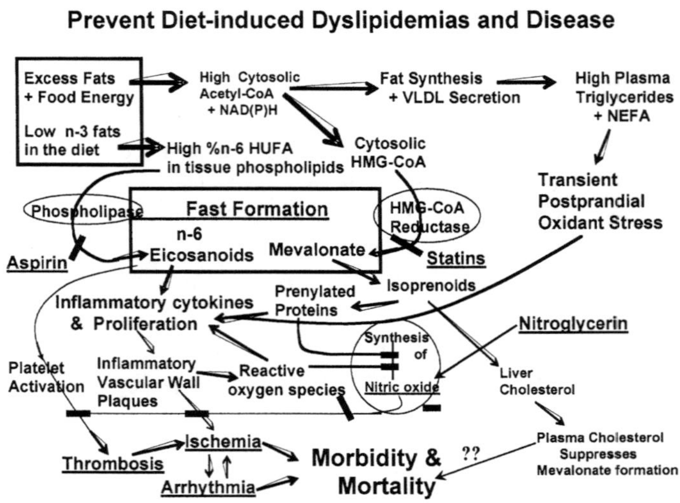

Fig. 5-3 Morbidity and mortality follow excessive actions of n-6 eicosanoids and prenylated proteins that are promoted by dyslipidemias caused by the two diet imbalances at the upper left. Sites of action of aspirin, statins and nitroglycerin are also noted. (Modified from Lands, 1993.)

peroxides away from damaging reactions with vulnerable tissue components (such as sulfhydryl groups in proteins or folate). Clinical nutrition studies have searched for protection by eating more of the antioxidants, vitamin C, vitamin E or carotenoids and vitamin A. For example, one large study in Italy failed to show a benefit of added vitamin E while supplements of fish oil did decrease deaths (GISSI, 1999).

Some think that drinking red wine (as in Mediterranean life-styles) gives antioxidants that might decrease vascular damage. In one study, wine was tested with subjects eating a fat-enriched breakfast that increased blood levels of triglycerides and increased activation of the pro-inflammatory nuclear transcription factor kappaB (NF-κB) in peripheral blood mononuclear cells (Blanco-Colio et al, 2000). Activation of NF-κB occurred in a time-dependent manner when triglyceride-rich VLDL was added to cultured mononuclear cells. That activation did not occur in the presence of two antioxidants from red wine, quercetin and alpha-tocopherol. However, intake of red wine induced a greater increase in postprandial triglycerides, particularly in VLDL, than seen after fat ingestion alone (Blanco-Colio et al, 2000). A widely held wish to find possible benefits of drinking red wine likely will lead to a continuing series of such studies, although the antioxidants are readily obtained from many other foods.

The evaluation of the different competitive interactions for polyunsaturated fatty acids in Chapter 14 gives insight into how dietary fish oils can impair atherogenic tendencies by affecting cellular events that are independent of serum cholesterol levels. The recognition of the biosynthesis of thromboxane as a necessary enzymatic process in platelet aggregation (see Chapter 6) permitted investigators to propose an effect of arachidonate (and other polyunsaturated acids) on platelet function which mediates thrombosis and atherogenesis (and also vasospasm; see Chapter 7). Thus, the correlation of prolonged bleeding times in Eskimos with their relative absence of atherosclerotic disease may be an external manifestation of the way in which platelet function participates in both processes, and the effect of a marine diet in diminishing this function of platelets. As noted by Harris and Connor (1980) and Harris et al. (1982), fish oils, with their characteristic high content of n-3 polyunsaturated fatty acids, lower the plasma lipoprotein (LDL and VLDL) content and also reduce thrombotic tendencies. These two events tend to diminish atherogenesis and the incidence of atherosclerotic disease in humans. These investigators found that (when compared to the typical average American diet rich in n-6 fatty acids) a diet high in n-3 fatty acids significantly reduced plasma triglyceride levels, improved fat tolerance, prolonged bleeding times, and decreased platelet adhesiveness.

They reported that diets containing 20 en% 18:2n-6 decreased the total plasma cholesterol from 191 to 174 in healthy adults, but failed to lower the plasma content of triglycerides. In contrast, diets with 12 en% 18:2n-6 and 8.0 en% of 20:5n-3 plus 22:6n-3 decreased both values significantly (Hams et al 1983). The decreased serum triglycerides seems due to a substantially lower flux of VLDL apoprotein B when the n-3 fatty acids are in the diet (Nestel et at., 1984; lllingworth et al., 1984). Sanders et al. (1981) demonstrated a slightly elevated level of HDL cholesterol in healthy young men receiving a supplement of fish oil. Elevating the HDL lipoproteins in blood and decreasing the LDL and VLDL lipoproteins are generally regarded as beneficial. Thus the n-3 fatty acids may prove helpful in the prevention of atherosclerosis.

Technical Details

Inflammation Can Become Too Extreme

Amplification is the key feature that makes inflammation move from normal physiology to pathology, such as occurs in atherosclerosis and other immune inflammatory diseases described in Chapter 10. When amplified, inflammatory signals can give pain and discomfort, resembling the positive feedback of a public address microphone placed in front of the loudspeaker. Fig. 5-4 maps some of the network of molecular and cellular signals with their multiple positive feedback loops that can amplify further release of inflammatory mediators and cause a normally transient localized immune cell response to give redness, heat, pain, and swelling and sometimes leads to loss of normal tissue function and even death.

The importance of EFA in inflammatory processes is evident in the fact that major anti-inflammatory drugs (aspirin, ibuprofen, Celebrex and Vioxx) inhibit prostaglandin formation from tissue EFA precursors (see Chapter 14). In addition, n-6 EFA are more active than n-3 EFA (Thies, 2003) in amplifying oxidant peroxide levels and inflammatory signals (Kulmacz and Lands, 1997; details in Fig. 5-4), and they drive normally reversible physiological events more rapidly toward undesired

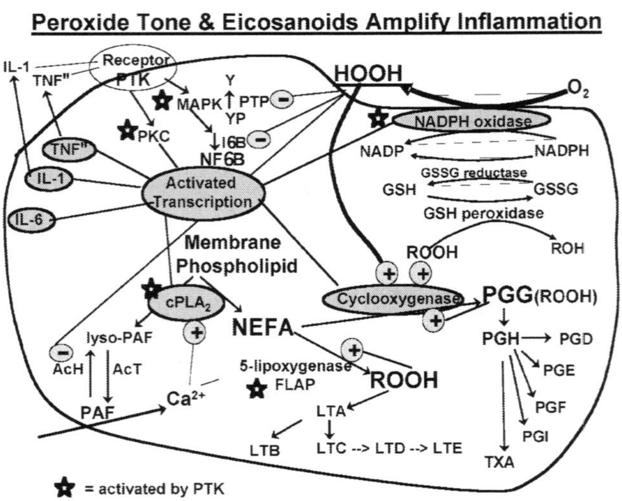

Fig. 5-4. Oxidant Stress Amplifies Inflammatory Signals Hydroperoxides (HOOH and ROOH) activate some processes (+) and inhibit others (-). Increased gene transcription gives more enzymes and cytokines that amplify signaling events. Steps activated by protein tyrosine kinases (PTK) are noted with a star. Abbreviations are noted in the text. (Modified from Kulmacz and Lands, 1997.)

inflammatory damage. Atherosclerotic inflammatory plaques accumulate in regions of blood vessels where eddy currents give the blood a longer residence time (Giddens, 1993) and allow accumulation and amplification of many inflammatory signals (e.g., hydrogen peroxide, HOOH, and platelet activating factor, PAF), cytokines (e.g., TNFa, IL-1, IL-6), calcium, phagocytic macrophages and their oxidative products (Ross, 1999; Libby, 2002). These local inflammatory signals are diluted as blood moves downstream, although acute phase reactants remain in the bloodstream as markers of the inflammatory/oxidant stress. In addition, activated leukocytes carry the inflammatory signals further downstream.

Oxidant Stress in Amplified Inflammation

The locally formed hydrogen peroxide (HOOH) and other reactive oxidant species (ROS) are both markers and mediators of inflammation. Their oxidant stress amplifies cytokine-enhanced protein tyrosine kinase (PTK) actions by stopping the protein tyrosine phosphatase (PTP) suppression of mitogen-activated protein kinase (MAPK) action as shown in Fig. 5-4. Oxidants also cut the IkB suppression of nuclear factor κB (NFκB), allowing greater NFkB action of activating the transcription and synthesis of more phospholipase (cPLA2) and cycloxygenase (COX-2), which produce increased amounts of NEFA, prostaglandins and leukotrienes. Greater NFkB action also increases transcription and synthesis of several inflammatory genes that further amplify the inflammatory signaling (upper left of Fig.5-4).

The combined events cause cells in the local area to make more NADPH oxidase activity that generates still more amplifying oxidants (upper right of Fig.5-4), making more inflammation. These oxidants also inactivate PAF acetylhydrolase (AcH in the lower left corner of Fig. 5-4), allowing accumulation of platelet-activating factor (PAF) that causes calcium to enter the cell and further amplify acute inflammatory and thrombotic conditions. The PAF acetylhydrolase (AcH in the lower left corner of Fig. 5-4) suppresses inflammation by hydrolyzing and inactivating PAF and related oxidized phospholipids. The PAF receptor also responds to oxidized phospholipids that are formed during oxidant stress (Zimmerman et al, 2002), further amplifying inflammatory and thrombotic events. That is one reason why the plasma HDL lipoproteins carrying PAF acetylhydrolase activity have beneficial anti-inflammatory action.

An alternate way to lower oxidative stress was shown for patients with CHD and high serum triglycerides who received twice a day 2 g of a concentrate of n-3 HUFA from fish oil. There was a sustained significant decrease in serum triglycerides by 20-30% ($p < 0.005$) and in very low density lipoprotein (VLDL) cholesterol by 30-40% ($p < 0.005$) at three, six, and 12 months compared either to baseline or placebo (Durrington et al, 2001). The arterial endothelium is injured in diabetes mellitus by inflammatory responses modulated by cytokines and growth factors such as platelet-derived growth factor (PDGF) and monocyte chemoattractant protein-1 (MCP-1). Ingestion of n-3 fats (but not n-6 or n-9 fats) by human volunteers lowered the inflammatory responses of gene activation for PDGF-A and -B and for MCP-1 (von Schacky et al, 2001).

Activated protein tyrosine kinase (receptor associated) increases as elevated oxidant levels cut protein tyrosine phosphatases activity (PTP), stimulating more events maked by asterisks. These further amplify inflammatory signaling by increasing cellular synthesis of PAF by activating the acetyltransferase activity (Sakamoto et al, 2002). Also, receptor associated PTK activates NADPH oxidase, increasing the HOOH signaling and further amplifying the oxidant signals. In addition, MAPK increases transcription and release of inflammatory mediators (IL-1, IL-6 and TNFalpha) and stress-reactive proteins. Finally, it directly activates phospholipase activity (cPLA2) that mobilizes arachidonate and its eicosanoid products (Pawliczak et al, 2002, Hayama et al, 2002), amplifying the intracellular peroxide tone (Kulmacz and Lands, 1997).

High glucose (25 mM) causes oxidant stress with protein kinase signaling (Hsieh et al, 2002), p38 MAPK phosphorylation, induction (mRNA gene expression) and secretion of angiotensinogen. Also, abundant non-esterified fatty acids prompt oxidant stress and inflammation (Aikawa et al, 2002) and inflammatory levels of hydrogen peroxide (10 μM) mimics the glucose effect (Hsieh et al, 2002). Lower vasodilatation and greater adhesion of leukocytes on vascular walls (Jagla and Schrezenmeir, 2001; Hyson et al, 2002) accompanies an impaired ability to produce and respond to the self-healing autacoid, nitric oxide (NO). Local inflammatory oxidants can destroy nitric oxide and form toxic peroxynitrite that damages vascular walls (Ceriello, 2002).

Antioxidants as Inhibitors of Oxidant Stress

Oxidant stress increases release of acute phase reactants, orosomucoid and C-reactive protein (CRP), which are markers that predict greater carotid plaque volume (Gronholdt et al, 2001). Both are positively associated with circulating levels of the triglycerides in the lipoproteins,VLDL, IDL, LDL, and they are negatively associated with HDL. Two markers of inflammation, C-reactive protein (CRP) and serum amyloid A (SAA), were significantly reduced by atorvastatin, but not by simvastatin (Wiklund et al, 2002). Both drugs (which were initially made to cut cholesterol formation) lowered the pro-inflammatory secretory phospholipase A2, although they made little change in other inflammatory mediators, IL-6 and ICAM-1. Nevertheless, such evidence is the beginning of recognizing how the mevalonate-forming enzyme that is blocked by statins has an important pathophysiological role in making isoprenoid products (esp. prenylated proteins with farnesyl and geranylgeranyl groups) other than cholesterol. For example, adding mevalonate prevented a statin-induced lowering of inflammatory NADPH oxidase activity (Bandoh et al. 2003).

Are Inflammation Markers Also Mediators?

Isoprostanes in blood or urine are sensitive markers of oxidative stress and injury (Morrow and Roberts, 2002). Lipid peroxidation in vivo was assessed by measurement of urinary excretion of F2-isoprostanes during two interventions, one providing daily fish meals and the other eicosapentaenoic acid (EPA, 20:5n-3) or docosahexaenoic acid (DHA, 22:6n-3), the two principal n-3 fatty acids in fish oils (Mori et al, 2000). Both trials showed urinary F2-isoprostanes were significantly reduced by 20-27%, indicating that n-3 HUFA may reduce oxidant stress in humans. Questions remain about the degree to which these isoprostane products of tissue injury may themselves cause further injury in the way that oxidized phospholipids do when they activate PAF receptors.

Higher levels of homocysteine ("de-methylated" methionine) in blood are associated with chronic oxidant stress and atherosclerosis, most likely due to oxidative loss of limited supplies of folate and vitamin B_{12} that are needed to maintain methyl group availability. Questions remain as to whether the elevated homocysteine observed in people with known vascular disease (Harker et al, 1974; McCully et al, 1996; Wang and Siow, 2000) caused the injury or whether it is only a marker for oxidant stress.

Added folic acid and vitamin B_{12} lowered the homocysteine levels, but did not prevent atherosclerosis or vascular dysfunction in monkeys (Lentz et al, 2001). Apparently, this elevated marker is not a major mediator of the underlying imbalance that causes the oxidative inflammatory disorder. People wanting to understand the cause of death need to carefully weigh evidence of whether an associated marker or predictive risk factor actually mediates death and disease or whether it is only a resultant marker of the disease processes. The current awareness of transient intercellular signaling will turn attention to how unwise food choices can amplify normally reversible signals and cause irreversible damage to vascular walls. People with adequate information could readily modify their food choices and prevent such imbalances.

Serum lipid levels should be considered as one of several factors promoting atherogenesis. However, recognition of the inflammatory cellular processes involved in atherogenesis makes it clear that serum lipids or serum cholesterol cannot be sole factors causing vascular damage and that imbalanced eicosanoid-mediated actions of cells resulting from imbalanced dietary intakes are important pathobiological factors.

References

Ahrens EH, Hirsch J, Peterson ML, et al. (1959). The effect of human serum-lipids of a dietary fat, highly unsaturated, but poor in essential fatty acids. *Lancet* 115:1 19, 1959.

Aikawa M, Sugiyama S, Hill CC, et al. Lipid lowering reduces oxidative stress and endothelial cell activation in rabbit atheroma. *Circulation* 106(11):1390-1396, 2002.

Bae JH, Bassenge E, Kim KB, et al. Postprandial hypertriglyceridemia impairs endothelial function by enhanced oxidant stress. *Atherosclerosis* 155:517-523, 2001.

Bandoh T, Sato EF, Mitani H, et al. Antioxidative potential of fluvastatin via the inhibition of nicotinamide adenine dinucleotide phosphate (NADPH) oxidase activity. *Biol Pharm Bull* 26(6):818-22, 2003.

Bang HO, Dyerberg J. Plasma lipids and lipoproteins in Greenlandic west coast Eskimos. *Acta Med Scand* 192:85-94, 1972.

Bang HO, Dyerberg J, Nielsen AB. Plasma lipid and lipoprotein pattern in Greenlandic west-coast Eskimos. *Lancet* 1:1143-1146, 1971.

Blanco-Colio LM, Valderrama M, Alvarez-Sala LA, et al. Red wine intake prevents nuclear factor-kappa B activation in peripheral blood mononuclear cells of healthy volunteers during postprandial lipemia. *Circulation* 102(9):1020-1026, 2000.

Brongeest-Schoute H C, van Gent CM, Luten JB, et al. The effect of various intakes of w3 fatty acids on the blood lipid composition in healthy human subjects. *Am J Gun Nun* 34:1752-1757, 1981.

Brown M. Editorial. *Lancet* 354:441-442, 1999.

Ceriello A. Nitrotyrosine: new findings as a marker of postprandial oxidative stress. *Int J Clin Pract Suppl* 129:51-58,2002.

Consensus Conference: Lowering blood cholesterol to prevent heart disease. *JAMA* 253:2080-2086, 1985.

Durrington PN, Bhatnagar D, Mackness MI, et al. An omega-3 polyunsaturated fatty acid concentrate administered for one year decreased triglycerides in simvastatin treated patients with coronary heart disease and persisting hypertriglyceridaemia. *Heart* 85(5):544-548, 2001.

Dyerberg E, Bang HO, Hjorne N. (1975). Fatty acid composition of the plasma lipids in Greenland Eskimos. *Am J Clin Nutr* 28:958-966, 1975.

Enos WF, Holmes RH, Beyer J. (1953) Coronary disease among United States soldiers killed in action in Korea. *JAMA* 152:1090-1093, 1953.

Feldman SA, Ho K.-J, Lewis LA, et al. Lipid and cholesterol metabolism in Alaskan Artic Eskimos. *Arch Pathol* 94:42-58, 1972.

Giddens DP, Zarins CK, Glagov S. The role of fluid mechanics in the localization and detection of atherosclerosis. *J Biomech Eng* 115(4B):588-594, 1993.

GISSI-Prevenzioni Group. Dietary supplementation with n-3 polyunsaturated fatty acids and vitamin E after myocardial infarction: results of the GISSI-Prevenzione trial. *Lancet* 354:447-455, 1999.

Goodnight SH Jr, Harris WS, Connor WE, et al. Polyunsaturated fatty acids, hyperlipidemia, and thrombosis. *Arteriosclerosis* 2(2):87-113, 1982..

Griendling KK, Sorescu D, Lassegue B, et al. Modulation of protein kinase activity and gene expression by reactive oxygen species and their role in vascular physiology and pathophysiology. *Arterioscler Thromb Vasc Biol* 20:2175-2183, 2000.

Gronholdt ML, Sillesen H, Wiebe BM, et al. Increased acute phase reactants are associated with levels of lipoproteins and increased carotid plaque volume. *Eur J Vasc Endovasc Surg* 21(3):227-234, 2001.

Harker LA, Slichter SJ, Scott CR, et al Homocystinemia, vascular injury and arterial thrombosis. *N Engl J Med* 291:537-543, 1974.

Harris WS, Connor WE. The effects of salmon oil upon plasma lipids, lipoproteins and triglyceride clearance. *Trans Assoc Am Physicians* 93, 148-155, 1980.

Harris WS, Connor WE, Goodnight SH Jr. Dietary fish oils, plasma lipids and platelets in man. *Frog Lipid Res* 20, 75-79, 1982.

Hams WS, Connor WE, McMurray MP. (1983). The comparative reductions of the plasma lipids and lipoproteins by dietary polyunsaturated fats: Salmon oil versus vegetable oils. *Metab Clin Exp* 32:179-184, 1983.

Hayama M, Inoue R, Akiba S, et al. ERK and p38 MAP kinase are involved in arachidonic acid release induced by H(2)O(2) and PDGF in mesangial cells. *Am J Physiol Renal Physiol* 282(3):F485-F491, 2002.

Hsieh TJ, Zhang SL, Filep JG, et al. Hgh glucose stimulates angiotensinogen gene expression via reactive oxygen species generation in rat kidney proximal tubular cells. *Endocrinology* 143(8):2975-2985, 2002.

Hyson DA, Paglieroni TG, Wun T, et al. Postprandial Postprandial lipemia is associated with platelet and monocyte activation and increased monocyte cytokine expression in normolipemic men. *Clin Appl Thromb Hemost* 8(2): 147-155, 2002.

Illingworth DR, Hams WS, Connor WE. Inhibition of low density lipoprotein synthesis by dietary omega-3 fatty acids in humans. *Arteriosclerosis* 4:270-275, 1984.

Jagla A, Schrezenmeir J. Postprandial triglycerides and endothelial function. *Exp Clin Endocrinol Diabetes* 109:S533-S547, 2001.

Kingsbury KJ, Morgan DM, Aylott C et al. Effects of ethyl arachidonate, cod-liver oil, and corn oil on the plasma-cholesterol level. *Lancet* 1:739, 1961.

Kris-Etherton PM, Harris WS, Appel LJ, for the Nutrition Committee. Fish consumption, fish oil, omega-3 fatty acids, and cardiovascular disease. *Circulation* 106:2747-2757, 2002.

Kulmacz RJ, Lands WEM. Peroxide tone in eicosanoid signaling. In HJ Forman, E Cadenas, (eds.*). Oxidative Stress and Signal Transduction.* New York: Chapman & Hall, pp. 134-156, 1997.

Lands WEM. Eicosanoids and health. In K.T. Lee, Y. Oike, T. Kanazawa (eds.). *The Third International Conference on Nutrition in Cardio-Cerebrovascular Diseases* New York:The New York Academy of Sciences, pp. 46-59, 1993.

Lands WEM, Pitt BW, Culp BR. Recent concepts on platelet function and dietary lipids in coronary thrombosis, Vasospasm and angina. *Hertz* 5:34-41, 1980.

Lentz SR, Piegors DJ, Malinow MR, et al Supplementation of atherogenic diet with B-vitamins does not prevent atherosclerosis or vascular dysfunction in monkeys. *Circulation* 103:1006-1011, 2001.

Libby P. Inflammation in atherosclerosis. *Nature* 420:868-874, 2002.

McCully KS. Homocysteine and vascular disease. *Nature Medicine* 2:386-389, 1996.

McGill HC Jr, McMahan CA, Zieske AW, et al. Associations of coronary heart disease risk factors with the intermediate lesion of atherosclerosis in youth. The Pathobiological Determinants of Atherosclerosis in Youth (PDAY) Research Group. *Arterioscler Thromb Vasc Biol* 20(8): 998-2004, 2000.

Mori TA, Puddey IB, Burke V, et al. Effect of omega 3 fatty acids on oxidative stress in humans: GC-MS measurement of urinary F2-isoprostane excretion. *Redox Rep* 5(1):45-46, 2000.

Mori TA, Watts GF, Burke V, et al. Differential effects of eicosapentaenoic acid and docosahexaenoic acid on vascular reactivity of the forearm microcirculation in hyperlipidemic, overweight men. *Circulation.* 102(11):1264-1269, 2000.

Morrow JD, Roberts LJ. The isoprostanes: their role as an index of oxidant stress status in human pulmonary disease. *Am J Respir Crit Care Med* 166: S25-S30, 2002.

Nelson A. Diet therapy in coronary disease-effect on mortality of high-protein, high-seafood, fat-controlled diet. *Geriatrics* 27:103, 1972.

Nestel PJ, Connor WE, Reardon NI et al. Suppression by diets rich in fish oil of very low density lipoprotein in man. *J.Clin. Invest* 74, 82-89, 1954.

Pawliczak R, Huang XL, Nanavaty UB, et al. Oxidative stress induces arachidonate release from human lung cells through the epithelial growth factor receptor pathway. *Am J Respir Cell Mol Biol* 27(6):722-731, 2002.

Peifer JJ. Hypocholesterolenic etlects induced in the rat by specific types of fatty acid unsaturation. *Nutrition* 88:351-355, 1966.

Peifer JJ, Janssen F, Muesing R, et al. The lipid depressant activities of whole fish and their component oils. *JAOCS* 39:292-296, 1962.
Ross R. Atherosclerosis–An inflammatory disease. *New Engl J Med* 340:115-126, 1999.
Ross R, Glomset JA. The pathogenesis of atherosclerosis. *New Eng. J Med* 295:369, 1976a.
Ross R, Glomset JA. The pathogenesis of atherosclerosis. *New Engl J Med* 295:420-425, 1976b.
Sakamoto H, Tosaki T, Nakagawa Y. Overexpression of phospholipid hydroperoxide glutathione peroxidase modulates acetyl-CoA, 1-*O*-alkyl-2-lyso-*sn*-glycero-3-phosphocholine acetyltransferase activity. *J Biol Chem* 277:50431–50438, 2002.
Sanders TAB, Vickers M, Haines AP. Effect on blood lipids and haemostasis of a supplement of cod liver oil, rich in eicosapentaenoic and docosahexaenoic acids, in healthy young men. *Clin Sci* 61:317-324, 1981.
Thies F, Garry JMC, Yaqoob P, et al. Association of n-3 polyunsaturated fatty acids with stability of atherosclerotic plaques: a randomised controlled trial. *Lancet* 361:477-485, 2003.
von Lossonezy T0, Ruiter A, Bronsgeest-Schoute HC, et al. The effect of a fish diet on serum lipids in healthy human subjects. *Am J Clin Nutr* 31:1340-1346, 1978.
von Schacky C, Baumann K, Angerer P. The effect of n-3 fatty acids on coronary atherosclerosis: results from SCIMO: An angiographic study, background and implications. *Lipids* 36:99-102, 2001.
Wang G, Siow YL. Homocysteine stimulates nuclear factor kappaB activity and monocyte chemoattractant protein-1 expression in vascular smooth-muscle cells: a possible role for protein kinase C. *Biochem J* 352:817-826, 2000.
Wiklund O, Mattsson-Hulten L, Hurt-Camejo E, et al.Effects of simvastatin and atorvastatin on inflammation markers in plasma. *J Intern Med* 251:338-347, 2002.
Wilber CG, Levine VE. Fat metabolism in Alaskan Eskimos. *Exp Med Surg* 8: 422-425, 2002.
Zimmerman GA, McIntyre TM, Prescott SM, et al. The platelet-activating factor signaling system and its regulators in syndromes of inflammation and thrombosis. *Crit Care Med* 30(5 Suppl): S294-S301, 2002.

2005 National Library of Medicine Search Results:

(http://www.ncbi.nlm.nih.gov/entrez/query.fcgi)
atherosclerosis = 90,088; atherosclerosis eicosanoid = 1,729; atherosclerosis fish = 464
atherosclerosis inflammation = 3,442; atherosclerosis endothelium = 8,507
inflammation = 152,907; inflammation eicosanoid = 5,857; inflammation essential fatty acid = 1,377; inflammation oxidant stress = 576; inflammation omega-3 = 332
endothelium = 93,523; endothelium adhesion = 14,205; endothelium eicosanoid = 5,739; endothelium inflammation = 5,739; endothelium fatty acid = 7,061; endothelium omega-3 = 241
oxidant stress = 9,937; oxidant stress MAPK = 396; oxidant stress fatty acid = 681
NADPH oxidase = 4,119; NADPH oxidase phox = 675; NADPH oxidase MAPK = 158
platelet activating factor = 10,155; platelet activating factor receptor = 1,217; platelet activating factor hydrolase = 498
prenylated proteins = 414

6—Heart Attack: Coronary Thrombosis

Two very different processes combine to stop the flow of blood (hemostasis) from a blood vessel: the clumping of platelets and the formation of a fibrin clot. The first event is a rapid assembling of platelets (thrombocytes) at a point of blood vessel injury which gives a plug that stops the loss of blood from that zone. Assembly of this plug is then followed by a more progressive appearance of insoluble fibrin fibers which form the network of a clot. The chemistry underlying these two processes is very different, and the process of assembling platelets to form a thrombus and their interactions with plasma proteins to form a blood clot appear to significantly involve the eicosanoids that are made from the polyunsaturated fatty acids. Primary attention on coronary thrombosis in this chapter is focused on platelet function affected by dietary polyunsaturated fatty acids, although recent studies indicate that some of the factors involved in fibrin formation or clotting may also be affected by the composition of dietary fatty acids.

Platelet Function

A major step forward in understanding the biochemistry of platelet aggregation followed the discovery by Smith and Willis (1971) that aspirin prevents the aggregation of platelets by inhibiting the formation of eicosanoids from arachidonate catalyzed by prostaglandin synthase. This discovery occurred at the same time that John Vane and his group discovered the action of aspirin in blocking prostaglandin formation in inflammatory events. The importance of arachidonate conversion to eicosanoids was stressed when Silver et al (1974) showed that injection of arachidonate, 20:4n-6 (but not 18:2n-6, 20:3n-6, 20:3n-3, 20:5n-3. or 22:6n-3) caused the death of rabbits within 3 minutes. Histological examination of all animals killed by this procedure showed the accumulation of platelet thrombi in the lungs. A paradox evolved when the prostanoid derivatives commonly recognized at that time were tested and found to have an insufficient effect on platelet function. Apparently the known prostanoids were not the way in which the arachidonate caused thrombosis.

The paradox was then elegantly resolved by Hamberg et al (1974a,b) when they demonstrated that a previously unknown derivative was formed by platelets from the endoperoxide intermediate of prostaglandin biosynthesis (PGH_2). The newly recognized compound, thromboxane A_2 (TXA_2), stimulated aggregation (Fig. 6-1) and had highly potent contracting activity on aortas. From these studies, it became apparent that aspirin exerted its antiaggregatory effect through the inhibition of PGH formation, just as it did in other recognized systems. However, in platelets the PGH was converted to *thromboxane,* rather than the previously known prostanoids. Thromboxane was then recognized to be the unstable rabbit aorta contracting substance that was released from guinea pig lungs after perfusion with antigen or by challenge with a slow reacting substance. Thus by 1975 a new concept of the regulation of blood flow had evolved based on the transformation of the PGH_2 endoperoxide intermediate to hemostatic aggregatory TXA_2 (Hamberg et al, 1974a,b; 1975).

Subsequent studies by Moncada et al (1976) showed that isolated aortas and other vascular tissues did not produce the contracting substance (thromboxane A_2) from the intermediate peroxide, PGH, but instead generated a vasodilating, antiaggregatory material. This latter substance was the major product formed from arachidonate in vascular tissues, and it was the most potent inhibitor of platelet aggregation known at the time (Fig. 6-2).

This compound, designated PGI_2 and frequently called prostacyclin, appears to be an important natural protecting agent (Moncada and Vane, 1981). The aggregatory action of thromboxane generated by platelets and the antiaggregatory action of prostacyclin generated by endothelial cells constitute a dramatic system for the control of hemostasis that depends on the biochemistry of the participating polyunsaturated fatty acids. Thus in 1976 there were three new revolutionary perceptions of the cellular (Ross and Glomset, 1976) and biochemical (Hamberg et al, 1974a,b; Moncada et al, 1976) processes by which dietary polyunsaturated acids influence the cellular interactions that underlie heart disease and heart attacks. The combined impact of these discoveries has been widely confirmed, but they have not yet been translated into routine daily nutritional applications in medicine. We have all been struggling to understand ways to diminish heart disease and heart attacks, but the molecules that regulate the

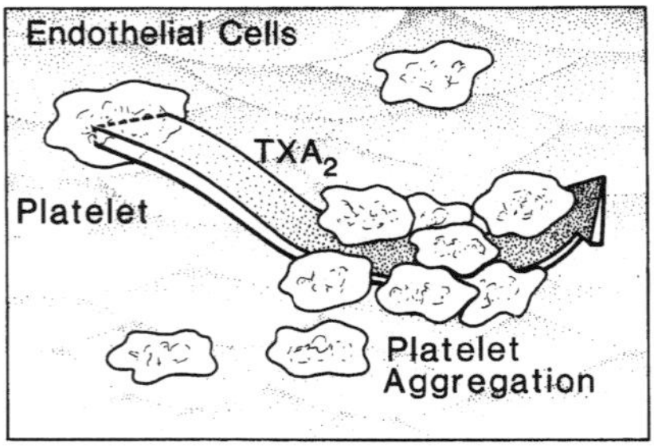

Fig. 6-1 Platelet aggregation

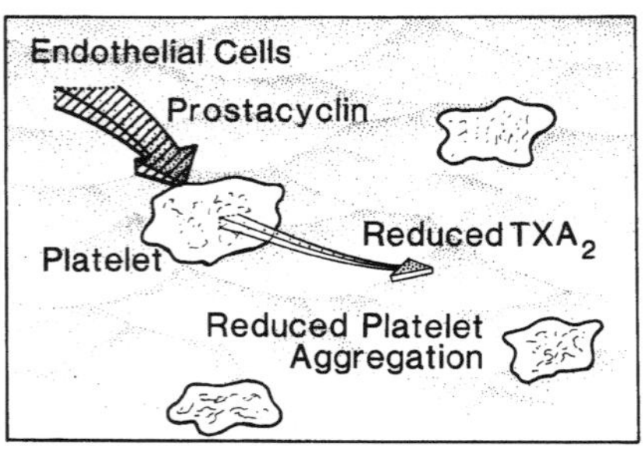

Fig. 6-2. Vessel walls make the anti-aggregatory eicosanoid, prostacyclin.

processes remain unfamiliar to many. Perhaps more important, the dietary sources of the precursors and antagonists are still not widely recognized. Many physicians are still unaware that they and their patients consume large amounts of the dietary n-6 precursors of prostaglandins and leukotrienes. It will take more time to assimilate the knowledge into effective primary prevention education.

Effects of Fish Oil

In 1978, Jorn Dyerberg and his colleagues joined with Salvador Moncada and John Vane (Dyerberg et al, 1978) to propose that the low incidence of acute myocardial infarction among Eskimos may be attributed in part to a conversion of one of the fatty acids in fish oil, eicosapentaenoic acid, (20:5n-3) into PGI_3. This hypothesis proposed that thromboxane A_3 is also formed but that it is relatively inactive as an aggregant, whereas the PGI_3 formed is active as an antiaggregating substance. The rationale was based in part on an earlier report (Raz et al, 1977) claiming that TXA_3 is not proaggregatory. It seemed reasonable to suggest that the observed lower platelet activity in people who ate lots of fish was due to the dietary polyunsaturated fatty acid 20:5n-3 forming trienoic prostaglandin derivatives (PGI_3, TXA_3, etc.) that had different properties from the dienoic derivatives (PGI_2, TXA_2, etc.) formed from 20:4n-6. An alternate mechanism that had been proposed earlier (Lands et al, 1973) was that the dietary n-3 fatty acids might block the formation of prostaglandin derivatives from arachidonic acid. This blocking inhibition was shown to reflect the selectivity of the prostaglandin-synthesizing enzyme (Lands et al, 1973).

A related study showed that feeding fish oil that contained high amounts of n-3 fatty acids could lower the amount of brain damage to cats undergoing cerebral ischemia (Black et al, 1979). Culp et al (1980) demonstrated that an experimental model for myocardial infarction was also sensitive to the presence of fish oil (menhaden) added to the diet. Following a standard thrombotic challenge, only about 3% of the left ventricle was infarcted in animals that had received a supplement of menhaden oil for 4 weeks, whereas control animals manifested an infarction volume of about 25%. The experiments could not determine whether the benefit was from the n-3 acids forming special trienoic eicosanoids or inhibiting an excessive production of dienoic eicosanoids from arachidonate. Regardless of the mechanism, the results from both the epidemiologic and laboratory animal studies clearly suggested the possible benefit of maritime foods in the diet.

To directly test the effect of maritime foods on platelet aggregation in humans, Siess et al (1980) demonstrated that 7 healthy men on a diet of 500-800 g of mackerel per day (representing a consumption of 7-11 g of eicosapentaenoic acid 20:5n-3) had significantly decreased platelet function. The decreased platelet aggregation correlated with an increased ratio of 20:5n-3/20:4n-6 in the platelet phospholipids. In 3 weeks, the ratio for these polyunsaturated fatty acids had shifted from 0 to a value of 0.52 for one subject. Eskimos have an even higher ratio of 20:5n-3/20: 4n-6 (approximately 1.0), and their platelet aggregation occurs less readily Supplementing an otherwise unchanged Western diet with 40 ml daily of cod liver oil (3 g 20:5n-3 and 5 g 22:6n 3) increased the bleeding times of 8 healthy males from 104 to 145 seconds and decreased the TXB_2 formed in response to collagen (Lorenz et al, 1983). The longer bleeding time may be due to lower amounts of proaggregatory substances (like thromboxane) or higher amounts of antiaggregatory material (like prostacyclin).

A detailed study by Hamazaki et al (1982) on the effect of orally administered ethyl eicosapentaenoate examined the ability of aortas to produce antiaggregatory materials. The ethyl ester of eicosapentaenoic acid enhanced the production of PGI_2-like material, but no evidence for derivatives of PGI_3 that would arise from n-3 precursors was detected. Incubation of 14C-eicosapentaenoic acid (20:5n-3) with aortas either from control rats or rats fed the eicosapentaenoate provided no detectable PGI_3 derivative. Thus the authors concluded that the antiaggregatory substance produced by rat aortas was most likely PGI_2 derived from 20:4n-6 and not derived from 20:5n-3.

A similar conclusion was provided by Needleman et al (1980), who noted the antagonism by 20:5n-3 of 20:4n-6 being converted to prostaglandin derivatives. Studies by Vas Dias et al (1982) showed a significant reduction in experimentally induced platelet aggregation in rabbits fed fish oil but not in those fed linseed oil, corn oil, or coconut oil. The change in platelet aggregation was associated with increased eicosapentaenoic acid and decreased arachidonate acid in the platelet lipids. Although the eicosapentaenoate content significantly increased in platelets with both linseed oil and fish oil diets the accumulation of eicosapentaenoic acid in aortic lipids occurred only in rabbits fed the fish oil diet. The difference between the two tissues can reflect differences in the distribution of dietary fatty acids in the relative activities of the desaturating enzymes and in the lipid synthetic specificities. Irrespective of differences in tissue acyl chain composition, both dietary 18:3n-3 and 20:5n-3 appeared to be equally antiaggregatory with isolated rabbit platelets that were challenged with collagen or thrombin.

Three studies confirmed the beneficial effect of added supplements of a fish oil concentrate or purified eicosapentaenoic acid (20:5n-3) in reducing risk factors. A double blind study with 12 volunteers included 2 g of 20:5n-3 daily for 4 weeks and decreased platelet aggregation (Nagakawa et al, 1983). A similar study with 8 subjects showed a significant decrease in platelet aggregation and an increase in red cell deformability and whole blood viscosity following 3.5 g of 20:5n-3 daily for 4 weeks (Terano et al, 1983). A long-term study of 107 subjects for periods of up to 2 years reported increased bleeding times and decreased frequency of anginal attacks that needed glyceryl trinitrate for relief (Saynor et al, 1984). In that study, the patients were asked to take 10 ml of fish oil twice daily with food, an amount equivalent to about 2 g of 20:5n-3 per day.

Heterogeneous Dietary Practices

The consistent correlation of lower myocardial infarction or thrombosis with higher dietary eicosapentaenoic acid led Lea and co-workers (1982) to estimate whether people without infarctions had somehow consumed more eicosapentaenoic in their daily diets. They analyzed the fatty acids of the red blood cells of 20 patients who had suffered myocardial infarctions and a group of 17 healthy age-matched controls. The content of the eicosapentaenoic acid in the cellular fatty acids of the two groups was significantly different: only 3.9% for patients who had experienced a myocardial infarction and 6.6% in the cellular lipids of control subjects. These results help emphasize that the average diet of a nation may not be that of all individuals, and that each person's health status should be evaluated with evidence of his/her polyunsaturated fatty acid intake (see examples in Chapter 17). The results also enforce those from animal experiments to suggest that the presence of n-3 polyunsaturated acids in the diet may help decrease the incidence of heart attacks (coronary thrombosis).

There is a need for more data to show how much difference occurs in the dietary intakes of n-3 and n-6 fatty acids by different individuals so that appropriate comparisons can be made among subsets of the study group rather than mix all the results from random populations. For example, in a study of 262 subjects, 14 had 13% of total erythrocyte fatty acids as 20:5n-3 and a 20:4n-6/20:5n-3 ratio of 0.2, whereas the overall average for the group was 2.3% 20:5n-3 and a ratio of 20:4n-6 to 20:5n-3 of 2.8 (Angelico and Amodeo, 1978.). The small subset of 14 individuals might be expected to have very different platelet functions compared with the rest of the group. More studies in which fatty acid analyses accompany clinical and physiological findings will be needed to reduce the "random noise" levels that are inherent in studies of independent, individualistic humans.

The amount of dietary n-3 fatty acid that can produce a significant change in the platelet function of subjects appears to be somewhere between 1.8 and 3.6 g daily from the results of Saynor and Verel (1982). This agrees with the limited results observed by Dyerberg who used 6 g of 20:5n-3 per day for 3 weeks with European volunteers and those of Kobayashi et al (1981) who used 1.4 g daily of 20:5n-3 with Japanese volunteers. The effective range was confirmed with six patients with peripheral vascular disease who were supplemented daily for one month with 10g of 20:5n-3, and platelet synthesis of thromboxane A_2 declined 58% with a coinciding increase in thromboxane A_3 (Knapp et al, 1986). Lowering the daily 20:5n-3 supplement to 1g did not maintain the decreased thromboxane A_2 synthesis. All our knowledge of lipid metabolism suggests that the daily supply of dietary n-3 and n-6 fatty acids compete with each other in maintaining the proportions of 20:4n-6 and 20:5n-3 stored in tissues and the customary daily supply of 15 grams of n-6 acids in foods requires high amounts of supplemental n-3 fats to decrease the availability of 20:4n-6 for platelet-endothelial cell signaling events.

It is important before concluding this summary of n-3 fatty acids and coronary thrombosis to note the results of Owren, who provided a series of papers which evaluated the effect of linseed oil as a possible preventive measure against coronary thrombosis (Owren et al, 1964; Owren, 1965, a,b). Linseed oil contains large amounts of the 18-carbon n-3 fatty acid, linolenic acid (18:3n-3), but none of the 20- or 22-carbon acids that are so abundant in fish. However, subsequent controlled clinical trials (e.g.,

Natvig et al, 1968) did not show any significant effect on platelet adhesiveness with daily dosages of 10 or 20 ml of refined linseed oil, and Dr. Owren noted that the results were insufficient to permit him to maintain his original concept and recommend the use of refined linseed oil as a possible preventive measure against coronary thrombosis. Platelet adhesiveness differs from aspects of platelet behavior which are regarded to be important in mediating thrombosis. Perhaps now the improved insight into the interactions of platelets with endothelial cells may lead to improved tests for platelet function. For example, using different amounts of collagen to induce platelet aggregation, workers showed that 60 ml of linseed oil per day for 6 weeks caused a striking decrease in the threshold for platelet sensitivity to collagen (Budowski et al, 1984). Dietary linolenate can decrease prostaglandin formation from arachidonate (Hwang and. Carroll, 1980; ten Hoor et al, 1980) so further study seems warranted. New understanding of the esterification, elongation and desaturation reactions for 18:3n-3, fed to humans and our better understanding of the biochemistry of platelet function may now permit us to reassess Owren's findings about dietary 18-carbon n-3 fats that are so much less effective than the 20-carbon n-3 HUFA.

Aspririn and Thrombosis

The 1986 edition of this book noted evidence that aspirin prevents thrombosis by blocking the platelet cyclooxygenase that catalyzes conversion of the n-6 arachidonate to the potent n-6 autacoid, thromboxane A_2. Nevertheless, much time lapsed before the biomedical community accepted the cyclooxygenase inhibitor, aspirin, as a preventive intervention in decreasing heart attacks. Looking back on the delays and the confusion shows that the biomedical community had an inadequate appreciation of the fact that aspirin irreversibly inactivates the cyclooxygenase.

Aspirin-treated platelets (without nuclear DNA with which to generate new active enzyme protein) remain unable to form the aggregatory n-6 autacoid, thromboxane, for their 7-14-day life, whereas endothelial cells rapidly recover their anti-aggregatory n-6 autacoid, prostacyclin, by forming new active cyclooxygenase within hours after aspirin treatment. It was clear at that time that intermittent, low-dose aspirin could block platelets from forming the aggregatory n-6 autacoid while permitting endothelial cells to continue forming the antiaggregatory autacoid, prostacyclin.

Eventually, three large trials, the Physicians' Health Study (1989; 1991), the Antiplatelet Trial Collaboration (1994, 2002), and the Thrombosis Prevention Trial (1998), showed the benefit of decreasing excessive n-6 thromboxane action to reduce the risk of ischemic heart disease (reviewed by Hennekens, 2002). The recognized importance of n-6 autacoid actions in ischemic heart disease led to the current almost universal use of low-dose aspirin in secondary prevention and adjunctive treatment of cardiovascular patients.

However, interindividual variability in platelet responses makes it important to not depend on aspirin treatment alone (Patrono et al, 2004). Despite clear mechanistic support for using low doses of aspirin to prevent n-6-thromboxane-mediated thrombotic events, there are many reasons against using such drugs (with their associated costs and harmful side effects) for primary prevention in large populations. Most importantly, drug treatments leave unaltered the original dietary imbalance in n-3 and n-6 EFA that supported excessive n-6 autacoid action. Over-attention to drug treatments has overlooked the simple fact that prevention of an imbalanced autacoid response in the body does not always require the use of drugs. The food we eat deserves closer attention.

Activated platelets mobilize a highly amplified hydrolytic release of the n-6 arachidonate and rapidly convert it to active autacoid, thromboxane A_2 (TXA_2), in much greater amounts than needed for aggregation. However, the unstable active TXA_2 spontaneously decomposes within seconds to the inactive thromboxane B2 (TXB_2), allowing only small amounts of active autacoid to bind to receptors in a vigorous but transient aggregation response. Following a few minutes of stimulation, platelets rapidly accumulate up to 550 ng/ml of the inactive degradation product, TXB_2, even though only 30-40 ng/ml of the active TXA_2 can give nearly full aggregation (Lands, 1985). That report showed widely diverse platelet responses for individuals, in part due to diverse food habits (see Fig. 6-3). Feeding n-3 HUFA clearly decreased platelet function in ways that reduce the risk of heart attack. However, the common practice of interpreting results with a linear statistical analysis of mean values obscures the effect of intervention on the hyperbolic non-linear platelet responses (Lands et al, 1985). Also, because cycloxygenase acts several-fold faster with the n-6 precursor compared to n-3 precursor (Chapter 14), the n-6 HUFA released from platelet membranes amplifies aggregation signals within seconds under conditions in

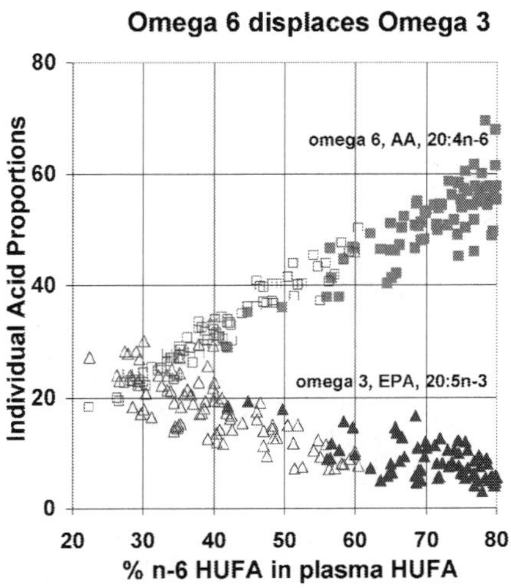

Fig. 6-3 Analyses from many different people show how higher proportions of n-6 in HUFA accompany lower n-3 HUFA in plasma HUFA. Open symbols are analyses from individual Japanese and closed symbols are from Americans.

which slower formation from the n-3 HUFA may accumulate little active autacoid at platelet receptors. These important kinetic aspects can be measured in small clinical studies of autacoid mechanisms with a few patients. Unfortunately, handling and storing the hundreds or thousands of blood samples needed in large clinical trials keeps clinical researchers from obtaining the needed rapid measurements (Park et al, 2002). New assays of platelet activation which are better suited to mass handling of samples are still needed to obtain better proof in clinical trials of the role of platelets in fatal heart attacks.

Several studies using dietary n-3 fats to decrease platelet function were described in the first edition of this book. However, the widespread awareness of benefits from cutting excessive n-6 eicosanoid (thromboxane A_2) actions with drugs like aspirin was not matched in the drug-oriented medical community by an equal appreciation that raising dietary n-3 fats also can decrease the relative intensity of n-6 eicosanoid responses. The community wanted epidemiological evidence confirmed by direct intervention clinical trials. Successful prevention of heart attacks by dietary changes became much more evident from two recent large secondary prevention trials, the Lyon Diet Heart Study (deLorgeril, 1999) and the GISSI-Prevenzione trial (1999), that confirmed results of the earlier DART trial (Burr, 1989). An interesting fact is that awareness of excess thromboxane action was so widespread by the 1990s, that the GISSI clinical trial to study fish oil in secondary prevention found that 92% of the cardiovascular patients enrolled in the study had already been advised to take antiplatelet drugs. Clearly, excessive platelet action (via excessive n-6 thromboxane) was accepted as a cause of death more than its diet-based origin. Sadly, some people with no fear of excess bleeding from using aspirin expressed such a fear from using n-3 supplements to decrease excessive tissue production of n-6 eicosanoids. Such fear of the unknown caused little to be done for nutritional steps in primary prevention of thrombosis.

Diverse Human Tissue HUFA

The first edition noted that people differ in their food choices that provide n-3 and n-6 EFA, and the results noted above for platelets reflect that diversity. Recent analyses show that the n-6 HUFA proportion of plasma phospholipid HUFA in free-living people eating their customary self-selected food choices can range from 15% to 90% n-6 in HUFA. Results from Americans in the right side of Figure 6-3 illustrate that diversity, with almost no overlap with the diverse values from individual Japanese at the left of the figure. Such HUFA diversity within populations predicts a likelihood of different thromboxane generation rates for individuals just as differences among population means in Fig 6-4 fit observed CHD mortalities.

Recent research provided a quantitative empirical equation that predicts how much dietary EFA supply may affect general tissue HUFA composition (Chapter 17). The n-3 and n-6 HUFA compete during entry and exit at the 2-position of tissue phospholipids. Thus, any food-based diversity in HUFA proportions will affect n-6 throm-

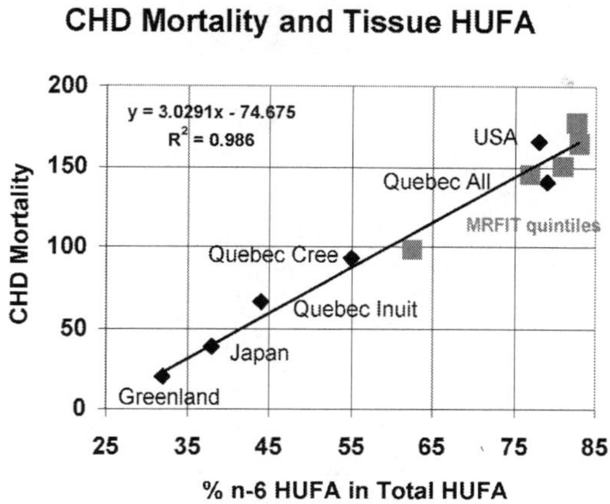

Fig. 6-4. The risk of a heart attack is greater when n-6 HUFA dominate the tissue HUFA.

boxane formation when activated platelet phospholipase releases HUFA with little or no selectivity between n-3 and n-6 HUFA (Weaver and Holub, 1986). As a result, platelet membranes with a lower proportion of n-6 HUFA in the total HUFA will release a lower proportion of the precursor of n-6 TXA_2 and provide a less intense aggregation response. Although Americans have a limited diversity in their tissue HUFA because of their typically high dietary n-6 EFA and relatively low dietary n-3 HUFA, the one quintile with the lowest proportion of n-6 HUFA had a significantly lower mortality from heart attacks in the MRFIT prospective longitudinal trial (Dolecek, 1991). Different proportions of n-6 HUFA autacoid precursor in tissues provides different intensities of the n-6 autacoid self-healing responses to stimuli, which is a likely cause of the closely associated cardiovascular mortality rates (Fig. 6-4).

The proportions of n-6 HUFA in tissue HUFA show a continuous gradient of risk in which there is no value completely free from risk. Chapters 17 and 19 examine the way that dietary intervention to improve the tissue balance of n-3 and n-6 HUFA can alter this readily modifiable risk factor during primary prevention efforts to improve the health of populations.

Technical Details

Results by Dyerberg and Bang (1978, 1979a,b) reaffirmed the decreased thrombotic tendency that was associated with a much greater threshold for ADP-induced platelet aggregation in Eskimos compared with Danes. Further evidence that the hemostatic function of Greenlanders was dominated by antiaggregatory prostaglandins was supported by the finding that aspirin gave a slightly shortened bleeding time for Eskimos rather than the lengthened bleeding time seen for Danes. The shift from 12.2 to 10.2 minutes following aspirin treatment still provided a time that was much greater than that characteristic of Danes (about 5 minutes).

A subsequent report by Hirai and co-workers (1980) demonstrated that residents of a fishing village in Japan had a lower tendency for platelet aggregation relative to a carefully matched population in a farming village. The threshold concentration of ADP for aggregation of platelets was 6.6 μM for fishing villagers whereas that for the farming villagers was 2.3 μM.

Thorngren and Gustafson (1981) indicated that the reduction of platelet-vessel wall interaction with diets rich in n-3 fatty acids seemed more complex than just a reduction in the susceptibility of platelets to aggregation by collagen or ADP. Thorngren et al (1983) noted that when aspirin was given to people supplementing their diets with extra amounts of fish, the inhibitory effect on platelet function was additive. Thus, antithrombotic therapy with drugs such as aspirin may be enhanced by selecting foods with higher n-3/n-6 ratios.

The mechanism whereby the increased dietary n-3 fatty acids exerted a beneficial effect seems likely to be an impaired conversion of arachidonate to thromboxane. The ratio of 20:5/20:4 in the platelet lipids of menhaden oil-supplemented dogs was changed from 0.06 to 1.8 with diet. The shift in the ratio of n-3 to n-6 acids from 0.04 to 0.31 was apparently not enough to reduce aggregation of rat platelets when supplements of eicosapentaenoic acid (20:5n-3) were added to a corn oil-based diet (Morita et al, 1984).

However when 20:5n-3 was added to a butter-based diet to shift the ratio from 0.05 to 0.70, significant inhibition of aggregation, occurred. Sanders et al (1980) reported that a daily supplement of cod liver oil for 6 weeks to healthy male subjects shifted the ratio of eicosapentaenoic to arachidonate in platelets from 0.02 to 0.13. This six fold change in ratio accompanied an elevation of bleeding time from 4.5 to 6.3 minutes. This shift in platelet function followed the daily ingestion of approximately 4 g of n-3 fatty acids, 1.8 g of 20:5n-3, and 2.2 g of 22:6n-3.

A brief study of 20 human volunteers receiving 10 ml of ethyl eicosapentaenoate daily for 3 weeks exhibited a significant fall in ADP-induced aggregation and an 11% greater bleeding time Dyerberg (1981). However, the author felt that the modest alterations obtained with 8 g of 20:5n-3 daily did not warrant far-reaching conclusions. Kobayashi et al (1981) noted the volunteers ingesting 1.4 g of eicosapentaenoic acid daily for 4 weeks had significantly lower blood viscosity although there was no significant difference in hematocrit levels. The basis for the decreased blood viscosity and platelet aggregability was not discussed in detail. Another prospective, controlled study in man (Goodnight et al, 1981) utilized diets containing salmon oil (60–90 ml per day) and salmon steaks (one pound per day). This provided about 15% of the calories as fat which contained approximately 10 g of the n-3 fatty acids. As the 20:5n-3/20:4n-6 ratio 'shifted from 0.004 in the control diet to 0.3 on the salmon diet, the bleeding time shifted from 6.7 to 10 minutes.

Another report by Hay et al (1982) illustrated altered platelet kinetics in patients with ischemic heart disease after they ingested fish oil. The nonlinear relationship between thromboxane production and aggregation (Lands et al, 1985) requires careful interpretation of data evaluating the effect of n-3 acids on platelets. Terano et al

(1982) administered 3.6 g of eicosapentaenoic acid daily to 8 healthy volunteers for 2-4 weeks, a statistically significant reduction in platelet aggregability was associated with decreased formation of thromboxane and a reduction in whole blood viscosity.

Increases in eicosapentaenoic acid content in erythrocyte membrane phospholipids were positively correlated with erythrocyte deformability. The authors suggested that the reduction in aggregation and the improved rheological properties of erythrocytes might be explained by the increased content of 20:5n-3 in the platelet and erythrocyte phospholipids. Rheological features of membranes illustrates one way in which the present awareness of the antithrombotic action of fish oil seems uncertain. In exploring further reduction in whole blood viscosity, workers found that there was no reduction in packed cell volume or plasma viscosity following fish oil supplementation, and the effect seemed due to changes in the red cell membrane (Woodcock et al. 1984). Feeding corn oil plus olive oil did not reduce whole blood viscosity. The reduced viscosity seems likely to be beneficial to patients with peripheral vascular disease, and more studies of this phenomenon seem likely.

Fibrin Formation

Stoffersen et al (1982) reported that Eskimos have a high level of plasma antithrombin III which may be a consequence, in part, of the high dietary intake of n-3 polyunsaturated fatty acids in contrast to Sanders' report (Sanders et at., 1981). Supplementation of the diet of 20 healthy Danish male volunteers for 3 weeks resulted in a significant increase in immunoreactive antithrombin III, although the increase in measurable biological activity of antithrombin III was insignificant. Nevertheless, the authors suggested that the Eskimo diet may result in a high level of antithrombin III which would increase the inhibition of activated coagulation factors and decrease the clotting tendency.

Subsequent work showed that plasma levels of antithrombin III were elevated by 10 g supplements of either fish or vegetable oil (Mortensen et al., 1983). Apparently both n-3 and n-6 polyunsaturated fatty acids can increase circulating amounts of this anticlotting protein. Thus, preliminary data suggest that not only platelet function but also fibrin clot formation may be decreased by including low amounts of maritime polyunsaturated fatty acids in the diet. The combined effects of the fish oil rich in n-3 were superior to those rich in n-6 acids alone. Such results stress the possible advantage of using dietary mixtures of polyunsaturated fatty acids in ways not commonly applied at the present.

Jakubowski et al (1982) reported that plasma factor 4 was significantly less in individuals receiving diets with polyunsaturated fat compared with those fed saturated fat diets. The secretion of these plasma clotting proteins from the liver may be influenced by different types of dietary polyunsaturated fatty acids in the same manner that the plasma lipoproteins are. Eating usual fat (but not medium-chain fat) induces postprandial lipaemia and elevates both Factor VII coagulant activity (FVIIc) and the activated form, FVIIa (Sanders et al, 1996). Increased intake of n-3 HUFA decreased circulating apoprotein AII concentrations, increased HDL2 cholesterol concentrations and resulted in less postprandial lipemia (Sanders et al, 1997). However, Factor VII coagulant activity (FVIIc) was higher and apoprotein AI concentration lower with a diet rich in n-3 compared with saturated fats. In contrast, plasma fibrinogen was significantly greater following the diet rich in n-6 than saturated fats.

A diet containing n-3 HUFA decreased postprandial lipemia, whereas a diet rich in alpha-linolenic acid did not (Sanders, 2003). Postprandial plasma triacylglycerol was greater following meals rich in oleate (5.8), elaidate (4.3) and palmitate (4.1) compared with stearate (2.0) and MCT (1.1) meals (Sanders et al, 2000). The increase in FVIIa at 7 h was greater after the oleate meal than after the stearate and MCT meals. These results do not support the hypothesis that dietary stearate and elaidate are responsible for the postprandial increases in FVII associated with high fat intakes. Eating unrandomized cocoa butter increased FVIIa 6 h later, but eating randomized cocoa butter did not. After randomization, the postprandial area under the curve for plasma triacylglycerol decreased by 41% ($P < 0.01$) and the proportion of oleic acid in the sn-2 position of the chylomicron triacylglycerol was reduced from 67.4 mol% to 35.9 mol% while the proportion of stearic acid rose from 9.2 mol% to 25.4 mol% (Sanders et al, 2003). Apparently the symmetrical stearic acid-rich triacylglycerol with oleic acid in the sn-2 position is absorbed more rapidly than are the natural asymmetrical triacylglycerols with long-chain saturated fatty acids in the sn-2 position, which leads to activation of FVII.

References

Angelico F, Amodeo P. Eicosapentaenoic acid and prevention of atherosclerosis. *Lancet* 2:531, 1978.

Antiplatelet Trialists' Collaboration. Collaborative overview of randomised trials of antiplatelet therapy. I. Prevention of death, myocardial infarction, and stroke by prolonged antiplatelet therapy in various categories of patients. *Brit Med J* 308:81–106, 1994.

Antiplatelet Trialists' Collaboration. Collaborative overview of randomised trials of antiplatelet therapy. II. Maintenance of vascular graft or arterial patency by antiplatelet therapy. *Brit Med J* 308:159–168, 1994.

Antiplatelet Trialists' Collaboration. Collaborative overview of randomised trials of antiplatelet therapy. III. Reduction in venous thrombosis and pulmonary embolism by antiplatelet prophylaxis among surgical and medical patients. *Brit Med J* 308:235–246, 1994.

Antithrombotic Trialists' Collaboration (2002). Collaborative meta-analysis of randomised trials of antiplatelet therapy for prevention of death, myocardial infarction, and stroke in high risk patients. *Brit Med J* 324:71-86, 2002.

Black KL, Culp B, Madison D, et al The protective effect of dietary fish oil on focal cerebral infarction. *Prostaglandins Med* 3, 257-268, 1979.

Budowskj ., Trostler N, Lupo M, et al Effect of linseed oil ingestion on plasma lipid fatty acid composition and platelet aggregability in healthy volunteers. *Nutr Res* 4:343-346, 1984.

Burr ML; Fehily AM; Rogers S, et al Diet and reinfarction trial (DART): design, recruitment, and compliance. *Eur Heart J* 10(6):558-567, 1989.

Collaborative overview of randomised trials of antiplatelet therapy: prevention of death, myocardial infarction, and stroke by prolonged antiplatelet therapy in various categories of patients. *Brit Med J* 308:81-106, 1994.

Culp BR, Lands WEM, Lucchesi BR, et al The effect of dietary supplementation of fish oil on experimental myocardial infarction. *Prostaglandins* 20:1021-1031, 1980.

deLogeril M, et al, The Final Report of the Lyon Diet Heart Study. *Circulation* 99:779-785, 1999.

Dolecek TA, Granditis G. Dietary polyunsaturated fatty acids and mortality in the Multiple Risk Factor Intervention Trial (MRFIT). *World Rev Nutr Diet* 66: 205216, 1991.

Dyerberg J. Platelet-vessel wall interactions. *Philos Trans R Soc London Ser B* 294:373-381, 1981.

Dyerberg J, Bang HO. Dietary fat and thrombosis. *Lancet* 1:152, 1978.

Dyerberg J, Bang HO.. Lipid metabolism, atherogenesis and haemostasis in Eskimos: The role of the prostaglandin-3 family. *Haemostasis* 8:227-233, 1979a.

Dyerberg J, Bang HO. Haemostatic function and platelet polyunsaturated fat acids in Eskimos. *Lancet* 2:433-435, 1979b.

Dyerberg J, Bang HO, Stoffersen E, et al Eicosapentaenoic acid and prevention of thrombosis and atherosclerosis. *Lancet* 2:117-119, 1978.

GISSI-Prevenzioni Group. Dietary supplementation with n-3 polyunsaturated fatty acids and vitamin E after myocardial infarction: results of the GISSI-Prevenzione trial. *Lancet* 354:447-455, 1999, plus an editorial by M. Brown, *Lancet* 1999; 354:441-442, 1999.

Goodnight SH Jr, Harris WS, Connor W. The effects of dietary w-3 fatty acids on platelet composition and function in man: A prospective, controlled study. *Blood* 58(5):880-885, 1981.

Hamazaki, T., Hirai, A., Terano, et al Effects of orally administered ethyl ester of eicosapentaenoic acid (EPA; C20:5, w-3) on PGI2-like substance production by rat aorta. *Prostaglandins* 23:557-567, 1982.

Hamberg M, Svensson J, Wakabayashi T, et al Isolation and structure of two prostaglandin endoperoxides that cause platelet aggregation. *Proc Natl Acad Sci USA*1:345-349, 1974a.

Hamberg M, SvenssonJ, Samuelsson B. Prostaglandin endoperoxides. A new concept concerning the mode of action and release of prostaglandins. *Proc Natl Acad Sci USA* 1:3824-3828, 1974b.

Hamberg M, Svensson J, Samuelsson B. Thromboxanes: A new group of biologically active compounds derived from prostaglandin endoperoxides. Pr*oc Natl Acad Sci USA* 72:2994-2998, 1975.

Hay CRM, Durber AP, Saynor R. Effect of fish oil on platelet kinetics in patients with ischaemic heart disease. *Lancet* 1:1269-1272, 1082, 1982.

Hennekens CH. (2002) Update on aspirin in the treatment and prevention of cardiovascular disease. *Am J Manag Care*. 22 (Suppl): S691-S700, 2002.

Hirai A, Hamazaki T, Terano T, et al Eicosapentaenoic acid and platelet function in Japanese. *Lancet* 2:1132-1133, 1980.

Hwang DH, Carrol AE. Decreased formation of prostaglandin derived from arachidonic acid by dietary linolenate in rats. *Am J Clin Nutr* 33:590-597, 1980.

Jakubowski JA, Ardlie NG, Morgan FJ, et al (1982). Further observations on the effects of dietary fatty acid composition on platelet reactivity and blood coagulation in man and the influence of methodology on findings. *Atherosclerosis* 41:285-294, 1982.

Knapp HR, Reilly IA, Alessandrini P, et al In vivo indexes of platelet and vascular function during fish-oil administration in patients with atherosclerosis. *N Engl J Med* 314:937-942, 1986.

Kobayashi S, Hirai A, Terano T, et al Reduction in blood viscosity by eicosapentaenoic acid. *Lancet* 2:197, 1981.

Lands WEM, LeTellier PR, Rome LH, et al Inhibition of prostaglandin biosynthesis. *Adv Biosciences* 9:15-28, 1973.

Lands WEM, Culp BR, Hirai A, et al (1985). Relationship of thromboxane generation to the aggregation of platelets from humans: Effects of eicosapentaenoic acid. *Prostaglandins* 30:819-825, 1985.

Lea EJA, Jones SP, Hamilton DV. (1982). The fatty acids of erythrocytes of myocardial infarction patients. *Atherosclerosis* 41, 363-369, 1982.

Lorenz R, Spengler U, Fischer S, et al (1983). Platelet function, thromboxane formation and blood pressure control during supplementation of the western diet with cod liver oil. *Circulation* 67, 504-511, 1983.

Moncada S, Vane JR. Prostacyclin: Its biosynthesis, actions and clinical potential. *Philos Trans R Soc London Ser* B 294:305-329, 1981.

Moncada S, Gryglewski R, Bunting S, et al An enzyme isolated from arteries transforms prostaglandin endoperoxides to an unstable substance that inhibits platelet aggregation. *Nature* 263, 663-665, 1976.

Morita I, Komeshinia N, Takahashi R, et al. (1984). A proposed method for exploring anti-aggregatory effects of eicosapentaenoic acid in the rat. *Prostaglandins, Leukotrienes Med* 14:123-129, 1984.

Mortensen JZ, Schmidt EB, Nielsen AH, et al. (1983). The effect of n-6 and n-3 polyunsaturated fatty acids on hemostasis, blood lipids and blood pressure. *Thromb Haemosrasjs* 50:543-546, 1983.

MRC General Practice Research Framework. Thrombosis prevention trial: randomised trial of low-intensity oral anticoagulation with warfarin and low-dose aspirin in the primary prevention of ischemic heart disease in men at increased risk. *Lancet* 351:233-241, 1998.

Nagakawa Y, Orimo H., Harasawa M, et al Effect of elcosapentaenojc acid on the platelet aggregation and composition of fatty acid in man. *Atherosclerosis* 47:71-75, 1983.

Natvig H, Borchgrevink CF, Dedichen J, et al (1968) A controlled trial of the effect of linolenic acid on incidence of coronary heart disease. The Norwegian vegetable oil experiment of 1965-66. *Scand J Clin Lab Invest Suppl* 105:1-20, 1968.

Needleman P, Whitaker MG, Wyche A, et al Manipulation of platelet aggregation by prostaglaridins and their fatty acid precursors: Pharmacological basis for a therapeutic approach. *Prostaglandins* 19:165-180, 1980..

Owren PA. Coronary thrombosis. Its mechanism and possible prevention by linolenic acid. *Ann Intern Med* 63:167-184, 1965a.

Owren PA. Linolenic acid and coronary thrombosis. *Ann Intern Med* 63:1160, 1965b.

Owren PA, Hellem AJ, Odegaard A. Linolenic acid for the prevention of thrombosis and myocardial infarction. *Lancet* 2:975-979, 1964.

Park Y, Schoene N, Harris W. Mean platelet volume as an indicator of platelet activation: methodological issues. *Platelets* 13:301-306, 2002.

Patrono C, Bachmann F, Baigent C. Expert Consensus Document on the use of antiplatelet agents: The Task Force on the Use of Antiplatelet Agents in Patients with Atherosclerotic Cardiovascular Disease of the European Society of Cardiology. *Eur Heart J* 25:166-181, 2004.

Physicians Health Study Research Group; Steering Committee. Final report on the aspirin component of the ongoing Physicians' Health Study. *N Engl J Med* 321:129-135, 1989.

Raz A, Minkes MS, Needleman P. Structural determinants for platelet aggregation and vasoconstriction. *Biochim Biophys Acta* 488:305-311, 1977.

Ridker PM, Manson JE, Buring JE, et al The effect of chronic platelet inhibition with low-dose aspirin on atherosclerotic progression and acute thrombosis: clinical evidence from the Physicians Health Study. *Am Heart J* 122:1588-1592, 1991.

Ross R, Glomset JA. The pathogenesis of atherosclerosis I. *N Engl J Med* 295:369-377, 1976.

Ross R, Glomset JA. The pathogenesis of atherosclerosis. II. *N Engl J. Med* 295, 420-425, 1976.

Sanders TA. Dietary fat and postprandial lipids. *Curr Atheroscler Rep* 5(6):445-451, 2003.

Sanders TA, Berry SE, Miller GJ. Influence of triacylglycerol structure on the postprandial response of factor VII to stearic acid-rich fats. *Am J Clin Nutr* 77(4):777-782, 2003.

Sanders TA, de Grassi T, Miller GJ, et al Influence of fatty acid chain length and cis/trans isomerization on postprandial lipemia and factor VII in healthy subjects (postprandial lipids and factor VII). *Atherosclerosis* 2000 149(2):413-420, 2000.

Sanders TA, Miller GJ, de Grass T, et al Postprandial activation of coagulant factor VII by long-chain dietary fatty acids. *Thromb Haemost* 76(3):369-371, 1996.

Sanders TA, Oakley FR, Miller GJ, et al Influence of n-6 versus n-3 polyunsaturated fatty acids in diets low in saturated fatty acids on plasma lipoproteins and hemostatic factors. *Arterioscler Thromb Vasc Biol* 17(12):3449-3460, 1997.

Sanders TA, Vickers M, Haines AP. (1981), Effect on blood lipids and haemostasjs of a supplement of cod liver oil, rich in eicosapentaenoic and docosahexaenoic acids, in healthy young men. *Clin Sci* 61:317-324, 1981.

Saynor R, Verel D. (1982). Eicosapentaenoic acid, bleeding time, and serum lipids. *Lancet* 2:72,1982.

Saynor R, Verel D, Gillott T. The long-term effect of dietary supplementation with fish lipid concentrate on serum lipids, bleeding time, platelets and angina. *Atherosclerosis* 50:3-10, 1984.

Siess W, Roth P, Scherer B, et al Platelet-membrane fatty acids, platelet aggregation, and thromboxane formation during a mackerel diet. *Lancet* 1:441-444, 1980.

Silver M., Hoch W, Kocsjs BB, et al Arachidonic acid causes sudden death in rabbits, *Science* 183:1085-1087, 1974.

Smith JB, Willis AL. Aspirin selectively inhibits prostaglandin production in human platelets. *Nature* 231:235-238, 1971.

Stoffersen E, Jorgensen KA, Dyerberg E. Antithrombin Ill and dietary intake of polyunsaturated fatty acids. *Scand J Clin Lab Inves*. 42, 83-86, 1982.

ten Hoor F, DeDeckere EAM, Haddeman E, et al Dietary manipulation of prostaglandin and thromboxane synthesis in heart, aorta and blood platelets of the rat. *Adv Prostaglandin Thromboxane Res* 8, 1771-1781, 1980.

Terano T, Hirai A, Hamazaki T, et al Effect of oral administration of a highly purified eicosanentaenojc acid on PG metabolism and blood viscosity in normal volunteers, In International Conference, p. 697. Florence Italy: Fondazione Giovanni Lorenzinj, 1982.

Terano T, Hirai A, Hamazakj T. Effect on oral administration of highly purified eicosapentaenoic acid on platelet function, blood viscosity and red cell deformability in healthy human subjects. *Atherosclerosis* 46:321-331, 1983.

Thorngren M, Gustavson A. Effects of 11-week increase in dietary eicosapentaenoic acid on bleeding time, lipids and platelet aggregation. *Lancet* 2, 1190-1193, 1981.

Thorngren M, Gustafson A, Wohlfart G. Effects of acetylsalicylic acid on platelet aggregation before and during increase in dietary eicosapentaenoic acid. *Haemostasis* 13, 244-247, 1983.

Vane JR, Bunting S, Moncada S. Prostacyclin in physiology and pathophysiology. *Int Rev Exp Patho.* 23:161-207, 1982.

Vas Dias EW, Gibney MJ, Taylor TG. The effect of polyunsatumted fatty acids of the n-3 and n-6 series on platelet aggregation and platelet and aortic fatty acid composition in rabbits. *Atherosclerosis* 43:245-257, 1982.

Weaver BJ, Holub BJ. The relative degradation of [14C]eicosapentaenoyl and [3H]arachidonoyl species of phosphatidylinositol and phosphatidylcholine in thrombin-stimulated human platelets. *Biochem Cell Biol* 64(12):1256-1261, 1986.

Woodcock BE, Smith E, Lambert WH, et al (1984). Beneficial effect of fish oil on blood viscosity in peripheral vascular disease. *Br Med J.* 288:592-594.

2005 National Library of Medicine Search Results:

(http://www.ncbi.nlm.nih.gov/entrez/query.fcgi)
thrombosis = 117,004; thrombosis eicosanoid = 1,609; thrombosis fish = 151; thrombosis aspirin = 3,870; thrombosis coronary = 3,428; thrombosis NSAID = 3,310; thrombosis omega-3 = 135

7—Vasospasm: Cardiac Output and Coronary Flow

Both the output of blood from the heart and the integrity of the blood vessels feeding the heart are needed to maintain an adequate delivery of oxygen and nutrients to the heart muscle. Saturated fatty acids in diets with too many calories have been implicated frequently in the progressive chronic onset of atherosclerosis with its resultant impaired blood flow described in Chapter 5. In contrast, polyunsaturated fatty acids of the n-6 type are associated more with the rapid aspects of hemostasis, thrombosis, and vascular spasm that involve thromboxane. Thromboxane A_2 derived from arachidonic acid (20:4n-6) may induce arterial spasm, and it has been implicated in Prinzmetal's angina. The fact that unstable angina and myocardial infarction can occur when a patient is at rest suggests that the primary cause of the problem was not a greater need for oxygen by an overexerting heart muscle, but a decreased delivery of oxygen to the heart muscle. The decreased oxygen supply could result from thrombus formation as described in Chapter 6 or from coronary vasoconstriction caused by either catecholamines or thromboxane.

Vasoconstriction, or spasm, is due to contraction of the smooth muscles lining the blood vessel, and it slows the delivery of oxygen and nutrients to the tissue. Repeated severe vasospasm of atherosclerotic vessels may also lead to rupture of atherosclerotic plaques. This would subsequently provoke more adhesion and aggregation of platelets, which would result in further release of thromboxane and cause more spasm and thrombus formation (Fig. 7-1). This complex interaction between the vascular smooth muscle and the platelets is another important area in which dietary fatty acids can have an impact on human health

The major prostaglandin formed by vascular tissue from arachidonate was identified by Vane and his associates as the vasodilating, antithrombotic prostacyclin, PGI_2. Nevertheless, arachidonic acid added to isolated perfused hearts caused coronary vasoconstriction followed by vasodilation. This vasoconstriction response was prevented by indomethacin or aspirin, which blocks the cyclooxygenase activity that forms prostaglandins. In fact, these drugs prevent both the constricting and the dilating responses caused by arachidonate. Thus, some vasoconstricting eicosanoid appears to be formed from arachidonate in the blood vessels. Talesnik and Hsia (1982) demonstrated that a slow infusion of docosahexaenoic acid also inhibited both the constricting and dilating responses of the coronary arteries to arachidonate. Thus the long-chain n-3 polyunsaturated fatty acid can function protectively in diminishing the amount of coronary vasospasm as well as the platelet aggregation. Both of these protective effects may be provided by the action of either 20:5n-3, 22:5n-3, or 22:6n-3 in inhibiting the generation of thromboxane by platelets. Local release of thromboxane in the coronary circulation was reported to

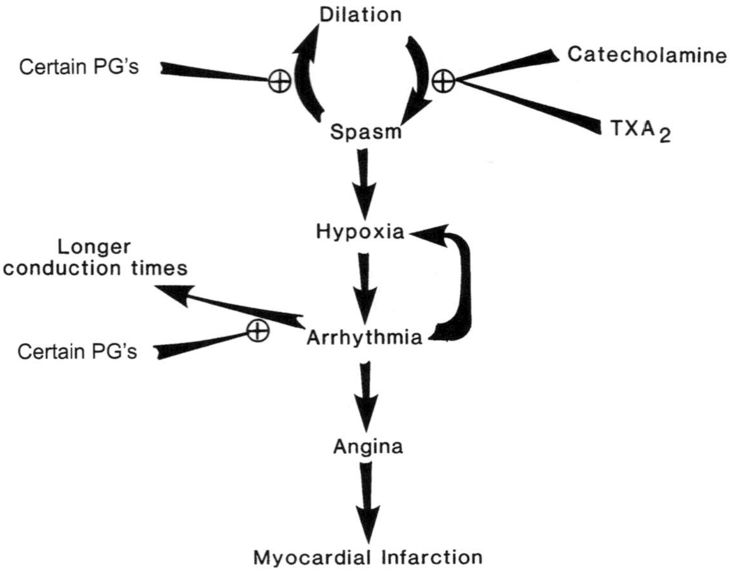

Fig. 7-1. Spasms and arrhythmias.

be associated with episodes of angina (Hirsh et al, 1981), but whether the elevated thromboxane was the cause of the angina or a subsequent effect of the anginal spasm on platelets remains unknown.

In studying the contractile effect of norepinephrine on rat aortic strips, Lockett et al (1982) concluded that the contraction is normally augmented by intrinsic prostaglandins, and that the augmentation can be diminished by a dietary intake of fish oil. Rats treated with fish oil supplements for 3 weeks demonstrated normal, unaltered contractile responses to potassium chloride and dilating responses to nitroprusside. Thus the general contractile action of the muscles was not altered by the diet. Also, vascular responses to added PGF_2 and PGE_2 were not altered. Thus, the decreased responsiveness to catecholamine challenge observed after feeding fish oil appeared to be due to a diminished generation of prostaglandins within the vessel walls. Earlier studies indicated that catecholamine-induced constriction of the mesenteric vessels was potentiated by PGE_2, although that in the splenic artery was inhibited (Kondo et al, 1978). The aortas of rats treated with fish oil had a 20:5n-3/20:4n-6 ratio of 2.8, whereas that of the untreated control rats was 0.36.

The significant reduction in vascular responsiveness to the catecholamine suggests that dietary intake of n-3 polyunsaturated acids may diminish the n-6 prostaglandins that enhance the responsiveness of coronary vessels to adrenaline, and thus n-3 acids could decrease the likelihood of severe coronary spasm during stressful conditions. This phenomenon seemed confirmed for humans when 8 volunteers were found to have reduced blood pressure responses to norepinephrine after their diet was supplemented with cod liver oil (Lorenz et al, 1983). In a special way, the sea may give us these polyunsaturated fatty acids and lessen our overreactions to the stresses in our lives on land. Again, we can question whether our average "Western industrial" diet has a polyunsaturated content that brings about overreactions to stressful stimuli. Are Eskimos less responsive than normal or are we hyper-responsive?

Extreme Heart Rhythms

Cardiac output depends on coronary vessels maintaining a flow of oxygen and nutrients to the heart muscle that pumps blood in response to a balance in sympathetic and parasympathetic (vagal) autonomic tone. A bias toward more sympathetic (adrenergic) activity is linked with a risk of cardiovascular death, and it is decreased by treatment with *alpha-* and *beta-*blockers.

During the 1980's, cardiologists blocked *alpha*-adrenergic signaling to decrease the ventricular arrhythmias that develop rapidly whenever blood flow to the heart is stopped and hypoxia develops (Heather, 1987). Increased adrenergic signaling with hypoxia is partly due to rapid reversible rises in adrenergic receptors, and an associated rise in intracellular calcium and release of nonesterified fatty acids from heart lipids.

Differing actions by n-3 and n-6 fatty acids were indicated when dietary fish oil prevented ventricular fibrillation following coronary artery occlusion (McLennan, 1988), apparently by decreasing *alpha*-adrenergic (but not *beta*-adrenergic) action (Reibel, 1988). After arrhythmias induced by impaired ion transport were prevented by n-3 HUFA, but not the n-6 HUFA, arachidonate (Hallaq, 1990), attention turned to calcium channels as a locus for the selective EFA action (Hallaq, 1992; Billman, 1994). Most nonesterified fatty acids with 2 or more double bonds can prevent arrhythmia, but the frequent arrhythmias with n-6 arachidonate depend on forming prostaglandins by cyclooxygenase (Kang and Leaf, 1994 and 2000; Xiao, 1997).

Arrhythmia-stimulating actions of n-6 arachidonate and its autacoids can be expected to be worse when tissue HUFA available for release have high proportions of n-6 HUFA (a condition that results from typical American diets). Cyclooxygenase products of the n-6 arachidonate are major arrhythmogenic autacoids, and products from the n-3 analog, eicosapentaenoate, seem much less active. Thus, the balance of n-3 and n-6 HUFA released from the tissue affects the extent of arrhythmogenic events.

Arrhythmogenic n-6 prostaglandins, especially PGF_2 and TXA_2, induce a concentration-dependent, reversible arrhythmia, although prostacyclin (PGI_2) acts through different receptors to signal protective actions (Li et al, 1997). The autacoids have parallel actions on vascular smooth muscle which acquires free calcium and contracts more with the n-6 PGF_2 and TXA_2 than with the corresponding n-3 autacoids. Overall, a diet-induced bias in tissue HUFA composition toward n-6 HUFA (and less n-3 HUFA) creates a bias in autonomic signaling toward sympathetic (and less parasympathetic) actions that result in vasospasm and arrhythmia accompanying a bias in platelet signaling toward thrombosis.

Interpreting Sudden Death

The rapid signaling events during platelet aggregation and heart rhythm dysfunction act together and make it difficult to distinguish the extent to which anti-thrombotic or anti-arrhythmic actions of fish oil prevent sudden death. Thus, reports of seafood or fish oil decreasing the incidence of "sudden death" in population studies or in clinical trials may be due to decreasing either or both thrombosis or arrhythmic death. Successful clinical intervention causing decreased mortality by increasing dietary n-3 intake has now been reported in three large trials (Burr, 1989; deLorgeril, 1999; GISSI group, 1999), and the decrease in sudden death was most dramatic. Also, the US Physicians Health Study reported that consumption of fish at least once per week may reduce the risk of sudden cardiac death in men (Albert, 1998; Sheard, 1998). Regardless of the cellular processes underlying the successful interventions, the results affirm the health benefit of shifting the bias of tissue HUFA away from excessive n-6 HUFA and toward more equal n-3 and n-6 HUFA.

Newly developed methods for continuous monitoring and analyzing rapid, transient changes of heart rate show high rate variability in healthy individuals, whereas low heart rate variability (due to excessive sympathetic adrenergic activity that decreases vagal tone) occurs with greater cardiac arrhythmic events and mortality (Curtis,2002). Beneficial maintenance of heart rate variability (HRV) by increasing dietary n-3 EFA was seen in a clinical trial of cardiovascular patients (Christensen, 1996). Also, healthy men had a positive relationship between their HRV and the n-3 HUFA in their red blood cells (Christensen, 1999). Continued studies of HRV with Holter monitor recorders has further confirmed the ability of increased dietary n-3 HUFA to shift autonomic tone away from a sympathetic bias and toward a parasympathetic bias with higher HRV that is associated with lower cardiovascular mortality (Christensen et al, 2001; Villa, 2002). By 2004, there is much evidence to support the benefit of eating n-3 HUFA to decrease risks of vasospasm and cardiac arrhythmia.

Technical Details

Bayer and Forster (1979) demonstrated that the n-6 fatty acids prolonged the conduction time and the functional refractory period for cat hearts *in situ*, whereas oleic and linolenic acid had only a weak effect. Pretreatment of the animals with indomethacin either diminished or abolished the action of the effective n-6 fatty acids. Apparently the n-6 acids exerted their effective antiarrhythmic action by being converted into certain prostaglandins. Depression of conduction in heart muscle and prolonging the refraction time are known to have antiarrhythmic effects.

These electrophysiological effects illustrate ways in which the n-6 fatty acids can have beneficial cardiovascular actions in contrast to the undesired actions of vasospasm and thrombosis associated with the n-6 acids participating in platelet function and thromboxane formation. The eicosanoids made by the heart muscle prevent that vital muscle from overreacting.

Gudbjarnason and Oskarsdottir (1975, 1977); Gudbjarnason and Hallgrimsson (1976), and Gudbjarnason et al (1978) reported changes in the composition of fatty acids in myocardial lipids associated with myocardial pathology. In 1975 Gudbjarnason and Oskarsdottir reported that the development of myocardial necrosis increases with a progressive replacement of linoleate and arachidonate by 22:6n-3. Interestingly, animals that had been fed a diet of cod liver oil did not show an alteration in the fatty acid composition of heart muscle phospholipid, and over-stimulation with isoproterenol did not produce any changes in the relatively high content of 22:6 in the membrane lipids of those animals. Subsequent studies with rats fed a standard commercial diet indicated that repeated challenge with norepinephrine significantly decreased the amount of 18:2n-6 and 18:ln-9 in heart phosphatidylcholine and increased the amount of 22:6n-3 in phosphatidylethanolamine (Emilsson and Gudbjarnason, 1981).

Serum PL of patients with CHD and of patients with acute, fatal MI contained significantly more arachidonic acid (20:4n6, AA) and docosahexaenoic acid (22:6n3, DHA) than serum PL of normal subjects (Skuladottir et al, 1985). Also, fatal ventricular fibrillation in rats and sudden cardiac death in man were accompanied by a high ratio of 20:4 n-6/22:6 n-3. The balance between n-6 and n-3 fatty acids in cellular phospholipids seem to play an important role in sudden cardiac death (Gudbjarnason, 1989). The incidence of ventricular fibrillation (VF) and sudden cardiac death induced by isoproterenol in adult rats fed different dietary fat was lowest in rats fed cod liver oil, with a low ratio of AA/DHA in cardiac phospholipids (Gudbjarnason et al, 1989). Mortality due to VF was highest in rats fed corn oil with the highest ratio of AA/DHA.

Using high levels of dietary linoleate, deDeckere and ten Hoor (1980) showed a positive relationship between the maximum left ventricular work and the amount of 18:2 in the diet. Presumably prostaglandins mediate the observed higher coronary flow rate and myocardial contractility. Similar studies in the presence and absence of indomethacin or some other cyclooxygenase inhibitor would be helpful in reaching further conclusions on the mechanism of this effect of high levels of dietary linoleate. In 1982, ten Hoor and deDekere noted that feeding rats a diet of 18 en% linoleic acid resulted in a 50% decrease in prostacyclin production of the isolated heart, but did not significantly influence the coronary flow or contractual force of isolated perfused hearts. In these experiments, previous injection of aspirin or indomethacin completely inhibited the release of prostacyclin and decreased the coronary flow, but had no effect on the contractual force. Thus the mechanisms whereby dietary fatty acids can modify myocardial effectiveness appear to be intricate.

References

Albert CM; Hennekens CH; O'Donnell CJ; et al Fish consumption and risk of sudden cardiac death. *JAMA* 279(1):23-28, 1998.

Bayer BL, Forster W. Actions of prostaglandin precursors and other unsaturated fatty acids on conduction time and refractory period in the cat heart in situ. *Brit J Pharmacol* 66:191-195, 1979.

Billman GE, Hallaq H, Leaf A. Prevention of ischemia-induced ventricular fibrillation by omega 3 fatty acids. *Proc Natl Acad Sci* 91(10):4427-4430, 1994.

Burr ML; Fehily AM; Rogers S; et al Diet and reinfarction trial (DART): design, recruitment, and compliance. *Eur Heart J* 10(6):558-567, 1989.

Curtis BM, O'Keefe JH Jr. Autonomic tone as a cardiovascular risk factor: The dangers of chronic fight or flight. *Mayo Clin Proc* 77(1):45-54, 2002.

Christensen JH, Gustenhoff P, Korup E, et al Effect of fish oil on heart rate variability in survivors of myocardial infarction: a double blind randomised controlled trial. *Brit Med J* 312:677-678, 1996.

Christensen JH, Christensen MS, Dyerberg J, et al Heart rate variability and fatty acid content of blood cell membranes: a dose-response study with n-3 fatty acids. *Am J Clin Nutr* 70:331-337, 1999.

Christensen JH; Skou HA; Fog L; et al Marine n-3 fatty acids, wine intake, and heart rate variability in patients referred for coronary angiography. *Circulation* 103:651-657, 2001.

deDeckere EAM, ten Hoor F. Influences of dietary fats on coronary flow rate and left ventricular work of the isolated rat heart: Sunflower seed oil versus lard. *Nutr Metab* 24:396-408, 1980.

deLorgeril M, et al, The Final Report of the Lyon Diet Heart Study. *Circulation* 99:779-785, 1999.

Emilsson A, Gudbjarnason S. Changes in fatty acyl chain composition of rat heart phospholipids induced by nonadrenaline. *Biochim Biophys Acta* 664:82-88, 1981.

GISSI-Prevenzione Group. Dietary supplementation with n-3 polyunsaturated fatty acids and vitamin E after myocardial infarction: results of the GISSI-Prevenzione trial *Lancet* 354:447-455, 1999

Gudbjarnason, S. Pathophysiology of long-chain polyene fatty acids in heart muscle. *Nutr Metab* 24:42-146, 1980.

Gudbjarnason S. Dynamics of n-3 and n-6 fatty acids in phospholipids of heart muscle. *J Intern Med Suppl* 225(731):117-128, 1989.

Gudbjarnason S, Benediktsdottir VE, Skuladottir G. Effects of n-3 polyunsaturated fatty acids on coronary heart disease. *Bibl Nutr Dieta* 43:1-12, 1989.

Gudbjarnason S., Oskarsdottir O. Changes in fatty acid composition of cardiac lipids accompanying myocardial necrosis. *Recent Adv Stud Card Struct Metab* 6:193-203, 1975.

Gudbjarnason S, Hallgrimsson J. The role of myocardial membrane lipids in the development of cardiac necrosis. *Acta Med Scand* 58:717-727, 1976.

Gudbjarnason S, Oskarsdottir O. Modification of fatty acid composition of rat heart lipids by feeding cod liver oil. *Biochim Biophy Acta* 487:10-15, 1977.

Gudbjarnason S, Oskarsdottir G, Doell B, et al Myocardial membrane lipids in relation to cardiovascular disease. *Adv Cardiol* 25:130-144, 1978.

Hallaq H, Sellmayer A, Smith TW, et al Protective effect of eicosapentaenoic acid on ouabain toxicity in neonatal rat cardiac myocytes. *Proc Natl Acad Sci* 87(20):7834-7838, 1990.

Hallaq H, Smith TW, Leaf A. Modulation of dihydropyridine-sensitive calcium channels in heart cells by fish oil fatty acids. *Proc Natl Acad Sci* 89(5):1760-1764, 1992.

Heathers GP, Yamada KA, Kanter EM, et al Long-chain acylcarnitines mediate the hypoxia-induced increase in alpha 1-adrenergic receptors on adult canine myocytes. *Circ Res* 61(5):735-746, 1987.

Hirsh PD, Hillis LD, Campbell WB, et al Release of prostaglandins and thromboxane into the coronary circulation in patients with ischemic heart disease. *N Engl J Med* 304:685-691, 1981.

Kang JX, Leaf A. Effects of long-chain polyunsaturated fatty acids on the contraction of neonatal rat cardiac myocyte. *Proc Natl Acad Sci* 91:9886-9890, 1994.

Kang JX, Leaf A. Prevention of fatal cardiac arrhythmias by polyunsaturated fatty acids. *Am J Clin Nutr* 71(1 Suppl):202S-207S, 2000

Kondo K, Misumi J, Okuno T, et al Effect of prostaglandin E2 on vascular reactivity to norepinephrine in isolated rat, 1978 mesenteric artery, hind limb and splenic artery. *Prostaglandins* 2:67-75, 1978.

Li Y, Kang JX, Leaf A. Differential effects of various eicosanoids on the production or prevention of arrhythmias in cultured neonatal rat cardiac myocytes. *Prostaglandins* 54(2):511-530, 1997.

Lockette WE, Webb RC, Culp BR, et al Vascular reactivity and high dietary eicosapentaenoic acid. *Prostaglandins* 24:631-639, 1982.

Lorenz R, Spengler U, Fischer S, et al Platelet function, thromboxane formation and blood pressure control during supplementation of the western diet with cod liver oil. *Circulation* 67:504-511, 1983.

McLennan PL, Abeywardena MY, Charnock JS. Dietary fish oil prevents ventricular fibrillation following coronary artery occlusion and reperfusion. *Am Heart J* 116(3):709-717, 1988.

Reibel DK, Holahan MA, Hock CE. Effects of dietary fish oil on cardiac responsiveness to adrenoceptor stimulation. *Am J Physiol* 254(3 Pt 2):H494-499, 1988.

Sheard NF. Fish consumption and risk of sudden cardiac death. *Nutrition Reviews* 56:177-179, 1998.

Skuladottir G, Hardarson T, Sigfusson N, et al Arachidonic acid levels in serum phospholipids of patients with angina pectoris or fatal myocardial infarction. *Acta Med Scand* 218(1):55-58, 1985.

Talesnik J, Hsja JC. Coronary flow reactions to arachidonic acid are inhibited by docosahexaenoic acid. *J Pharm* 80:255-258, 1982.

ten Hoor F, deDeckere EAM. Essential fatty acids, prostaglandins and heart function. *Prog Lipid Res* 20:423, 1982.

Villa B, Calabresi L, Chiesa G, et al Omega-3 fatty acid ethyl esters increase heart rate variability in patients with coronary disease. *Pharmacol Res* 45:476-478, 2002.

Xiao, Y-F., Gomez, A.M., Morgan, J.P., Lederer, W.J. and Leaf, A. Suppression of voltage-gated L-type Ca2+ currents by polyunsaturated fatty acids in adult and neonatal rat ventricular myocytes. Proc Nat Acad Sci, USA 1997; 94: 4182-4187.

Yunyuan Li, Kang XJ, Leaf A, differential effects of various eicosanoids on the production or prevention of arrhythmias in cultured neonatal rat cardiac myocytes. *Prostaglandins* 54(2):511-530, 1997.

2005 National Library of Medicine Search Results:

(http://www.ncbi.nlm.nih.gov/entrez/query.fcgi)
vasospasm = 7,833; vasospasm eicosanoid = 432; vasospasm thromboxane = 264
cardiac output = 64,456; cardiac output eicosanoid = 1,055
arrhythmia = 119,701; arrhythmia eicosanoid = 455; arrhythmia fish = 144
heart rate = 139,876; heart rate eicosanoid = 1,964; heart rate adrenergic = 13,512
heart rate variability = 7,854; heart rate fish = 509

8—Strokes

Some strokes (or *cerebrovascular accidents*) are caused by events similar to those for heart attacks or cardiovascular accidents. Strokes and heart attacks occur more often when there has been a progressive reduction of the diameter of the blood vessel due to atherogenesis and an acute blockade of blood flow due to either thrombosis or arterial spasm. In addition to these three features, investigators who study strokes have to consider a fourth possible event that occurs in the brain: vascular rupture.

All four events can impair the flow of blood to the brain. In some populations, rupture of brain vessels and subsequent loss of blood into the tissue (hemorrhage) have been more common than the blockade of blood flow from thrombosis or spasm (see Chapter 1, Figs. 1-1, 1-2). The tendency for vessel rupture is increased by hypertension, so among Eskimos and in some districts of Japan where diets included high salt intake there was a higher rate of occurrence of cerebral hemorrhage (apoplexy) than of thrombotic or vasospastic incidents. A decreased rate of hemorrhagic stroke in Japan followed a decrease in salt intake and an accompanying lower hypertension. In Japan, the old way of preserving food with dry salt is steadily yielding to refrigerators and freezers, with important reductions in hypertension, stomach cancer, cerebral bleeding, and cerebrovascular death. Unfortunately, thrombotic stroke continues to be the major type of stroke in USA, and it now seems to be rising in Japan as diet habits become "Americanized" with higher proportions of n-6 relative to n-3 fats.

The 79,839 women in the Nurses' Health Study (aged 34 to 59 years in 1980) were studied for 14 years (Iso et al, 2001). After 1,086,261 person-years of follow-up, 574 incident strokes were documented, including 119 subarachnoid hemorrhages, 62 intraparenchymal hemorrhages, 303 ischemic strokes (264 thrombotic and 39 embolic infarctions), and 90 strokes of undetermined type. A significantly lower relative risk (RR) of thrombotic stroke (0.49) was found among women who ate fish two or more times per week (Iso et al, 2001).

Women in the highest quintile of intake of long-chain n-3 polyunsaturated fatty acids had lower risk of total stroke and thrombotic infarction, with RRs of 0.72 and 0.67, respectively. Women with higher fish or n-3 polyunsaturated fatty acid intake had no greater risk of hemorrhagic stroke, indicating that the intensity of platelet action that prevents blood vessel leakage is well below the level that causes thrombosis.

Hypertension also causes edema that can increase the severity of a stroke that was caused by blockade of blood vessels in the brain by either thrombosis or spasm. This makes hypertension another important health risk factor that we need to understand, and it too may be affected by our dietary habits. Hypertension will be considered in greater detail in Chapter 9.

Swelling due to edema can have serious consequences for the microcirculation network of microscopic vessels that distribute the oxygen and nutrients to all parts of our tissues. These vessels do not have the thick, strong muscular walls that enclose the high pressures of the major arteries. Instead, the microcirculation operates with a very low pressure differential so that when edema occurs, the flow in the microvessels can be slowed by the pressure of the surrounding swollen tissue.

This situation resembles, to some degree the way in which an inflatable pressure cuff is used in routine measurements of blood pressure. The cuff is expanded with increased air pressure until blood flow stops, and then the air is released. The squeezing effect of edema cannot be relieved as readily, and if the decreased blood flow is too prolonged, damage to the tissue may occur (Fig. 8-1). Such a problem is particularly severe in the brain where damaged cells cannot be replaced or repaired as readily as they can be in many other tissues.

Stopping Strokes

The importance of the n-6 fatty acid, arachidonate (20:4n-6), in *thrombotic* stroke was illustrated by Furlow when he showed that unilateral cerebrovascular occlusion was produced within 60 seconds after injection of sodium arachidonate into the carotid artery (see Furlow and Bass, 1975). Microscopic examination revealed complete obstruction of the cerebral hemispheric microcirculation by platelet aggregates. In this experimental model, heparin was used to diminish the involvement of the clotting process, and the microthrombi that killed the animals were predominantly formed by platelet aggregation rather than by fibrin generation.

Platelet aggregation is enhanced by arachidonate (20:4n-6), although "megadose" amounts of linoleate (18:2n-6) have been reported to antagonize this aspect of platelet function. Black et al, (1979) demonstrated that ligation of the middle cerebral artery produced a greater cerebral infarction in cats on a standard diet than in cats on diets with supplemental fish oil (menhaden) at 8 en% for 18-24 days. The authors suggested that moderate dietary supplements of fish oil with its n-3 fatty acids might be beneficial in the prophylactic treatment of ischaemic cerebral vascular disease.

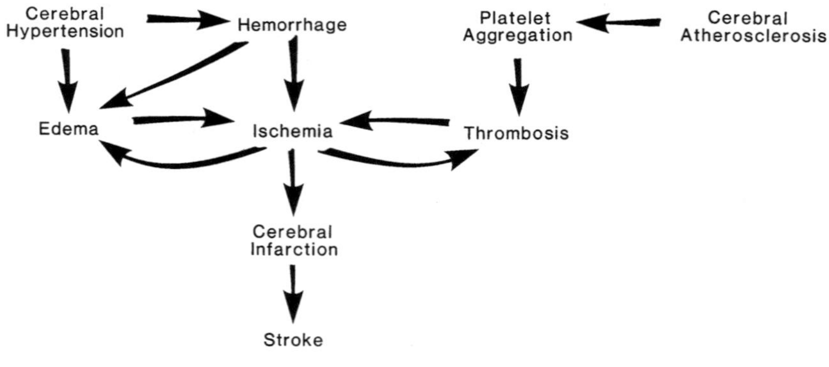

Fig. 8-1. Types of strokes and TIA.

The dramatic 42% decrease in the incidence of death from strokes in the United States during the decade 1972-1982 indicates that some significant change in causal factors or therapy occurred. Was the main effect due to changes in "life-style," in diet or smoking habits, in medications for hypertension, or in increased use of coronary care units? The change occurred also during a time when Americans shifted their average intake of dietary linoleate from about 8 g per day to more than 20 g per day (see Chapter 17).

Many medical experts feel that most of the decline in hypertension was due to progress in successfully treating high blood pressure, which reduced the risk of brain damage during ischemic conditions. A recent prospective nested case-control study of 7450 Japanese 40 to 85 years of age concluded that, compared with controls, hemorrhagic (n=75) and ischemic (n=122) stroke patients had in their total serum lipids similar proportions of n-3 polyunsaturated fatty acids, lower proportions of linoleic and arachidonic acids, and higher proportions of saturated and monosaturated acids (Iso et al, 2002). The authors inferred diet intakes from proportions of acids in the serum mixture of triglycerides, cholesterol esters and phospholipids, and their conclusions differ from those of Iso et al (2001). More data are needed.

The relationship between fish consumption and stroke is controversial. A significantly lower risk of thrombotic stroke (relative risk, 0.49) was observed among women who ate fish at least two times per week compared with women who ate fish less than once per month, after adjustment for age, smoking, and other cardiovascular risk factors (Skerrett and Hennekens, 2003). No association was observed between consumption of fish or fish oil and hemorrhagic stroke, supporting the hypothesis that consumption of fish several times per week reduces the risk of thrombotic stroke and does not increase the risk of hemorrhagic stroke.

However, a population-based case-control study with 440 incident cases of stroke and 473 controls between the ages of 40 and 85 found the risk of stroke was higher with higher consumption of fish (Caicoya, 2002). Although misclassification of exposure and residual confounding by unmeasured factors cannot be ruled out, high fish consumption was associated with a higher risk of stroke and cerebral infarction in this study. In contrast, the 1,086,261 person-years of follow-up in the Nurses' Health Study (Iso et al, 2001) showed that women who ate more fish had a lower risk of total stroke, with multivariate relative risks (RRs), adjusted for age, smoking, and other cardiovascular risk factors, of 0.93 for fish consumption 1 to 3 times per month, 0.78 for once per week, 0.73 for 2 to 4 times per week, and 0.48 for 5 or more times per week. Women who ate fish two or more times per week had significantly lower risk of thrombotic infarction (multivariate RR, 0.49).

There was no association between fish or omega-3 polyunsaturated fatty acid intake and risk of hemorrhagic stroke. Also, in a study of 43,671 men aged 40 to 75 years, the multivariate relative risk for men who consumed fish at least once per month compared with those who ate fish less than once per month was 0.56 (95% CI, 0.38-0.83) for ischemic stroke and 1.36 (95% CI, 0.48-3.82) for hemorrhagic stroke (He et al, 2002). Careful distinction between the two different types of stroke will be needed as medical researchers continue defining the impact of different dietary EFA.

References

Black KL, Culp B, Madison D, et al. (1979). The protective effect of dietary fish oil on focal cerebral infarction. *Prostaglandins Med* 3:257-268, 1979.

Caicoya M. Fish consumption and stroke: a community case-control study in Asturias, Spain. *Neuroepidemiology* 21(3):107-114, 2002.

Ellis EF, Nies AS, Oates JA. Cerebral arterial smooth muscle contraction by thromboxane A2. *Stroke* 8:480, 1977.

Furlow TW Jr, Bass NH. Stroke in rats produced by carotid injection of sodium arachidonate. *Science* 187, 658, 1975.

He K, Rimm EB, Merchant A, et al. Fish consumption and risk of stroke in men. *JAMA* 288(24):3130-3136, 2002.

Iso H, Rexrode KM, Stampfer MJ, et al. Intake of fish and omega-3 fatty acids and risk of stroke in women. *JAMA* 285(3):304-312, 2001.

Iso H, Sato S, Umemura U, al. Linoleic acid, other fatty acids, and the risk of stroke. *Stroke* 33(8):2086-2093, 2002.

Skerrett PJ, Hennekens CH. Consumption of fish and fish oils and decreased risk of stroke. *Prev Cardiol* 6(1):38-41, 2003.

2005 National Library of Medicine Search Results:

(http://www.ncbi.nlm.nih.gov/entrez/query.fcgi)
stroke = 90,152; stroke hypertension = 11,304; stroke thrombosis = 5,882; stroke thromboxane = 256; stroke eicosanoid = 520; stroke fish = 234

9—Hypertension

More than 95% of patients with hypertension are regarded to have essential hypertension, which develops in a slow, progressive manner with adaptive imbalances in the many control mechanisms that usually keep blood pressure normal (Frohlich, 1982). This chronic imbalance has some features that are similar to what can happen during normal acute changes in blood pressure, but the prolonged chronic aspect of hypertension distinguishes it from many experimental models. To study hypertension in more detail, medical researchers have found special genetic strains of laboratory animals that develop a form of spontaneous hypertension resembling the disorder in humans (Trippodo and Frohlich, 1981), Because these animals respond favorably to some drugs used to help humans, their study may help us find better ways of treating people with hypertension.

When there is increased resistance to blood flow in the small vessels of tissues, the overall blood pressure in larger arteries increases, and the heart works harder to force the blood through the system. This greater workload represents a strain on the heart muscle and more oxygen and nutrients are needed. The greater pressure that is developed can also increase the risk of fluid leakage into tissues (edema and swelling) and of rupture of the vessel (hemorrhage). We need to learn what causes chronic increased resistance to blood flow.

Proper treatment of high blood pressure must decrease the appropriate underlying cause to decrease the risks noted above. There are so many different compensatory regulatory signals that seem to help keep the blood pressure at a constant level that it may be hard to sort out which one was involved initially in creating the imbalance. In some people, hypertension can result from greater dietary salt intake and the resulting greater volume of water in the circulatory system.

If the original cause was a high salt intake more rapid than its excretion, a simple approach would be to restrict nutritionally the salt intake and, if needed, to stimulate pharmacologically greater salt excretion until a balance was restored. The high incidence of apoplexy and hemorrhagic stroke in Japanese and Eskimos may be very much related to their custom of using high salt concentrations in their diets. Interestingly, some eicosanoids can influence salt and water excretion, some can cause contraction or dilation of small blood vessels or alter the contractions induced by catecholamines, and others can cause edema. Because eicosanoids are formed from dietary fats, possible approaches to lowering hypertension risk might involve some aspect of polyunsaturated fatty acid nutrition.

Preventing the Need for Treatment

Applying this idea to an experimental model, Schoene et al (1981) showed that the production of prostaglandins was lower in homogenates of kidney medullae and cortices from rats fed a mixture of 4% menhaden oil plus 1% corn oil than from controls fed 5% corn oil. Animals fed the fish oil-supplemented diet had significantly lower systolic blood pressures after 12 and 20 weeks (Schoene and Fiore, 1982). Reductions in hypertension similar to those observed were known to diminish appreciably the incidence of stroke in a stroke-prone strain of spontaneously hypertensive rats. Thus, it seemed that a breakthrough was made on a type of diet therapy even though the mechanism of the disease and of the dietary benefit was still uncertain.

Because the catecholamine hormone, epinephrine (adrenaline), can cause constriction of blood vessels, it can also increase blood pressure. This type of constriction could result from greater hormone release, more tissue receptors to the hormone, or a more exaggerated response of the receptors to a moderate amount of hormone. Long-term increases in this type of constriction might lead to the adaptive imbalances of essential hypertension. The ability of fish oil to diminish the prostaglandin enhancement of catecholamine-induced contractions suggests that fish oil supplements might have lowered the hypertension in rats by a similar mechanism. Perhaps these experimental rats were hypertensive because of a prostaglandin-induced hyperresponsiveness to catecholamines. More careful studies might give us an answer.

At this point in my reading about hypertension, I found a distracting story about the spontaneously hypertensive strain of rats (SHR) that changed my attitude toward the subject. In the summer of 1984, Schoene reported at an international conference that the SHR strain of rats widely used as a model for human hypertension was believed to develop hypertension as a result of some defect in their immune system (Bendich et al, 1981, 1983). Perhaps an autoimmune disorder (Chapter 10) was the cause of the hypertension.

This idea opened a totally different approach to the causes of hypertension and suggested a different way in which the dietary fish oil may have its beneficial effect. It may have functioned in some way to suppress the autoimmune events that caused the spontaneous hypertension in the special experimental model. Another report demonstrated that chronic immunosuppression could attenuate hypertension and supported the concept of an autoimmune etiology for the laboratory model (Khraibi et al, 1984). Apparently fish oil supplements were achieving a result similar to immune suppression in these animals.

Since the 1986 edition, further studies with humans confirmed the lowering of hypertension by eating fish with n-3 fats. For example, n-3 HUFA supplementation tended to normalize blood pressure of hypertensive patients without affecting normotensive patients (Knapp & FitzGerald, 1989; Knapp, 1996). Treatment with n-3 fatty acids prevented a long-term continuous rise in blood pressure after heart transplantation, and it may have a direct or indirect protective effect on kidneys, making n-3 fatty acids a potentially attractive treatment for post-transplant hypertension (Holm et al, 2001).

Omega-3 fatty acids (3 g/d) reduced blood pressure by decreasing systemic vascular resistance (presumably by changing prostaglandin profiles), and they were used as an adjuvant for the treatment of hypertension in cyclosporine-treated cardiac transplant recipients (Ventura et al, 1993). Postoperative daily administration of 4 g of n-3 fatty acids in heart transplant recipients was effective as hypertension prophylaxis, depending on increases in serum eicosapentaenoic and docosahexaenoic acids.

Treatment with n-3 fatty acids gave a more pronounced vasodilation response to forearm skin ischemia, indicating preservation of microvascular hypotensive endothelial function (Andreassen et al, 1994). The close interaction between the central nervous system, endocrine organs, cytokines and exercise with dietary n-3 fatty acids may explain why dietary n-3 fatty acids could also benefit management of conditions such as septicemia and septic shock, Alzheimer's disease, Parkinson's disease, inflammatory bowel diseases, diabetes mellitus, essential hypertension and atherosclerosis (Das, 2000).

Regular consumption of dietary fish and n-3 fatty acids of marine origin can lower blood pressure (BP) levels and reduce cardiovascular risk (Bao et al, 1998). Dietary fish and weight loss had significant independent and additive effects on 24-hour ambulatory BP and ambulatory heart rates. Combining a daily fish meal with a weight-reducing regimen gave additive effects on ambulatory BP and decreased heart rate. The reduced heart rate seen with dietary fish suggests a cardiac/autonomic component, as well as vascular effects, of increased consumption of n-3 fatty acid from fish.

Unfortunately, many clinical trials of n-3 HUFA supplementation were designed with no controlled records of the ingested competing n-6 fats. Nevertheless, diet supplementation of individuals with untreated hypertension gave clinically relevant reductions (Appel et al, 1993). A total of 36 clinical trials showed the antihypertensive effect of fish oil (median dose: 3.7 g/day) with reduced blood pressure tending to be greater in older (>45 years) and in hypertensive populations (Geleijnse et al, 2002).

Is human hypertension caused by high salt intake and fluids in the body, by some over responsive behavior of blood vessels to catecholamines, or by some autoimmune event that impairs our adaptive responses? Here again one realizes that medical scientists are still struggling to understand each disease and its multiple mechanisms. How can one prove that some new therapeutic approach is going to be beneficial when the cause of the disease remains unknown? We had seen evidence that fish oil added to the diet did keep hypertension under control. Could someone find a way to show how that worked? Did it affect the salt balance, the catecholamine responses, or the autoimmune events? Were there three different kinds of hypertension in different people? No one knew.

Immune Markers

Some of the evidence for a monogenetic basis for essential hypertension in humans was summarized by Kristensen (1979) who noted that there were higher circulating levels of antinuclear antibodies in hypertensive patients. The levels were twice as high in patients with the HLA-B15 gene as in B15-negative patients. It is interesting to note that such autoantibodies (as well as the genes designated B15 and B8) are also associated with systemic lupus erythematosis (see Chapter 10) and insulin-dependent diabetes (see Chapter 10).

The possibility exists that the antibody-forming system of individuals who develop essential hypertension responds more vigorously to infections than the system in normotensive subjects (Kristensen et al, 1982). This hyperresponsive tendency may cause problems. Such consideration led to the hypothesis that components of the vascular system may be stimulating IgG production in patients with hypertension (Kristensen arid Solling, 1983). At the present time, the circulating immunoglobulins in humans may be regarded as markers of vascular damage, but future work may clarify whether they may also be involved in the process of developing the vascular damage and hypertension as they seem to do in the SHR rat model.

Two clinical research studies in Finland showed that a diet low in fat content and high in its ratio of polyunsaturated to saturated fatty acids could significantly reduce blood pressure (Puska et al, 1983). Similar changes associated with a vegetarian diet gave a distinct lowering of pressure that seemed more related to the composition of the fat rather than to dietary sodium or potassium (Rouse et al, 1983). These results, focusing on the possible role of dietary polyunsaturated fatty acids and their resultant eicosanoids in hypertension, make it increasingly important to learn how the balance between n-3 and n-6 fatty acids can influence this disorder. If there were three separate types of hypertension, would increasing the balance of n-3 to n-6 polyunsaturated acids be helpful in each type?

Technical Details

The blastogenic responses of lymphocytes from SHR rats to phytohemagglutinin and concanavalin A were less than one-fifth that of the parent strain W/Mk rats (Takeichi et al, 1980). When the immune function of the SHR animals was restored by thymus grafts or extracts from normal animals, the development of periarteritis anodosa and hypertension was significantly suppressed (Ba et al, 1982). This finding introduced the possibility that the development of hypertension in this genetic strain of animals was caused by some depression of the immune system that could be treated. Other work in this laboratory (Takeichi et al, 1981) confirmed that possibility by showing the development of a thymocytotoxic autoantibody in the SHR rats that was very similar to that observed in NZB mice that are widely studied because of their similarity to the autoimmune disorder, systemic lupus erythematosis. The disorder appears to be associated with a progressive loss of suppressor T cells. Restoration of the suppressor T-cell function may help constrain the antibody-forming responses that lead to the undesired autoimmune (anti-self) responses, More detail on the immune recognition and attack of "non-self" and "self" materials is given in Chapter 10.

Following a rationale that renal prostaglandins have hypotensive effects, Blond et al (1980) fed rapeseed oil containing 9.5% 18:3n-3 (and 21% 18:2n-6) in anticipation that it would lead to a diminished conversion of l8:2n-6 to 20:4n-6 and thus diminish the levels of prostaglandins formed. However, no noticeable effect on arterial pressure was observed during the 2- to 3-month period of the study. In this context, Schoene et al (1981) demonstrated that feeding spontaneously hypertensive rats a diet that was deficient in both n-3 and n-6 fatty acids made the eventual development of hypertension more severe. This result suggested that some prostaglandin biosynthesis might help diminish this form of hypertension. However, rats deficient in essential fatty acids have many health problems likely related to inadequate eicosanoids for balanced autacoid responses.

Lorenz et al (1982) demonstrated a reduction of blood pressure and a blunted pressor response to pressor hormones in human subjects ingesting a mackerel-rich diet. The effects were associated with high plasma renin levels. The phenomenon might reflect greater generation of vascular PGI_2. Daily supplements of 40 ml cod liver oil (ca. 3 g 20:5n-3 and 5 g 22:6n-3) were also reported to decrease the blood pressure in 8 normotensive men, and the supplemented diet seemed to blunt the increase in blood pressure following norephinephrine infusion (Spengler et al, 1982; Lorenz et al, 1982).

Singer et al (1983) reported that 2 weeks on a diet rich in mackerel (known to contain lots of n-3 fatty acids) gave markedly lower systolic and diastolic blood pressure in association with lower levels of circulating plasma noradrenaline. Thus the decreased blood pressure may have been caused by a reduction of transmitter release. Again we must wait for the medical scientists to unravel the underlying mechanisms for the disease before we can understand when diet changes can have consistent effects. Nevertheless, something beneficial seems to come from eating the n-3 HUFA in fish oil.

In another study, difficulty in seeing a diet-induced attenuated blood pressure change in spontaneously hypertensive rats (Hoffmann et al, 1982) was overcome by feeding pregnant rats and their offspring a diet rich in either 18:2n-6 or 18:3n-3 (relative to a diet deficient in polyunsaturated fatty acids) before studying the offspring. In this case, the male offspring supplemented with polyunsaturated fatty acids showed significantly lower blood pressure, and the values for the animals supplemented with 18:3n-3 were slightly lower at 16 weeks of age than for those fed 18:2n6.

The variable results obtained for dietary effects on hypertension may reflect differences among breeding strains of rats. Apparently conflicting results were reported in a comparison study of the effects of 18:3n-3 and 20:5n-3 (Scherhag, et al, 1982). In that report, dietary administration of 2 en% of either of these acids to rats receiving 5 en% 18:2n-6 was associated with higher arterial blood pressure and unchanged thromboxane formation during blood clotting. Again, addition studies are needed to define the conditions suitable for interpreting the relationships between the different dietary acids.

Although Tamura et al (1982) noted that 20:5n-3 enhanced the release of PGI_2-like material from arterial walls, later studies showed strain differences with little dietary effect on the hypotensive material released from thoracic aorta of SHR-SP strain of Wistar rats, and decreased amounts of hypotensive PGI_2-like material were released from the mesenteric artery (Tamura et al, 1982). Similarly, Kondo et al (1978) had previously reported that the modulating contribution of endogenous prostaglandins on vascular reactivity to norepinephrine was different in different vascular beds. Thus the effects on vascular tone noted by Lockette et al (1982) may differ in different vessels, and no single unified story on hypertension is evolving from the few studies that have been done so far with fish oil. Perhaps any polyunsaturated fat may have beneficial effects by a complex set of mechanisms not yet understood (Iacono et al, 1982).

References

Andreassen AK, Hartmann A, Offstad J, et al. Hypertension prophylaxis with omega-3 fatty acids in heart transplant recipients. *J Am Coll Cardiol* (6):1324-1331, 1997.

Appel LJ, Miller ER, Seidler AJ, et al. Does supplementation of diet with 'fish oil' reduce blood pressure? A meta-analysis of controlled clinical trials. *Arch Intern Med* 153(12):1429-1438, 1993.

Ba D, Takeichi N, Kodama T,et al. Restoration of T cell depression and suppression of blood pressure in spontaneously hypertensive rats (SHR) by thymus grafts or thymus extracts. *J Immunol* 128:1211-1216, 1982.

Bao DQ, Mori TA, Burke V, et al. Effects of dietary fish and weight reduction on ambulatory blood pressure in overweight hypertensives. *Hypertension* 32(4):710-717, 1998.

Bendich A, Blisole H, Strausser HR, et al. Immune system modulation and its effect on the blood pressure of the spontaneously hypertensive male and female rat. *Biochem Biophys Res Commun* 99: 600-607, 1981.

Blond JP, Poisson JP, Lemarchal P. Acide α-linolenique alimentaire et pression artérielle chez le rat. *Arch Int Physiol Biochim* 88:147-153, 1980.

Bendich A, Gabriel E, Machlin LJ. Effect of dietary level of vitamin E on the immune system of the spontaneously hypertensive (SHR) and normotensive Wistar Kyoto (WKY) rat. *J Nutr* 113, 1920-1926, 1983.

Das UN. Beneficial effect(s) of n-3 fatty acids in cardiovascular diseases: but, why and how? *Prostaglandins Leukot Essent Fatty Acids* (6):351-362, 2000.

Frohlich ED. Hemodynamic factors in the pathogenesis and maintenance of hypertension. *Fed Proc* 41:2400-2408, 1982.

Geleijnse JM, Giltay EJ, Grobbee DE, et al. Blood pressure response to fish oil supplementation: metaregression analysis of randomized trials. *J Hypertens* 20(8):1493-1499, 2002.

Hoffmann P, Forster W, Markov CM. Attenuation of blood pressure increase in spontaneously hypertensive rats by diets enriched with polyunsaturated fatty acids. *Prostaglandins Leukotrienes Med* 8:151-156, 1982.

Holm T, Andreassen AK, Aukrust P, et al. Omega-3 fatty acids improve blood pressure control and preserve renal function in hypertensive heart transplant recipients. *Eur Heart J* 22(5):428-436, 2001.

lacono JM., Judd JL, Marshall MW, et al. The role of dietary essential fatty acids and prostaglandins in reducing blood pressure. *Prog Lipid Res* 20:349-364, 1981.

Khraibi AA, Norman RA Jr, Dzjelak DJ. Chronic immunosuppression attenuates hypertension in Okarnoto spontaneously hypertensive rats. *Am J Physiol* 247:H722-H726, 1984.

Knapp HR. n-3 fatty acids and human hypertension. *Curr Opin Lipidol* 7(1):30-33, 1996.

Knapp HR, FitzGerald GA. The antihypertensive effects of fish oil. A controlled study of polyunsaturated fatty acid supplements in essential hypertension. *N Engl J Med* 320(16): 1037-1043,1989.

Kristensen BO Autoantibodjes in untreated and treated essential hypertension: relationship to histocompatability leucocyte antigen-B15 and vascular complications. *Clin Sci* 57:287S-290S, 1979.

Kristensen BO, Solling K. Serum concentrations of immunoglobulins and free light chains before and after vascular events in essential hypertension. *Acta Med Scand* 213:15-20, 1983.

Kristensen,BO, Andersen PL, Vestergaard BF, et al. Herpesvirus antibodies and vascular complications in essential hypertension. *Acta Med Scand* 212:375-377, 1982.

Lockette WE, Webb RC, Culp BR, et al. Vascular reactivity and high dietary eicosapentaenoic acid. *Prostaglandins* 24, 631-639, 1982.

Lorenz R, Spengler U, Siess W, et al. Membrane fatty acids, platelet aggregation and thromboxane formation on dietary cod liver oil supplementation. In *Prostaglandins. Vth International Conference.* Florence, Italy: Fondazione Giovanni Lorenzini, 1982, p 695.

Puska P, Nissjnen A, Vartjajnen E, et al. Controlled, randomised trial of the effect of dietary fat on blood pressure. *Lancet* 1:1-5, 1983.

Rouse IL, Beilin LJ, Armstrong BK, et al. (1983). Blood-pressure lowering effect of a vegetarian diet: Controlled trial in normotensive subjects. *Lancet* 1:5-10, 1983.

Scherhag R, Kramer HJ, Busing R. Dietary administration of eicosapentaenoic and linolenic acid increases arterial blood pressure and suppresses vascular prostacyclin synthesis in the rat. *Prostaglandins* 23:369-382, 1982.

Schoene NW, Fiore D. Effect of a diet containing fish oil on blood pressure in spontaneously hypertensive rats. *Prog Lipid Res* 20:569-570, 1982.

Schoene NW, Ferretti A, Fiore D. Production of prostaglandins in homogenates of kidney medullae and cortices of spontaneously hypertensive rats fed menhaden oil. *Lipids* 16:866-869, 1981.

Singer P Jaeger W, Wirth M, et al. Lipid and blood pressure-lowering effect of mackerel diet in man. *Atherosclerosis* 49:99-108, 1983.

Spengler U, Lorenz R, Weber PC. Effects of Indomethacin or n-3 polyunsaturated fatty acids on blood pressure, pressor response and levels of vasoactive hormones. In *Prostaglandins-5th International Conference.* Florence, Italy: Fondazione Giovanni Lorenzini, 1982, p 696.

Takeichi N, Suzuki K, Okayasu T, et al. Immunological depression in spontaneously hypertensive rats. *Clin Exp Immunol* 40:120-126, 1980.

Takeichi N, Ba D, Kobayashi H. Natural cytotoxic autoantibody against thymocytes in spontaneously hypertensive rats. *Cell Immunol* 60:181-190, 1981.

Tamura Y, Hirai A, Terano T, et al. (1982). Effect of eicosapentaenoic acid (EPA) on prostaglandin metabo lism of platelet and vascular wall of stroke-prone spontaneously hypertensive rats. In *Prostaglandins-5th International Conference.* Florence, Italy: Fondazjone Giovanni Lorenzini, 1982, p 693.

Trippodo NC, Frohlich ED. Similarities of genetic (spontaneous) hypertension: Man and rat. *Circ Res* 48:309-319, 1981.

Ventura HO, Milani RV, Lavie CJ, et al. Cyclosporine-induced hypertension: Efficacy of omega-3 fatty acids in patients after cardiac transplantation. *Circulation* 88(5 Pt 2):281-285, 1993.

2005 National Library of Medicine Search Results:

(http://www.ncbi.nlm.nih.gov/entrez/query.fcgi
hypertension = 234,924; hypertension adrenergic = 10,742; hypertension fish = 443; hypertension prostaglandin = 4,571; hypertension eicosanoid = 4,503; hypertension omega-3 = 288

10—Immune Responses

The human body responds to foreign materials in two major ways: *innate immunity* and *adaptive immunity*. Innate immunity operates rapidly after exposure to one of a fixed set of about a thousand "foreign" molecular structures that are recognized by genetically coded receptors. This fast innate interaction is the initial response to infectious agents like bacteria and viruses. In contrast, adaptive (acquired) immunity involves multi-cellular mechanisms that often take many days to develop protection against foreign materials. The adaptive system also interacts with cells of the innate immune system while developing an increased repertoire throughout a person's life. This slow adaptive system is involved in the chronic immune inflammatory diseases that seem to occur with lower frequency and intensity among families eating foods from the sea.

The low incidence of immune inflammatory disorders reported for Eskimos (Chapter 1, Fig. 1-1) provided a hint that perhaps some diseases with disorders in the immune system depend on eicosanoid formation similar to heart disease and heart attacks (Chapters 5 and 6). The network of cellular signals that maintains immune responses has much that remains unknown, but eicosanoids are known to participate. Therefore EFA are also involved.

Thrombocytes (platelets), lymphocytes and monocytes are derived from common precursor cells in our bone marrow, and they have important eicosanoid-modulated functions mediated by various eicosanoid receptors (see Chapter 14). At this time, the complex cellular interactions that produce immune events is still becoming recognized, and the manner in which the many eicosanoids modulate these events are still poorly understood. Nevertheless, there is a good possibility that actions of n-3 eicosanoids through eicosanoid receptors may differ from those of n-6 eicosanoids. This chapter examines some of the research data and notes the difficulty of finding suitable experimental animal models related to the human disorders.

Adaptive Systems Also Use Innate Reponse Mediators

Adaptive immune responses have two major aspects, humoral immunity and cell-mediated immunity, that will be discussed in relation to their early and late events. Humoral immunity involves the production of antibodies by B-lymphocytes after exposure to an antigen. In contrast, cell-mediated immunity does not involve antibody production, but involves effector cells (cytotoxic T-lymphocytes, macrophages and natural killer cells) that respond to an antigen with the release of various eicosanoids and cytokines. The early adaptive events lead from an initial provocation by antigen that produces activated effector cells and antibody (Fig. 10-1).

This is followed by later events in which antigen-antibody complexes and activated effector cells release mediators that induce the inflammatory symptoms of immune responses. These late events with effector cells produce the well-recognized symptoms associated with asthma (and even the common cold) and with chronic immune or inflammatory reactions in rheumatoid arthritis, systemic lupus erythematosis, psoriasis, allergic encephalomyelitis, and multiple sclerosis. Conversion of arachidonate to various n-6 eicosanoids may be important in amplifying the symptoms of all of these disorders.

One therapeutic approach in treating patients with these diseases is to block pharmacologically the eicosanoid-modulated responses of different effector cells in order to diminish the painful and undesired symptoms that they produce. Many drugs used to treat inflammatory disorders provide relief by treating only the symptoms and not the early initiating causes. A reduction of inflammatory symptoms certainly is better than no treatment, but it is not a cure for the underlying disorder. The chances remain that the patient will need to return repeatedly to the use of the medicine unless a true cure is somehow achieved. Of course, once excessive immune sensitivities develop, they can still be moderated by decreasing exposure to the challenging antigens. The comments in this chapter, however, focus on how different dietary EFA balance tissue HUFA and moderate excessive n-6 eicosanoid actions in immune inflammatory events.

Targets for Intervention

Approaches to a successful intervention pose difficult conceptual problems. We may wish to suppress the early stages of activating effector cells and forming antibodies, but indiscriminate approaches to this tactic would leave us immunologically defenseless and vulnerable to infection. We need to make moderate changes that leave the basic defense system intact but that diminish the specific aggressive overreaction that causes so much distress. The problem (like that of thrombosis) is how to slow down overreactions while permitting needed ones. Will fish oil diminish immune overreactions as it does platelet overreactions? Are early events in developing adaptive immune responses more important than the later events of releasing mediators from effector cells? The reported lower incidence of immune inflammatory diseases in Eskimos might reflect a depressed level of both early and late immune events. If so, a lower incidence of asthma and autoimmune disease might be expected to be associat-

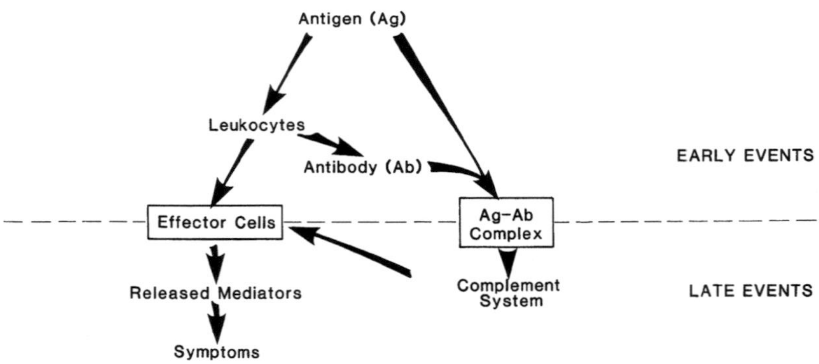

Fig. 10-1. Adaptive immune responses.

ed with a high incidence of infection. However, it is difficult to distinguish this result from that expected from inadequate anti-infective medical care. The point of interest for this chapter is "How did it come to pass that the incidence of asthma, diabetes, psoriasis, and thyrotoxicosis among Eskimos was less than among Danes?"

Autoimmune disorders may originate in an overzealous immune system attacking "self" cells rather than only "foreign" cells. Our immune system seems designed to recognize, attack and destroy foreign material, and its signaling networks encourage the defensive response while simultaneously starting to dampen the response and moderating such aggressive behavior toward our own tissues. For example, once the triggering stimulus is removed, healthy inflammatory processes tend to return to a quiescent state as further self-healing signaling resolves the inflamed condition. This important biphasic defense depends on well-balanced self-healing signals that are still slowly being understood.

As medical scientists gain more experience with organ graft tolerance and rejection, they develop immune suppressive strategies to carry the patient through a critical transition period in which the transplanted tissue gradually becomes tolerated and accepted by the patient's immune defenses. Tolerance may occur when the immune balance is shifted in favor of suppressor mechanisms (Charpentier et al, 1983). The suppressor cells involved in this process appear to have a prostaglandin-dependent mechanism (Thomas et al, 1983). Blocking their ability to make prostaglandins can enhance lymphocyte proliferation to mitogens. The response has a complicated relationship to the amount of each prostaglandin available and its action at specific prostaglandin receptors. A stimulatory effect of PGE on host versus graft reactions occurs with relatively small amounts of endogenously generated prostaglandins, whereas a suppressive effect occurs with high concentrations of PGE as well as with the removal of all PGE by selective antibodies (Merlin et al, 1984). Such dose-dependent effects on cell-mediated immunity may have significance in experimental models of lupus.

A little more detailed description of the defense network that our leukocytes provide can help illustrate the delicate complexity of the control system for our immune inflammatory responses. We may have relatively normal health when only one of the many control signals is faulty, but with imbalances in more than one signal, destructive processes can occur. Thus patients with an autoimmune disease often have close relatives who have some of the imbalanced aspects in their immune responses, even though they have no clinically evident symptoms (Shoenfeld and Schwartz, 1984). The special strains of experimental animals used to express hypertension and other immune disorders in laboratory studies were obtained by extensive inbreeding until the combination of defects occurred. The combination of defects in these strains of laboratory animals allows scientists to study the onset of the disease and to try to develop ways to prevent it.

The experimental animal models might have parallels in human medicine with some small tribes of people that have had many inter-cousin marriages. Eskimos are reported to have such customs, and they may have different genetic patterns than customarily found in Western nations. Nevertheless, they appear to have less rather than more immune inflammatory type disease. This may be due more to dietary habits than to genetic factors. If early adaptive immune events are critical to this type of disease in humans, then successful primary prevention in the United States may need to include more n-3 acids in the diet from birth as the Eskimos do. If the later effector cell actions that produce the symptoms are critical to the disease, some beneficial effects may still be obtained with dietary n-3 acid supplements later in life as a form of secondary prevention.

T-Helper and T-Suppressor Cells

The first steps in the early adaptive response are recognition and processing of an antigen that signals the T-helper lymphocyte cells to stimulate the multiplication of antibody-forming B cells (see Fig. 10-2). The sophisticated signaling by which T-suppressor lymphocyte cells edit and govern the process is vital. Overzealous or indiscriminate actions by T-helper cells would have the immune defenses mobilized to every material around and lead to a general self-destruction. However, too much editing or censoring of signals could suppress antibody formation to a degree that would permit foreign invasion. Dietary polyunsaturated fatty acids take on a new importance when we recognize that they form prostaglandins and leukotrienes that play a role in linking the actions of T-suppressor cells with those of T-helper cells. In the dialog between these cells in the antibody-forming network, we need to better understand how diet-based eicosanoids affect the decision to go ahead with the defensive response. The fact that a diet rich in n-3 acids when given from the time of weaning could delay the fatal expression of the autoimmune defect in SHR rats just as thymic transplants do suggests an important role for eicosanoids in autoimmune disease. The n-3 acids likely help maintain an important balance between suppressor and helper cells not achieved by n-6 acids alone (Fig. 10-3).

Once a specific clone of antibody-forming cells has proliferated, the antibodies that are formed will bind the corresponding antigen and stimulate the cascade of mediators (see Fig. 10-4) that spread the alarm signals throughout the body. In this situation, signaling by n-3 and n-6 eicosanoids may have different effects on different eicosanoid receptors on different cells. Our current therapeutic strategies in immune

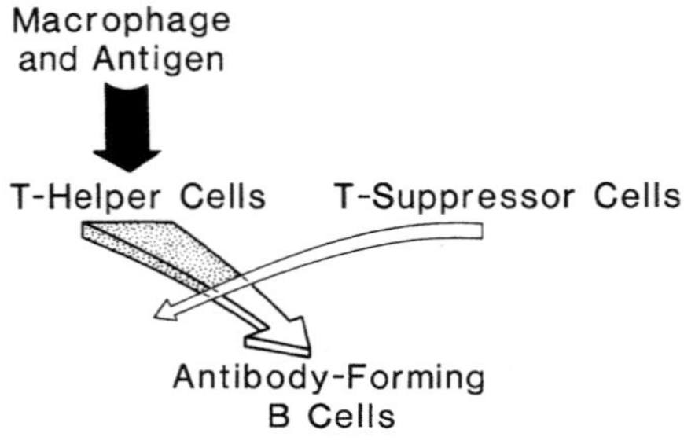

Fig 10-2. Helper cells and suppressor cells.

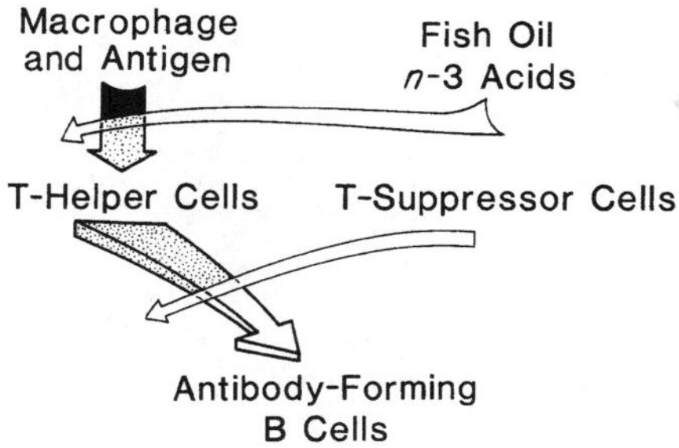

Fig 10-3. Possible action of n-3 acids.

disorders are few, and the general attempts that we make to diminish eicosanoid synthesis with aspirin-like drugs offer a convenient and common tactic to at least reduce outward symptoms of the disorder. The fact that Eskimos appear to have less severe immune-related disorders suggests that dietary n-3 fatty acids might diminish excessive n-6 eicosanoid signaling. This action of diets may be an especially useful tactic during early phases of chronic immune disorders when the inflammatory actions of effector cells may promote more antibody production and cause greater response. Some technical details later in this chapter suggest that the n-3 acids may be more beneficial in cell-mediated disorders than in immune globulin-mediated disorders.

Having large proportions of n-3 HUFA in our tissues throughout life represents a simple intervention that is unmatched by any drug research. With the continued use of fish-rich diets, fishing villagers have for years maintained eicosanoid responses that differ from those of many other people. However, few reports have examined this mode of primary prevention. At this time, we can only speculate on the possible impact made by chronic antagonism of eicosanoid production throughout one's entire childhood and adult life.

Certainly early phases of antibody production would be affected as well as subsequent expression of the allergic symptoms. For such conditions, we should reconsider whether the daily intake of dietary fatty acids of the fishing villagers is suppressing diseases below "normal" or whether American diets thought to be typical (see Chapter 17) are enhancing diseases above "normal". Since immune surveillance can also destroy abnormal tumor cells, there is a narrow distinction between the desired recognition and removal of tumor cells and the undesired development of chronic autoimmune responses to a tissue that is temporarily damaged and in the process of repair. We need to carefully define the biological events that are acceptable and those that are unacceptable in defining new therapeutic tactics and in evaluating the desirability of the current U.S. diet.

Recognizing Multiple Mediators

At the time of the first edition of this book, autacoid actions of prostaglandins and leukotrienes had created a renaissance in understanding immune inflammatory

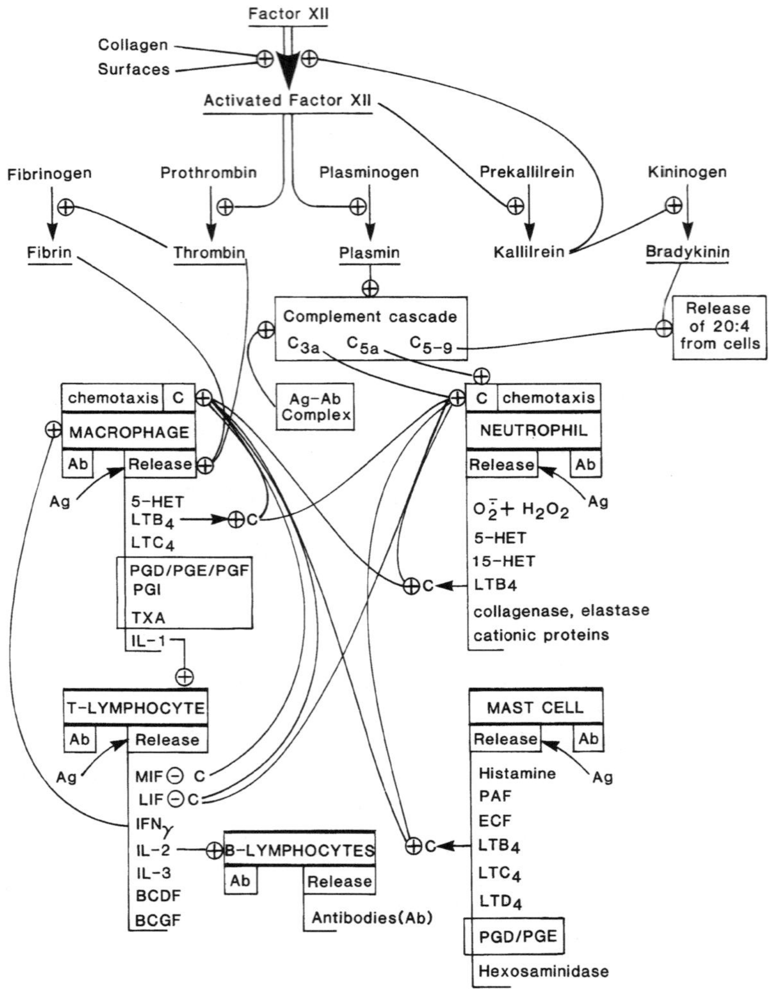

Fig. 10-4. Interactions of effector cells and effector molecules.

processes. Worldwide success with non-steroidal anti-inflammatory drugs (NSAIDs) continues to illustrate a clear proof of principle that n-6 eicosanoids are key mediators in immune inflammatory diseases. Since 1986, newly recognized cellular signaling interactions during immune events (briefly sketched in Figure 10-4) have expanded to where even a brief summary diagram of intercellular and intracellular signaling actions of the immune system would cover several pages. However, what remains unchanged (and further strengthened) is evidence that chronic actions of n-6 eicosanoids amplify and extend the normally transient immune signals beyond levels desired for healthy lives.

Immune signaling systems now include a large number of intercellular events facilitated by cytokines and adhesion molecules that bring cells together and change tissue physiology. These events at cell surface receptors then activate a complex intracellular signaling network of kinase and phosphatases actions that signal the cell nucleus and regulate the expression of genes that further alter the cellular response to changing external conditions. Recognizing how the readily modified intake of dietary n-3 and n-6 eicosanoid precursors can decrease the incidence and severity of over-amplified immune inflammatory processes remains the focus of this chapter. That recognition can ensure better attention to changing the still poorly informed food choices that continue to drive a wide range of diseases and disorders and impair the quality of life of our friends and families.

Almost any disease with an immune inflammatory aspect (e.g., Alzheimer's disease) is now being tested for possible moderation by dietary n-3 fats, and many new published reports are listed at the National Library of Medicine PubMed site. The technical details in this chapter illustrate how dietary n-3 fats may diminish excessive n-6 eicosanoid actions in autoimmune disorders such as arthritis, lupus, multiple sclerosis, encephalomyelitis, asthma and diabetes noted earlier in Chapter 1, Figs. 1-1, 1-2.

In animal models of autoimmune diseases, diets high in n-3 fatty acids from fish oil increase survival and reduce disease severity in spontaneous autoantibody-mediated disease, whereas n-6 linoleic acid-rich diets seem to increase disease severity (Ergas et al, 2002). Fish oil has only a limited effect on acute inflammation, and it is effective in chronic inflammatory disorders only after several weeks. Nevertheless, even a mild effect (by altering T cell signaling) might prevent relapse to active inflammation states. In the milder inflammation of IgA nephropathy, fish oil may slow or prevent disease progression. Perhaps, a constant life-long consumption of n-3 fatty acids may suppress early proliferation of autoreactive (or hyper-reactive) T cells. However, high n-3 fat consumption might be less beneficial once there is already an active immune disease.

Overall, n-3 fatty acids can be recommended to a general healthy population to prevent development of atherosclerosis, thrombosis, arrhythmia and also reduce the risk of increased autoimmune conditions. The important aspect, as emphasized in Chapter 5, is to begin effective balancing of dietary EFA early enough to prevent amplified actions BEFORE cellular changes and tissue damage occur in an irreversible way. Atherosclerosis has finally become acknowledged as a condition of localized vascular inflammation that comes from an imbalance in otherwise normal general immune processes. That recognition is a very important step forward in identifying and preventing the dietary causes for the disease.

Technical Details

The biochemistry of immune responses is much too detailed to fit in this chapter. For convenience, five immune-related diseases are reviewed: arthritis, lupus, multiple sclerosis, asthma, and diabetes. Information presented here helps evaluate the possible effects of having greater amounts of n-3 fatty acids in the diet. This may help us decide how lessons learned from life in the coastal villages might be applied to our lives. Results obtained with Eskimo villagers led us to wonder if dietary n-3 acids suppressed some immune functions. In addition, Friend et al (1980) reported that a diet with megadose 18:2n-6 (about 21% of the daily calories) reduced the ability of guinea pigs to form antibody in response to an antigen, and thereby decreased the allergic delayed hyper sensitivity response. Medical scientists need to examine such situations to determine whether such "megadose" levels of linoleate are suppressing or stimulating eicosanoid production and whether such supplementation is useful for humans.

Four major types of mediators and modulators of immune responses noted in Fig. 10-4 are prostaglandins, leukotrienes, complement peptides and cytokines. Some of the modulators are not derived from diets and are noted merely to help the reader recognize ways in which the agents can be involved. Many activated peptides noted at the top of the figure are mobilized during tissue injury, and they stimulate chemotactic and secretory responses of the macrophage and neutrophil leukocytes. Similarly, antigens ("foreign" proteins) combine with antibodies to stimulate either the complement cascade or the release of modulators from the different leukocytes. The ability of the late components of complement (C5-9) to stimulate the release of arachidonate from cell membranes (Betz and Hansch, 1984) provides a link between the complement cascade and the eicosanoid cascade. Many of the modulators in the figure influence the disease symptoms of which we tend to be most aware. For example, histamine is a self-healing autacoid released from mast cells, and many people take antihistamines to antagonize its action when it is being secreted in undesired amounts. Similarly, taking aspirin can diminish the release of prostaglandin autacoids from mast cells and macrophages and thereby diminish some of the undesired symptoms. We need to learn more about the effects of diet on the release and actions of these modulators.

Rheumatoid Arthritis

One dietary approach to understanding the role of eicosanoid precursors in immune inflammatory disorders is the removal of all polyunsaturated precursors and antagonists from the diet to obtain a deficiency of essential fatty acids (Bonta and Pamham, 1982). This experimental approach impairs the formation of eicosanoids, but it also causes many other defects. It seems unlikely to be applicable to any mode of treatment of any human cases.

However, this extreme approach shows that dietary n-6 fatty acids have a role in certain experimental models of inflammatory disorder. Prostaglandins acting at different cellular receptors can have both anti-inflammatory and proinflammatory actions. Awareness of the dual actions of prostaglandins is important, but it does not indicate the dietary strategy to follow in treating inflammation. Indeed, one expert summary of many years of experience with diet treatment of arthritis concluded that three possible diets might be considered for use in treating rheumatoid arthritis, although success is not certain and evaluating the results is extremely difficult (Ziff, 1983).

The three possible approaches were: (1) eliminate all polyunsaturated fat from the diet; (2) use a diet very rich in n-6 fatty acid; (3) use a diet rich in eicosapentaenoic acid, 20:5n-3 found in sea foods. Presumably, medical researchers will evaluate all three options in the coming years. The options are discussed again in Chapter 19.

Eicosapentaenoic acid with human leukocytes formed a leukotriene B_5 that had much less biological effect than the leukotriene B_4 formed from arachidonic acid (Prescott, 1984). In fact, the LTB_5 was reported to bind 500 times less firmly to the high affinity receptors of neutrophils than did the LTB_4 (Goldman et al, 1983). This difference could be the basis for fish oil in the diet significantly decreasing certain inflammatory conditions. The effects are not all simple to interpret, however, since studies with an experimental model of polyarthritis in rats showed enhanced susceptibility to collagen-induced arthritis when fish oil was fed (Prickett et al, 1984).

This paradoxical effect was observed also when the widely used immunosuppressive agent, cyclosporin A, was used to treat rats with collagen-induced arthritis (Kaibara et al, 1983). When the agent was present only during the induction phase of the experiment, it successfully suppressed the development of arthritis as well as the delayed type hypersensitivity responses to collagen.

However, when cyclosporin was added after the onset of the disease, there was a significant enhancement of the disease. Apparently the agent was suppressing a population of T-suppressor cells which resulted in an enhanced T-cell-mediated helper effect. A principal action of cyclosporin may be in blocking the production of messenger RNA for interleukin-2 (IL-2) (Elliott et al:, 1984) which thus prevents the signal that would have stimulated the proliferation of the T-helper cells and shifts the immunological balance in favor of the T-suppressor cells (Kupiec-Weglinski et al, 1983).

When Is Intervention Best?

The ability of dietary fish oil to diminish eicosanoid-mediated immune inflammatory events was examined in rats. The induction of the formation of IgE and IgG antibodies in response to foreign protein was four- to eightfold greater in rats fed fish oil compared with those receiving beef tallow (Prickett et al, 1982).

This finding might reflect a diminished functioning of the immune suppresor T cells in the absence of an adequate synthesis of eicosanoids from arachidonate. Such a lack of suppression in animals fed fish oil may have permitted greater production of antibody, and several experimental systems showed enhanced antibody production (Prickett et al, 1982). This finding parallels the report that pharmacologic inhibition of prostaglandin synthesis may enhance secondary antibody synthesis in humans (Goodwin et al, 1978).

However, the secretion of antibody by purified samples of B lymphocytes can be either increased or decreased by similar inhibitors depending on the timing of the pharmacologic treatment after exposure to antigen (Zimecki and Webb, 1976). Thus prostaglandins likely play opposing roles at different stages of the immune cell response. When 17 patients with rheumatoid arthritis were studied in a 12-week controlled dietary intervention with supplemental fish oil (equivalent to 1.8 g of eicosapentaenoate per day) there was reported improvement with decreased morning stiffness and the number of tender joints, but the variance of the measurements was too great to permit a consistently rigorous interpretation from control patients (Kremer et al, 1985).

In one approach to adjuvant-induced polyarthritis, supplementation of rat diets with primrose oil for two weeks prior to adjuvant challenge significantly diminished the arthritic index from 34 to 17 (Kunkel et al, 1982). The primrose seed oil contained 71.5% 18:2n-6, 8.6% 18:3n-6, and 0.3% 20:4n-6 with no n-3 fatty acids.

Many questions remain unanswered regarding the mechanism whereby this change in dietary acids suppressed the development of polyarthritis in this model. If the effect was due to the 8.6% 18:3n-6 in the oil, was it achieved by diminishing the conversion of 18:2n-6 to 20:4n-6 or by converting the 18:3n-6 to 20:3n-6, which then formed some "ameliorative" monoenoic prostaglandins? Did the results with this oil differ from those obtainable with any vegetable oil containing 70—80% 18:2n-6? Would tests with oils rich in n-3 fatty acids be more effective? Are the results with this model applicable to human disease? To answer these questions, further study is needed. How will we be able to develop effective evidence that lifelong prophylaxis with a moderate immune suppressor may have health benefits when the suppressor harms those who are already afflicted?

Consistent evidence from double-blind, placebo-controlled clinical trials indicates that dietary n-3 fats supplied as fish oil have modest beneficial effects in rheumatoid arthritis. Although the size and extent of benefit seemed blunted by high n-6 polyunsaturated fat diets and concurrent anti-inflammatory drug use, there is a potential for increased intake of n-3 fats and decreased intake of n-6 fats to have drug-sparing effects (James and Cleland, 1997). A small clinical study in patients with rheumatoid arthritis showed that fish oil supplementation at a daily dose of 40 mg n-3 fatty acids per kg body weight/day, with dietary n-6 fatty acid intake below 10 g/day, gave substantial improvement in clinical status (Volker et al, 2000).

Supplements of n-3 fatty acids consistently reduced both the number of tender joints and the amount of morning stiffness in patients with rheumatoid arthritis (Kremer, 2000). A minimum daily dose of 3 g eicosapentaenoic and docosahexaenoic acids consumed for at least 12 wk gave clinical benefits and gave lower release of inflammatory mediators; leukotriene B4 (LTB_4) from stimulated neutrophils and of interleukin-1 (IL-1) from monocytes. As a result, rheumatoid arthritis patients taking n-3 supplements could lower their daily doses of nonsteroidal antiinflammatory drugs or disease-modifying antirheumatic drugs.

Overall, beneficial anti-inflammatory effects of dietary fish oils in rheumatoid arthritis were seen in randomized, double-blind, placebo-controlled trials (Cleland et al, 2003). Importantly, fish oils have protective clinical effects also in cardiovascular disease for which arthritis patients are also at high risk. The clinical use of anti-inflammatory fish oil doses in these patients had good compliance, particularly when a biomarker of n-3 intake was used to provide helpful feedback reports to patients that attainment of target levels was being monitored.

So far, suppression of the oxidant stress and inflammation of rheumatoid arthritis with n-3 supplements has had more success than blocking tissue damage from mediators of osteoarthritis. Nevertheless, supplementation with n-3 PUFA, and not n-6 PUFA, decreased both degradative and inflammatory aspects of chondrocyte metabolism in tissue from patients with osteoarthritis while not affecting normal tissue physiology (Curtis et al, 2002a).

The n-3 supplementation reduced expression of mRNA from genes for ADAMTS-4, MMP-13, and MMP-3 (but not TIMP-1, -2, or -3). Also, n-3 PUFA supplementation abolished the expression of mRNA for mediators of inflammation (cyclooxygenase 2, 5-lipoxygenase, 5-lipoxygenase-activating protein, tumor necrosis factor alpha, IL-1alpha, and IL-1beta) without affecting the expression of message for genes of several other proteins involved in normal tissue physiology (Curtis et al, 2002b). As in all chronic inflammatory diseases, the difficulty of reversing all of the cellular changes in a fully developed auto-immune disorder following years of imbalanced amplified tissue responses is much greater than in preventing the early stages of amplifying the initial triggering immune events.

This book focuses on primary prevention of the dietary imbalances that drive such disorders to irreversible pathology that then requires lifelong medication. If preventive action is not taken early enough, then drug treatment to suppress aggressive effector cells that cause severe clinical signs becomes a major remaining option.

Systemic Lupus Erythematosis

Systemic lupus erythematosis in humans represents a puzzling chronic immune disorder. The disease is an autoimmune disorder that damages the blood vessels and leads to fatal damage of the kidneys. A similar condition that occurs spontaneously in certain strains of mice is often used to examine details of the disease process and to test various therapeutic strategies.

Degenerative vascular disease associated with circulating immune complexes can lead to deposits of leukocytes and immune complexes in the walls of the medium and small arteries and cause medial degeneration. The vascular damage may occur either with or without significant cellular inflammation. Vascular changes of this type resemble some events associated with essential hypertension, and they are frequently associated with myocardial infarction in experimental animals. Some researchers noted that myocardial infarction was reported with higher frequency in patients with long-standing systemic lupus erythematosis (Accinni and Dixon, 1979). Interpreting the mechanism of such degenerative vascular change associated with immune complexes is complicated. For example, an antigen can cause inflammatory lesions in acute serum sickness and non-inflammatory changes in chronic serum sickness. Such results suggest that long-term chronic expression of immune reactions may lead to a depletion of some essential mediator of inflammation (Accinni and Dix on, 1979) or to the greater expression of some anti-inflammatory process.

New Zealand B/W hybrid mice spontaneously develop an autoimmune disease in which antibodies to DNA and nuclei are produced. Apparently this mating causes a combination of genetic defects responsible for the progressive immune disorder. Immune complexes deposit in the renal glomerulus and along the junction of the dermis with epidermis, and all the animals generally acquire glomerulonephritis by 9 months of age and die by 12 months (Hurd et al, 1981).

All the disease manifestations were strikingly diminished when a diet deficient in polyunsaturated fatty acids was used. Of the animals deficient in essential fatty acid, 78% survived for 16 months. Even at 20 months, 55% of the mice on polyunsaturated deficient diets were still alive. At age 10 months, only 7% of the control mice that received n-6 fatty acid had survived, and none survived by 16 months. Adding more n-6 eicosanoid precursors did not seem to help in this model, since diets with 16% 18:2n-6 by weight (about 30%) failed to protect the mice.

Intervention with Omega-3

To examine the ability of dietary n-3 acids to diminish n-6 mediated responses in this model of autoimmune disease, Prickett et al (1981, 1983) compared the effects of diets containing either menhaden oil or beef tallow, The serum lipids of the mice on the latter diets contained 14.6% 18:2n-6, 14.9% 20:4n-6, and had less than 0.05% 20:5n-3, whereas those of mice on fish oil diets contained 3.2% 18:2n-6, 9.9% 20:4n-6, and 18.4% 20:5n-3. Severe proteinuria progressively occurred between 6 and 12 months in animals on the tallow diet and two-thirds died by 14 months. In contrast to this, none of the animals receiving fish oil exhibited appreciable proteinuria, and all survived for 14 months. If the special diets were initiated 4 months after birth, similar results were obtained with some proteinuria and death occurring after 14 months of age.

The disease trends were more distinct if the special diet was delayed until 5 months of age. In those cases, significant progressive onset of the disease apparently occurred even though the symptoms were not detected until later. Levels of circulating antibodies to nuclear DNA were low at 8 months in animals receiving fish oil from birth, whereas they were several times higher in animals receiving the fish oil after 4 or 5 months of age. This parallels the greater antibody formation in animals fed fish oil described in the Rheumatoid Arthritis Section.

Antibody formation, therefore, does not always correlate with disease. Apparently different balances of rate limiting events occur in the different disease models. This suppression of disease symptoms by fish oil may give an altered eicosanoid balance as in the SHR animals. Would thymic transplants provide a cure by introducing T cells that do not need this alteration in eicosanoids to keep a healthy balance? When patients with IgA nephropathy were treated for 1 year with 2.6 g of n-3 fatty acids daily, there was a significant arrest in the progressive deterioration of renal function (Hamazaki et al, 1984). Untreated patients had further loss of function during the same time period. Although fish oil helped stop deterioration, the previous damage was not repaired in treated patients.

Karmali et al, (1982) reported that supplements of an oil rich in n-6 fatty acids did not retard the development of this type of autoimmune disease in mice, and that levels of undesired antinuclear antibodies were high in both control and oil-fed mice. Comparison of this result with that obtained in the model for arthritis (described previously) illustrates the manner in which eicosanoids can have very different effects in complex immune signaling events. These results provide a useful illustration of the complex interactions of the immune system that may be expected to be influenced by dietary lipids. No single simplistic summary can indicate that prostaglandins are "good" or "bad" for us, and thus no single summary will suffice for the n-3 polyunsaturated antagonists of n-6 prostaglandin formation.

A scenario can be created in which antagonizing the conversion of 20:4n-6 to prostaglandins might either diminish certain features promoting cell response and proliferation and diminish antibody production or diminish other suppressive cell responses and increase antibody production. The immune system will not readily submit to oversimplified experiments with dietary fatty acids, and the current animal models of disease are poor imitations of the human conditions.

In patients with lupus nephritis, dietary supplementation with fish oil decreased some mechanisms and symptoms involved in the inflammatory and atherosclerotic vascular disease, but it did not decrease immune complexes, anti-DNA antibody titer or albuminuria linked to lupus pathology (Clark et al, 1989). In another study, patients with moderately active SLE were clinically and serologically improved during the first 3 months with n-3 HUFA supplements (relative to patients with olive oil control supplements), but the beneficial effect was short-lived, and there was no difference at 6 months. (Westberg and Tarkowski , 1990).

Multiple Sclerosis/Experimental Allergic Encephalomyelitis

Some evidence indicates that multiple sclerosis may be an immune-related disorder involving some autoimmune processes. Without suitable animal models for the disease, only a small amount of information is available. One experimental model of this type of disease is experimental allergic encephalomyelitis (EAE) which has provided insight into the mechanisms of this type of disease and helped explore some ways to diminish its severity.

The EAE can be induced by a single subcutaneous injection of emulsified material from the central nervous system, especially myelin basic protein. (This resembles, in part, the approach to collagen-induced arthritis discussed previously) The immunological inflammatory condition that develops can later be transferred to control animals by transferring cells from the lymph nodes or spleen of affected animals. Apparently normal thymic function does not prevent the expression of this disease as it does in the SHR model, and it is not due to a genetic imbalance of suppressor and helper cell function. The severity of the disease in the recipients can be increased if the transferred cells are cultured for 72 hours with a T-cell mitogen before the transfer is completed. This incubation presumably changes the balance of suppressor to helper cells of the spleen that favors the helper cell functions.

Feeding plant oil rich in n-6 fatty acids causes smaller numbers of lymph node cells to be sensitized to the myelin basic protein in this experimental model, and it suppresses the symptoms of the disorder (Stackpoole and Mertin, 1982). Apparently the T-cell-mediated suppressive events involve prostaglandins, because administering indomethacin prior to the n-6 fatty acids prevents the oil-induced suppression of the symptoms. When the animals have their spleen removed, the suppressive effect of the supplemental plant oil does not occur. Mattingly et al (1979) showed that the ability of certain cells in the spleen to function as suppressor cells depended on their PGH synthase activity.

The suppression by prostaglandin forming spleen cells resembles that noted for the arthritis model. Presumably, n-3 fatty acids will have limited benefit in these models once the helper/suppressor cell ratio has been altered, since one of their major actions may be to influence earlier events that lead to tolerance. Perhaps a reversal of pathological effects may require the removal or inactivation of the undesired helper T cells with selective antibodies as reported recently by Waldor et al (1985). Nevertheless, the investigation of the ability of n-3 fatty acids to influence helper/suppressor ratios has a strong possibility of providing new understanding for medical science.

Studies with EAE still leave unanswered the immunoregulatory role of n-6 fatty acids and eicosanoids in this experimental model. A spontaneous encephalomalacia occurs in chicks deficient in vitamin E, and this disorder appears to be induced by dietary l8:2n-6 and diminished by 18:3n-3 (Budowski, 1981). Prevention of this phenomenon by vitamin E may reflect, in part, a role for lipid peroxides in this damage and the action of cyclooxygenase in amplifying peroxide levels more rapidly with n-6 than n-3 acids (see Chapter 14).

Results with Patients

In 20 patients with multiple sclerosis, a double-blind crossover trial showed that lymphocyte agglutination was greater for those receiving 16 g of 18:2n-6 daily (Untermohlen et al, 1982). Also, the monocytes exhibited a direct migration inhibition that was abrogated by indomethacin, suggesting that there could be an effect of prostaglandins (and thus dietary lipids) on the behavior of these immune-mediating cells. The significance of these findings is unclear, and attempts to interpret the role of dietary fatty acids in multiple sclerosis have not yet succeeded. No widely accepted dietary recommendation for patients with multiple sclerosis is available at the time of this writing.

Loss of fine motor coordination (spasticity) is a complicating sign in multiple sclerosis that also develops in a mouse model of chronic relapsing experimental autoimmune encephalomyelitis, and the tremor and spasticity are decreased with signaling through cannabinoid receptors (see Chapter 2). Elevated levels of the endocannabinoids, anandamide (arachidonoylethanolamide) and 2-arachidonoyl glycerol, and of the anandamide analog, palmitoylethanolamide, were detected in areas associated with nerve damage, suggesting that the impaired tissue was mobilizing self-healing responses (Baker et al, 2001). In addition, selective inhibitors of endocannabinoid re-uptake and hydrolysis significantly decreased spasticity as did added potent cannabinoid receptor agonists.

The results indicate the EFA-derived endocannabinoids suppress spasticity and raise the question of whether n-3 and n-6 derivatives have equal actions. If different, then food choices may alter the progression of multiple sclerosis and other neuromuscular diseases modulated by endocannabinoid levels and actions. More research is needed to know if dietary n-3 and n-6 levels make a difference. Some MS patients had lower linoleic and arachidonic acids in the lipids of cerebrospinal fluid (CSF), most pronounced in cholesterol esters (Neu, 1983).

Asthma

This immune-mediated disease has characteristically severe bronchoconstriction in response to antigen challenge. Again, no good animal model mimics the human disease, making it difficult to study potentially useful new drugs before applying them to humans. Asthma symptoms appear to be due to the responses of effector cells that generate leukotrienes and thromboxane (TXA_2). We know that anticyclooxygenase drugs do not appreciably reduce the symptoms of asthma, and prostaglandins may not be major mediators. Some researchers believe that leukotrienes are significant mediators of bronchoconstriction in humans. Thus considerable attention is focused on finding therapeutic antagonists to the lipoxygenase pathway that synthesizes leukotrienes (see Chapter 16). The relatively low incidence of asthma among Eskimos may reflect an action of dietary n-3 fatty acids that either lowers the activity of antibody generation, lowers the degree of effector cell response to antigen, or lowers the activity of the eicosanoids released in that response.

The effect of dietary n-3 fatty acid on the ability of mast cells to form leukotriene products of the lipoxygenase pathway was described by Murphy et al (1981). Relatively equal amounts of 20:4n-6 and 20:5n-3 in the lipids of the mast cells led to 10 times greater amounts of LTC_4 than LTC_5. Since LTC_5 was also less effective than LTC_4 in binding to receptors (Goldman et al, 1983) and in causing smooth muscle contraction (Hammarström, 1980), there is likely to be decreased expression of symptoms with the eicosanoids released from n-3 supplemented cells. Possibly the high 20:5n-3 in the Eskimo diet may partially be the basis for the low incidence of asthma among Greenland natives.

When immunologically sensitized guinea-pigs were challenged with antigen to create an asthma-like response, pretreatment with an aspirin-like medicine made the response more severe (Lee et al, 1984). That result suggests that some prostaglandins are serving to help keep the bronchi dilated. Diet supplements of menhaden oil also intensified the constrictor response with these animals in contrast to their action on vascular muscle. The constriction with this model system makes it difficult to understand how fish oil supplements might benefit individuals already sensitized to antigens. Perhaps Eskimos benefit from having the n-3 acids in their diets continuously from birth (and even before). Supplements of fish oil may have a greater effect in decreasing the earlier stages of asthma in which eliciting antibody formation is the primary event. At that stage of the immune response, the events may be more sensitive to the balance between the n-3 and n-6 fatty acids.

T-Helper Cells and Cytokines

Asthma is a chronic immune disease with intermittent periods of inflammatory conditions in the respiratory airways, characterized by bronchial airway inflammation with greater mucus production and airway hyper-responsiveness and episodes of wheezing, coughing, and shortness of breath. The early pathophysiology seems due to inadequately regulated CD4+ T-cell immune response with overactive T-helper 2 (Th2) immune responses while T-helper 1 (Th1) activity (corresponding more to cell-mediated immunity) is dampened (Miller, 2001).

The Th2 subset produces cytokines interleukin-4 (IL-4), IL-5, IL-6, IL-9, IL-10, and IL-13, which stimulate the growth, differentiation, and recruitment of immune cells (mast cells, basophils, eosinophils, and B-cells) that mediate immunity, inflammation, and allergic responses. The n-3 HUFA, especially eicosapentaenoic acid, appear to down-regulate Th1-type responses linked to chronic inflammatory disease (Calder et al, 2000). The fatty acid composition of lymphocytes and other immune cells affects the capacity of those cells to produce immunoregulatory eicosanoids, such as prostaglandin E_2. The evidence for beneficial effects of fish oil is strongest for rheumatoid arthritis, but there is some evidence for benefit in asthma and related diseases. Neonates whose mothers had fish oil supplementation had significantly lower plasma IL-13 compared to the control group (Dunstan et al, 2003). The neonatal cell membranes also had a significant inverse relationship between their levels of n-3 PUFA and levels of IL-13 released to plasma.

A report of 30%-50% lower incidence of childhood asthma with exclusive breastfeeding for three months or with eating fish regularly (i.e., a high intake of n-3 fatty acids) suggests that major modifiable dietary environmental risk factors for childhood asthma are lack of breastfeeding and low intake of n-3 fatty acids (Mellis , 2002). In contrast, nine randomised controlled trials conducted between 1986 and 2001 gave little evidence to recommend that established asthma could be moderated by supplements of marine n-3 fatty acids (Woods et al, 2002). However, there also was no evidence that patients are at higher risk if they do so. Japanese have a higher intake of fish and a lower incidence of asthma than people in western countries. Although many past clues suggest possible benefits of eating n-3 fats, a recent study of Japanese children described a higher prevalence of asthma for those who ate fish one to two times a week than among those who ate fish one to two times a month (Takemura et al, 2002). The reason for less observed asthma among Eskimos remains a puzzle.

Diabetes

Diabetes mellitus was reported in Eskimos at a frequency much lower than expected for a similar group of Danes (Chapter 1). In examining the nature of the disease to understand the role that diet might play, important features need emphasis. Two very different forms of diabetes occur: type I (or juvenile-onset diabetes), and type II (or maturity-onset diabetes). They are very different, just as thrombotic and hemorrhagic stroke are very different types of stroke.

The symptoms of type II diabetes mellitus are controlled by a careful choice of diet. Thus patients with this disorder are often advised on ways to select foods that can be handled adequately by their limited amount of insulin activity. Apparently, the secretion and action of insulin in these people progressively declines until at some mature age the symptoms of diabetes become evident. Usually some insulin is mobilized by these patients, and they are regarded to be insulin "independent."

In contrast, patients with type I diabetes have lost the ability to secrete insulin and are dependent on insulin added from outside sources. This lost function appears due in part to an aggressive autoimmune reaction that damages the insulin-secreting cells of the pancreas. Why don't Eskimos seem to have either of these common forms of disease? The reports of a greater incidence of diabetes mellitus among Eskimos who adopted food habits of Western industrialized nations gives a useful clue to the puzzle.

Oxidant Stress from Diets and Immune Responses

Apparently the traditional Eskimo diet with its high content of meat from the maritime food chain and low amount of refined carbohydrates provides the dietary control needed to suppress the symptoms of type II diabetes in aging individuals who are vulnerable to the progressive onset of that type of inadequate hormone action. When these individuals adopt Western-style foods, symptoms then appear.

On the other hand, how did Eskimos avoid type I diabetes, a disease that attacks young individuals and makes them dependent on external supplies of insulin for the rest of their lives? Type I diabetes mellitus has particularly tragic consequences in that its victims are subject to continual risk of damage to the blood vessels, resulting in stroke, blindness, or loss of limbs or organs, such as kidneys. The Eskimos are indeed fortunate to have a low incidence of this disease. Could the relative lack of this type of diabetes also be attributed to moderated immune action as a result of their diet? If so how could that information be applied to other people?

Medical researchers have evidence that the juvenile onset diabetes is a form of autoimmune disease. Apparently an imbalance in the white cells causes them to generate antibodies and effector cells that can promote an attack on the insulin-forming cells of the pancreas. This selective destruction of these cells is a result of several parts of the immune system going out of balance, as occurs in other autoimmune diseases. Blood samples from newly diagnosed patients with type I diabetes had abnormally elevated numbers of lymphocytes bearing specific antigens that were not detected in patients with type II diabetes (Pozzilli et al, 1983). Lymphocytes from patients with type I diabetes were markedly impaired in developing normal suppressor cell function when preincubated with concanavalin A (Con A), whereas cells from type II patients were normal (Lederman et al, 1981). The hypofunction of supressor cell responses was noted with challenges by either the general, nonspecific antigen, ConA, or the specific antigen derived from the insulin-secreting tissue (Fairchild et al, 1982).

The autoimmune processes that destroy the insulin-secreting cells are not identical in all patients with type I diabetes, so that even this one type of disease contains different subsets. If diets rich in n-3 polyunsaturated fatty acids could so dramatically suppress the function of platelets, could they also shift the balance between the functions of T-suppressor and T helper cells derived from the same stem cell, as are platelets? As with other examples of autoimmune diseases noted earlier in this chapter, a special strain of laboratory animal (the BB rat) has been found that spontaneously develops a form of Type I diabetes (Marliss et al, 1982). These animals appear to have an imbalance in the interactions of their T lymphocytes which can be corrected with transfusions of lymphocytes from closely related donors (Rossini et al, 1984). Is this comparable to the thymic transplants in SHR animals? This corrective approach may not be a very suitable form of therapy at this time for humans. It will be interesting to learn whether fish oil might moderate this autoimmune disorder if provided early enough in the disease process. Cyclosporin could only defer the onset of symptoms (Stiller et al, 1983).

One interesting attempt to treat type-1 patients with the immunosuppressive agent, cyclosporin showed that 16 of 30 patients who were treated within 6 weeks of diagnosis improved and became insulin independent (Stiller et al, 1984). However, with those for which therapy began 8-44 weeks after diagnosis, only 2 of 11 achieved that state. Apparently once the original immune imbalance occurs, medicine does not reverse the imbalance. Also of concern in this situation is the likelihood that withdrawal of the medicine may cause the disease to reappear. This is a particularly troublesome consideration because continued long-term treatment with such an immunosuppressor seriously compromises the immune surveillance system and increases the vulnerability of the patient to infection or cancer. Some milder and selective approach to correcting the immune imbalance is needed, perhaps by having less aggressive n-6 eicosanoid responses.

The recent epidemic rise in type-2 diabetes associated with imbalances in energy intake and expenditure in the USA includes a serious diabetes-associated risk of inflammatory cardiovascular damage described in Chapter 5 linked with its resultant thrombosis and arrhythmia. Sustaining a dietary balance in n-3 and n-6 EFA may decrease risks in both type-1 and type-2 diabetes. Moderate daily intake of n-3 fatty acid ethyl esters by 935 patients with hyper-triglyceridemia (55% had either impaired glucose tolerance or type 2 diabetes (non-insulin-dependent diabetes mellitus; NIDDM) led to lowered triglyceride (triacylglycerol) concentrations without any worsening of glucose tolerance (Sirtori et al, 1997).

A reduced fat diet incorporating one daily fish meal reduced serum triglycerides and increased HDL2 cholesterol in patients (Dunstan et al, 1997). Fish consumption reported by patients was strongly related to the content of n-3 HUFA in their platelets. Furthermore, patients with type 1 diabetes also had a close positive association between the content of n-3 HUFA in platelets and 24-h HRV, but the association was not statistically significant in the group of patients with type 2 diabetes (Christensen et al, 2001). In type 2 diabetes patients with hypertriglyceridemia, moderate amounts of fish oil induce a long-term significant reduction in plasma triglycerides, VLDL triglycerides, and NEFA and a significant enrichment in the red blood cell phospholipid content of long-chain n-3 fatty acids, without deteriorating blood glucose control (Rivellese et al, 1997). Importantly, discussions of diabetes often focus on blood glucose levels, whereas the enhanced death rate of diabetes involves cardiovascular events described in Chapters 5, 6 and 7. Higher consumption of fish and long-chain n-3 fatty acids was clearly associated with a lower CHD incidence and total mortality among diabetic women (Hu et al, 2003). Compared with women who ate less than 1 fish serving/mo, the relative risks of CHD were 0.70 for fish consumption 1 to 3 times per month, 0.64 for 2 to 4 times per week, and 0.36 for 5 or more times per week.

References

Accinni L, Dixon FL. Degenerative vascular disease and myocardial infarction in mice with lupushke syndrome. *Am J Pathol* 96:477-492, 1979.

Baker D, Pryce G, Croxford JL, et al Endocannabinoids control spasticity in a multiple sclerosis model. *FASEB J* 15(2):300-302, 2001.

Betz M, Hansch GM. Release of arachidonic acid: A new function of the late complement components. *Immunobiology* 166:473-483, 1984.

Bonta IL, Parnham MJ. Prostaglandins, essential fatty acids and cell-tissue interactions in immune-inflammation. *Prog Lipid Res* 20:617-623, 1982.

Budowski P. Review: Nutritional effects of w-3 polyunsaturated fatty acids. *Isr J Med Sci* 17:223-231, 1981.

Calder PC, Yaqoob P, Thies F, et al Fatty acids and lymphocyte functions. *Br J Nutr* 87(Suppl 1): S31-S48, 2002.

Charpentier BM, Bach M-A, Lang P, et al Expression of OKT 8 antigen and receptors by suppressor cells mediating specific unresponsiveness between recipient and donor in renal-allograft-tolerant patients. *Transplantations* 36:495-501, 1938.

Christensen JH, Skou HA, Madsen T, et al Heart rate variability and n-3 polyunsaturated fatty acids in patients with diabetes mellitus. *J Intern Med* 249(6):545-552, 2001.

Clark WF, Parbtani A, Huff MW. Omega-3 fatty acid dietary supplementation in systemic lupus erythematosus. *Kidney Int* 36(4):653-660, 1989.

Cleland L, James M, Proudman S. The role of fish oils in the treatment of rheumatoid arthritis. *Drugs* 63(9): 845-532, 2003.

Curtis CL, Rees SG, Cramp J, et al Effects of n-3 fatty acids on cartilage metabolism. *Proc Nutr Soc* 61(3): 381-389, 2002a.

Curtis CL, Rees SG, Little CB, et al Pathologic indicators of degradation and inflammation in human osteoarthritic cartilage are abrogated by exposure to n-3 fatty acids. *Arthritis Rheum* 46(6):1544-1553, 2002b.

Dunstan JA, Mori TA, Barden A, et al Maternal fish oil supplementation in pregnancy reduces interleukin-13 levels in cord blood of infants at high risk of atopy. *Clin Exp Allergy* 33(4): 442-448, 2003.

Dunstan DW, Mori TA, Puddey IB, et al The independent and combined effects of aerobic exercise and dietary fish intake on serum lipids and glycemic control in NIDDM. A randomized controlled study. *Diabetes Care* 20(6): 913-921, 1997.

Elliott JF, Lin Y, Mizel SB, et al Induction of interleukin 2 messenger RNA inhibited by cyclosporin A. *Science* 226:1439-1441, 1984.

Ergas D, Eilat E, Mendlovic S, et al n-3 fatty acids and the immune system in autoimmunity. *Isr Med Assoc J*4(1):34-38, 2002.

Fairchild RS, Kyner JL, Abdou NI. Specific immunoregulation ábnormality in insulin-dependent diabetes melitus. *J Lab Clin Med* 99:175-186, 1982.

Friend JV, Lock SO, Gurr MI, et al Effect of different dietary lipids on the immune responses of Hartley strain guinea pigs. *Int Arch Allergy Appl Immunol* 62: 292-301, 1980.

Goldman DW, Pickett WC, Goetzl EJ. Human neutrophil chemotactic and degranulating activities of leukotriene B5 (LTB5) derived from eicosapentaenoic acid. *Biochem Biophys Res Commun* 117:282-283, 1983.

Goodwin JS, Selinger DS, Messner RP, et al Effect of indomethacin in vivo on humoral and cellular immunity in humans. *Infect Immun* 19:430-433, 1978.

Hamazaki T, Tateno S, Shishido H. Eicosapentaenoic acid and IgA nephropathy. *Lancet* 1: 1017-1018, 1984.

Hammarström S. Leukotriene C5: A slow-reacting substance derived from eicosapentaenoic acid. *J Biol Chem* 255: 7093-7094, 1980.

Hu FB, Cho E, Rexrode KM, et al Fish and long-chain omega-3 fatty acid intake and risk of coronary heart disease and total mortality in diabetic women. *Circulation* 107(14): 1852-1857.

Hurd ER, Johnston JM, Okita JR. (1981). Prevention of glomerulonephritis and prolonged survival in New Zealand black/New Zealand white F1 hybrid mice fed an essential fatty acid-deficient diet. *J Clin Invest* 67: 476-485, 1981.

James MJ, Cleland LG. Dietary n-3 fatty acids and therapy for rheumatoid arthritis. *Semin Arthritis Rheum* 27(2): 85-97, 1997.

Kaibara N, Hotokebuchi T, Takagishi K, et al Paradoxical effects of cyclosporin A on collagen arthritis in rats. *J Exp Med* 158: 2007-2015, 1983.

Karmali RA, Hanrahan R, Volkman A. Prostaglandins and essential fatty acids in regulation of autoimmunity and development of antibodies of DNA in NZB >< NZW F1 mice. *Prog Lipid Res* 20:655-661, 1982.

Kremer JM. n-3 fatty acid supplements in rheumatoid arthritis. *Am J Clin Nutr* 71(1 Suppl): 349S-351S, 2000.

Kremer JM, Michalek AV, Lininger L. Effects of manipulation of dietary fatty acids on clinical manifestations of rheumatoid arthritis. *Lancet* 1: 184-186, 1985.

Kunkel SL, Ogawa H, Ward PA, et al Suppression of chronic inflammation by evening primrose oil. *Prog Lipid Res* 20: 885-888, 1982.

KupiecWeglinskj JW, Lear PA, Bordees-Azoar J. Acute rejection in cyclosporin A-treated graft recipients occurs following abrogation of suppressor cells. *Transplant Proc* 15: 531-534, 1983.

Ledemian MM, Elmer IJ, Rodmati HM. Defective suppressor cell generation in juvenile onset diabets. *J Immunol* 127: 2051-2055, 1981.

Lee TFL, Lewis RA, Robinson D. The effects of a diet enriched in menhaden fish oil on the pulmonary response to antigen challenge. *J Allergy Clin Immunol* 73: 150, 1984.

Lim M, Steinman L. Reversal of experimental allergic encephalomyelitis with monoclonal antibody to a T-cell subset marker. *Science* 227:415-417, 1985.

Marliss EB, Nakhooda AF Poussier P, et al The diabetic syndrome of the 'BB' Wistar rat: Possible relevance to type I (insulin-dependent) diabetes in man. *Diabetologia* 22: 225-232, 1982.

Mattingly JA, Eardley D, Kemp D, et al Induction of suppressor cells in rat spleen: Influence of microbial stimulation. *J. Immunol* 122: 787-790, 1979.

Merlin J, Stackpoole A, Shumwa SL. Prostaglandins and cell-mediated immunity. *Transplantation* 37:396-402, 1984.

Mellis CM. Is asthma prevention possible with dietary manipulation? *Med J Aust* 16:177. Suppl:S78-S80, 2002. Plus comment in: *Med J Aust* 2003 Mar 17;178(6):303; and author reply 303-304, .

Miller AL. The etiologies, pathophysiology, and alternative/complementary treatment of asthma. *Altern Med Rev* 6(1): 20-47, 2001.

Murphy RC, Picken WC, Culp BR, et al Tetraene and pentaene leukotriences: Selective production from murine mastocytoma cells after dietary manipulation, *Prostaglandins* 22(4): 613-622, 1981.

Neu IS. Essential fatty acids in the serum and cerebrospinal fluid of multiple sclerosis patients. *Acta Neurol Scand* 67(3): 151-163, 1983.

Pozzilli P, Zuccarini O, Lavicoli M. Monoclonal antibodies defined abnormalities of T lymphocytes in type I (insulin-dependent) diabetes. *Diabetes* 32: 91-94, 1983.

Prescott SM. The effect of eicosapentaenoic acid on leukotriene B production by human neutrophils. *J Biol Chem* 259: 7615-7621, 1984.

Prickett JD, Robinson DR, Block KJ. Enhanced production of I5E and IgG antibodies associated with a diet enriched in eicosapentaenojc acid. *Immunology* 46: 819-826, 1982.

Prickett JD et al Enhanced production of IgE and IgG antibodies associated with a diet enriched in eicosapentaenoic acid. *Immunology* 46: 819-826, 1982.

Piickett JD, Robinson DR, Steinberg AO. Effects of dietary enrichment with eicosapentaenojc acid upon autoimmune nephritis in female NZB x NZW F/F1 mice. *Arthritis Rheum* 26:133-139, 1983.

Prickett JD, Trentham DE Robinson DR. Dietary fish oil augments the induction of arthritis in rats immunized with type II collagen. *J Immunol* 132:725-729, 1984.

Rivellese AA, Maffettone A, Iovine C, et al Long-term effects of fish oil on insulin resistance and plasma lipoproteins in NIDDM patients with hypertriglyceridemia. *Diabetes Care* 19(11):1207-1213, 1996.

Rossini AA, Faustman D, Woda B, et al Lymphocyte transfusions prevent diabetes in the biobreeding/ Worcester rat. *J Clin Invest* 74:39-46, 1984.

Shoenfeld Y, Schwartz S. Immunologic and genetic factors in autoimmune diseases. *Immun Gen Auto* 311:1019-1029, 1984.

Sirtori CR, Paoletti R, Mancini M. N-3 fatty acids do not lead to an increased diabetic risk in patients with hyperlipidemia and abnormal glucose tolerance. Italian Fish Oil Multicenter Study. *Am J Clin Nutr* 65(6):1874-1881, 1997.

Spitzer K, Tomasso J, Boyar A. Unsaturated fatty acids and human mononuclear cell function. *Prog Lipid Res* 20: 739-741, 1982.

Stackpoole A, Merlin S. The effect of prostaglandin precursors in in vivo models of cell-mediated immunity. *Prog Lipid Res* 20: 649-654, 1982.

Stiller CR, Laupacis A, Keown PA, et al Cyclosporine: Action, pharmacokinetics, and effect in the BB rat model. *Metab Clin Exp* 32: 69-72, 1983.

Stiller CR, Dupre S, Gent M, et al M. 5. Effects of cyclosporine immunosuppression in insulin-dependent diabetes mellitus of recent onset. *Science* 223:1362-1367, 1984.

Takemura Y, Sakurai Y, Honjo S, et al The relationship between fish intake and the prevalence of asthma: the Tokorozawa childhood asthma and pollinosis study. *Prev Med* 34(2): 221-225, 2002.

Thomas S, Carver M, Foil FM, et al Role of prostaglandin-dependent suppressor cells in the immunosuppressive action of rabbit antithymocyte globulin. *Transplant Proc* 5: 1770-1772, 1983.

Untermohlen, V., Coniglio, J., Mao, D., Sierra, J., Smith, R., Benser, G., Hutchins, S., Spitzer, K., Tomasso, J., and Boyar, A. Unsaturated fatty acids and human mononuclear cell function. *Prog. Lipid Res.* 20, 739-741, 1982.

Volker D, Fitzgerald P, Major G, Garg M. Efficacy of fish oil concentrate in the treatment of rheumatoid arthritis. *J Rheumatol* 27(10): 2343-2346, 2000.

Waldor MK, Sriram S, Hardy R, et al Diet in the treatment of rheumatoid arthritis. *Arthritis Rheum* 26:457-461, 1983.

Westberg G, Tarkowski A. Effect of MaxEPA in patients with SLE. A double-blind, crossover study. *Scand J Rheumatol* 19(2):137-143, 1990.

Woods RK, Thien FC, Abramson MJ. Dietary marine fatty acids (fish oil) for asthma in adults and children. *Cochrane Database Syst Rev* (3):CD001283, 2002.

Zimecki M, Webb OR. The regulation of the immune response to 1-independent antigens by prostaglandins and B cells. *J Immunol* 117:2158-2164, 1976.

2005 National Library of Medicine Search Results:

(http://www.ncbi.nlm.nih.gov/entrez/query.fcgi)
immune = 266,849; immune inflammation = 13,144; immune eicosanoid = 2,810; immune fish = 2,053
arthritis = 148,009; arthritis eicosanoid = 1,546; arthritis fish = 234
lupus = 46,143; lupus eicosanoid = 263; lupus fish = 92
multiple sclerosis = 30,275; multiple sclerosis eicosanoid = 152; multiple sclerosis fish = 35
encephalomyelitis = 15,390; encephalomyelitis eicosanoid = 51; encephalomyelitis fish = 20
asthma = 85,376; asthma eicosanoid = 2,512; asthma fish = 197
diabetes = 229,568; diabetes eicosanoid = 1,779; diabetes fish = 510

11—Cell Proliferation and Cancer

Rapid growth (or proliferation) of a selected set of cells occurs during the amplification of antibody-producing lymphocytes in a stimulated immune response, during wound healing, or during malignant tumor growth. The first two processes are generally regarded to be desired events, whereas malignant growth of tumors is not. The intricate cellular interactions that promote all these proliferative processes appear to be mediated by several types of chemical signals that are to some extent common for most living cells. We thus need to have a highly selective control device to permit desired signals and prevent undesired proliferative signals.

The detailed blueprint for cell life is contained in the DNA of each cell. At different times in the life of a cell the blueprint is "read" to form new parts or replacement parts. Some of these parts regulate the switches and circuits that control cell growth and division. When some signal causes these parts to keep working when they normally would be resting, the cells keep multiplying or proliferating too fast for good health. Whenever eicosanoids formed from cellular polyunsaturated fatty acids have an influence on these signals, we can expect that dietary intakes of EFA might have some impact on the proliferative events. Some data suggest that the type and amount of polyunsaturated fat in the diet can influence some cancers that depend on inflammatory proliferative processes.

An important consideration of cancer as a disease is that there is a high probability that oxidative damage of cellular DNA which provides the initiation of new tumor cells may be a widespread occurrence. If the damage is repaired before the mistake is propagated to the daughter cells, no tumor will occur. However, if a cell replicates when the mistake is still not repaired, the error is perpetuated (see Fig 11-1). Initiation of damage may be faster in the presence of elevated amounts of peroxides that are associated with inflammatory events and enhanced formation of n-6 eicosanoids.

Although many isolated cells with abnormal DNA may occur individually in the body, their presence would still not be clinically evident until one of them proliferates out of control and spreads invasively in a tissue. Is the proliferative, invasive state aided by eicosanoids formed from the n-6 acids? Sometimes, decades might pass before the initial events that altered the cellular DNA are converted into the final invasive and proliferative events of a detectable tumor in a tissue. Sometimes an unusual antigen on the surface of the abnormal cell may be recognized as "alien" by the immune surveillance system and the cell is eliminated. Thus, modulation of immune responses by eicosanoids can also affect the development of tumors. The various cellular interactions are too complex and too poorly understood to permit a single generalization of the impact of n-3 and n-6 fatty acids on diverse types of cancers.

At this time, our current limited level of knowledge on tumor proliferation parallels the limited state of knowledge on heart disease and heart attacks that medical sci-

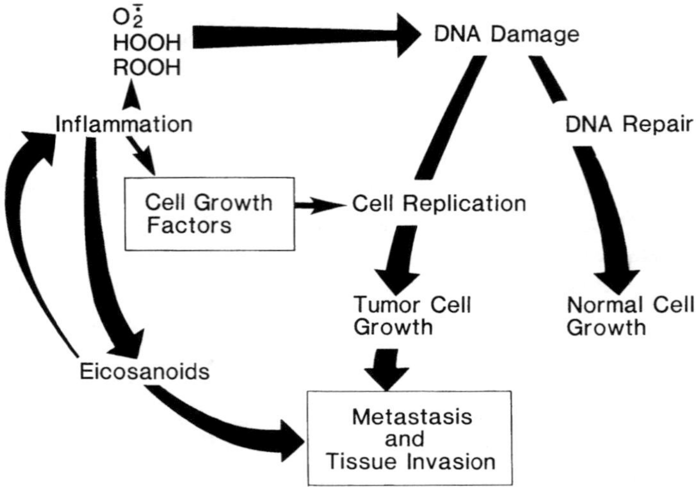

Fig. 11-1 Eicosanoids, peroxides, and cancer.

entists had several decades ago. We have not yet experienced the discoveries of biochemical modulators of tumors to parallel the discoveries by Samuelsson and by Vane for vascular thrombotic and antithrombotic events. However, early evidence suggests that the release of factors from platelets (aggregation) during atherosclerotic and thrombotic events can also participate in tumor invasiveness that leads to fatal development of dispersed secondary tumors.

Mediators of Metastasis

The biochemistry of metastasis seems crucial to understanding the control of cancer (Rawls, 1985). Eicosanoids derived from n-6 acids have been hypothesized to play a key role in facilitating the metastatic invasiveness of some tumors (Honn et al, 1983). In this hypothesis prostacyclin (PGI_2) plays an antimetastatic role (Honn et al, 1981), whereas the aggregation of platelets with thromboxane (TXA_2) is regarded to be prometastatic. Karmali et al (1983) reported that human breast cancers had higher production of thromboxane (TXB_2) associated with tumor size and metastasis at axillary lymph nodes and distant sites.

Prevention of prostaglandin formation from arachidonate has been beneficial in cutting the proliferation of some tumors (Narisawa et al., 1981; Bennet, 1982). The successful use of antioxidant compounds to prevent implantation and proliferation of tumor cells is another clue that may relate to the actions of fatty acid oxygenases in forming eicosanoids that promote tumor growth. The antioxidants tend to inhibit radical-mediated reactions, and they can inhibit the proliferation of peroxide-initiated reactions such as those of the oxygenases. The oxygenase reaction that forms prostaglandins is activated by very small amounts of peroxide, and more readily amplifies their concentration when acting with the n-6 type of fatty acids than with the n-3 type (see Chapter 14). Finding that high dietary amounts of vegetable oils (containing n-6 acids) significantly increased tumor formation (Broitman et al, 1977; Rogers, 1983) makes it important to recognize a role of the prostaglandin-forming oxygenase in tumor development.

This concept was confirmed by the finding that tumor growth-promoting effects of diets containing 10 and 20% fats rich in n-6 acids were completely abrogated by treatment with indomethacin (Kollmorgen et al, 1983). Similar studies with dibenzanthracene-induced tumors showed that the stimulated tumorigenesis with corn oil (>50% n-6 acid) was blocked by indomethacin although the drug had no effect in rats fed a standard rat diet (Carter et al, 1983). The inhibition of enhanced tumor development by inhibiting the prostaglandin-forming oxygenase as noted above suggests that the oxygenase-catalyzed reaction facilitates tumor growth when diets are rich in n-6 fatty acids. Fig. 11-2 displays some of the detailed data published by Ip et al, 1985 (reviewed by Lands, 1991) which shows that mammary tumor development was proportionately increased by dietary linoleate in the range of 0.5 to 4.4%. Ip (1997) later commented further on how linoleic acid availability enhances tumor growth whereas a suppressive response is observed with n-3 PUFA.

A different aspect of prostaglandin biosynthesis during the spread of tumors is the reported ability of tumor cells to produce compounds derived from n-6 acids that subvert the immune system and allow escape from immune surveillance by the host

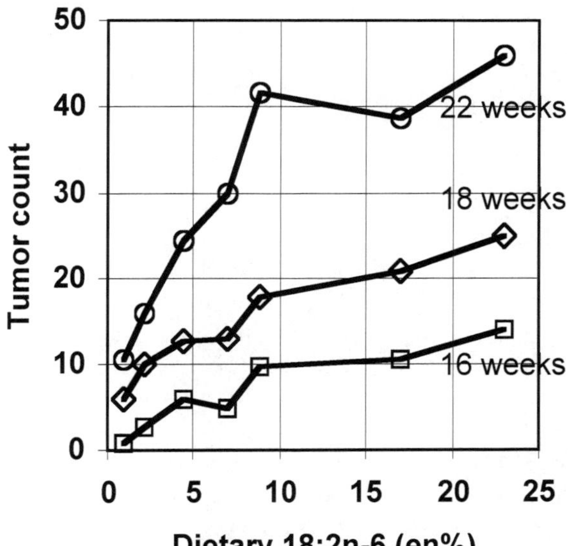

Fig. 11-2. Dietary linoleate enhances tumor growth. Detected tumors increased steadily over the weeks following carcinogen treatment .

(Plescia et al, 1975). In this situation, the tumors may exert an immunosuppressive activity that leads to "tolerance" rather than cytotoxic defense reactions. Much more needs to be done in selecting appropriate animal models and diet regimens to test these hypotheses.

Cross-Country Comparisons

One epidemiological summary of cancer in various countries merits a careful analysis by scientists interested in dietary fats. In a manner very similar to the earlier strong positive correlation of coronary heart disease to the total dietary fat intake, there was a strong positive correlation for the incidence of breast cancer and total dietary fat intake (Carroll et al, 1982). The correlation was also clear for the intake of animal fat, but not very evident for vegetal fat intake (which tends to occur at lower average amounts per day). The types of fatty acids in vegetal fats can vary widely, and the results obtained may reflect varied proportions of n-3 and n-6 acids in the diets. Colon cancer incidence increased since the early 1970s with more than one-third of the cases associated with imbalances in the Western diet (Roynette et al, 2004), and n-3 PUFA may be useful in colon cancer prevention.

The evidence clearly suggests the advisability of keeping the intake of fat at much lower levels than it currently is in "developed" Western nations. No evidence supports the ingestion of 30-40% of calories as fat as being a nutritionally beneficial activity, even though this is the amount typically consumed by Americans. Although Eskimos eat appreciable amounts of meat and fat, the much higher amounts of n-3 fats in the food may moderate the overall impact. Certainly chronic maintenance of intakes of 18:2n-6 at "megadose" levels should be viewed with caution, and efforts to cut also the total dietary fat while supplementing with the 20:5n-3, 22:5n-3, and 22:6n-3 seem desirable and beneficial.

Since 1986, much epidemiologic and experimental evidence indicates that n-3 HUFA in fish oils protect against breast, colon and prostate cancers, likely by inhibiting the production and action of n-6 eicosanoids (Rose and Connolly, 1999). The protection involves decreases in tumor and blood vessel growth and increases in tumor death. Patients whose colonic epithelial cells were proliferating too much had a strong correlation of the n-6/n-3 ratio with the percent of dividing cells (Huang et al, 1996). Also, when patients with stage 1 or stage 2 colon carcinoma or adenomatous polyps consumed 9 g/d n-3 fatty acid capsules for 12 months, polyps were no longer found, indicating that n-3 fatty acids may have a useful chemopreventive action.

Bagga et al (2002) concluded that n-6 EFA may contribute to the high risk of breast cancer in the United States and that n-3 HUFAs derived from fish oils seem protective. Apparently, dietary patterns in the USA give effects of n-6 fats relatively unopposed by dietary n-3 HUFAs, and breast cancer risk is associated with total n-6 EFA intake. In Sweden, a large, nationwide case-control study (709 cases and 2,888 controls) showed consumption of fatty fish was inversely associated with endometrial cancer risk (Terry et al, 2002). The multivariate odds ratio was 0.6 for the highest quartile (median, 2 servings per week) compared to the lowest (median, 0.2 servings per week). In contrast, the corresponding odds ratio was 1.0 for the highest to lowest quartile of lean fish. In a different population-based prospective cohort of 6,272 Swedish men, those who ate no fish had two- to three-fold higher frequency of prostate cancer than did those who ate moderate to high amounts (Terry et al, 2001).

Technical Details

Numerous studies show that greater action of cyclooxygenase-2 (COX-2) in tumor cells gives excess prostaglandins (PGE and PGF) that signal through specific receptors (EP4 and FPb) and enhance cell proliferation (Fujino and Regan, 2003). Ironically, PGE_2 acting through EP4 receptors on macrophages has a potentially beneficial anti-inflammatory action (Takayama et al, 2002). Treatment of colon cancer cells with docosahexaenoic acid (DHA; 22:6n-3) down-regulated the expression of genes for cyclooxygenase 2 and prostaglandin family genes as well as several cell cycle-related genes, whereas it up-regulated caspases 5, 8, 9, and 10 that act in tumor cell destruction (Narayanan et al, 2003). Treatment with DHA also down-regulated iNOS, which forms nitric oxide that activates the cyclooxygenase 2 enzyme, a pivotal mediator in the progression of colon cancer via prostaglandin synthesis and angiogenesis. Human colon carcinoma tissue put into athymic nude mice (Kato et al, 2002) grew more with mice fed n-6-rich corn oil (2,302 mg) than with menhaden oil that has much n-3 HUFA (782 mg) or an algal oil with DHA (223 mg). Dietary omega-3 fatty acids, especially docosahexaenoic acid, have significant tumor suppressing properties.

Feeding fish oil, compared with corn oil, decreases activation and localization on colon cell membranes of the growth promoting oncogene Ras and decreases tumor formation in an experimental rat model (Collett et al, 2001). The major n-3 EFA constituent of fish oil, DHA (22:6n-3), compared with n-6 linoleate (18:2n-6), decreases Ras localization to the plasma membrane and decreases GTP binding to Ras and the downstream p42/44(ERK)-dependent signaling that would support cell proliferation. Tumors induced in laboratory rats had increasingly high levels of COX-2 (but not COX-1) with advancing stages of colon tumorigenesis, which was enhanced by dietary corn oil (an n-6 fat) and decreased by fish oil with its n-3 fats (Singh et al, 1997), correlating with the incidence and multiplicity of grossly visible colon tumors.

A case-control study involving 402 colorectal cancer cases and 668 population-based controls showed a greater risk associated with arachidonic acid (AA) (odds ratio = 2.0) among males and with the n-6/n-3 ratio (odds ratio=1.5; $p = 0.001$) among females (Nkondjock et al, 2003a). Arachidonic acid was linked with up to fivefold greater risk (odds ratio=5.3) among men with high vitamin C intake. A review of published literature concluded that higher concentrations of short-chain fatty acids (SCFAs) and eicosapentaenoic acid (EPA) seem to protect against colorectal cancer, whereas higher medium-chain fatty acids (MCFAs) and arachidonic acid (AA) might be associated with higher risk (Nkondjock et al, 2003b).

A procarcinogenic signaling axis (PKC beta II → COX-2 → TGF-beta) within the colonic epithelium, provides a molecular mechanism by which dietary n-3 fatty acids and nonsteroidal antiinflammatory agents suppress colon carcinogenesis (Yu et al, 2003). The n-3 fatty acid eicosapentaenoic acid (EPA; 20:5n-3) inhibits PKC beta II activity and colon carcinogenesis. PKC beta II promotes colon cancer through induction of Cox-2, suppression of TGF-beta signaling, and establishment of a TGF-beta-resistant hyperproliferative state in the colonic epithelium. In contrast, a selective COX-2 inhibitor restores expression of TGF-beta RII both in vitro and in vivo and restores TGF beta-mediated transcription in RIE/PKC beta II cells.

Eating fish more than three times per week (compared with less than twice per month) was associated with a lower risk of prostate cancer (Augustsson et al, 2003). The strongest association was for metastatic cancer with each additional daily intake of 0.5 g of marine fatty acid from food associated with a 24% lower risk (multivariate relative risk, 0.56). During 12 years of follow-up of the 47,882 men participating in the Health Professionals Follow-up Study, 2,482 cases of prostate cancer were diagnosed (617 advanced including 278 metastatic), and men with high consumption of fish had a lower risk of prostate cancer.

Both DHA and EPA inhibit androgen-stimulated growth of prostate cancer cells (Chung et al, 2001). Also, androgenic induction of prostate-specific antigen (PSA) protein was repressed by DHA and EPA in a dose-dependent manner, and mRNA levels of five androgen up-regulated genes, were also decreased with DHA treatment in the presence of androgens. Interestingly, the proto-oncoprotein c-jun was increased by DHA treatment, and c-jun inhibited androgen receptor transactivation activity. Thus, the inhibition by n-3 polyunsaturated fatty acids of androgen receptor-mediated growth is due, at least in part, to an increase in c-jun protein.

Fatty acids levels in breast adipose tissue suggest a protective effect of n-3 fatty acids on breast cancer risk and support the hypothesis that dietary n-3 fats diminish and n-6 fats enhance breast cancer (Maillard et al, 2002). Women in the upper third of alpha-linolenic acid (18:3 n-3) intake had an odds ratio of 0.39 compared to women in the lowest third. In a similar way, women in the highest third of DHA had an odds ratio of 0.31. Women in the highest third of the long-chain n-3/total n-6 ratio had an odds ratio of 0.33 compared to women in the lowest third.

The n-3 DHA markedly inhibited TPA- and EGF-induced cell transformation by inhibiting AP-1 transactivation. Treatment with the n-3 EPA also inhibited TPA-induced AP-1 transactivation and cell transformation but had no effect on EGF-induced transformation (Liu et al, 2001). Although the n-6 AA had no effect on either, it prevented the inhibitory actions of DHA. The inhibitory effects of n-3 fatty acids on tumorigenesis are more significant for DHA than for EPA and are related to an inhibition of AP-1. Because AA blocks the beneficial effects of DHA, the dietary ratio of n-6 to n-3 fatty acids may be a significant factor in mediating tumor development.

References

Augustsson K, Michaud DS, Rimm EB, et al A prospective study of intake of fish and marine fatty acids and prostate cancer. *Cancer Epidemiol Biomarkers Prev* 12(1):64-67, 2003.

Bagga D, Anders KH, Wang HJ, et al. Long-chain n-3-to-n-6 polyunsaturated fatty acid ratios in breast adipose tissue from women with and without breast cancer. *Nutr Cancer* 42(2): 180-1855, 2002.

Bennet A. Prostaglandins, tumor invasiveness and treatment with inhibitors of prostaglandin synthesis. *Prog Lipid Res* 20:677-679, 1982.

Broitman SA, Vitale JJ, Vavrousek-Jakuba E, et al Polyunsaturated fat, cholesterol and large bowel tumorigenesis. *Cancer* 40:2455-2463, 1977.

Carroll KK, Hopkins GJ, Kennedy TG, et al (1982). Essential fatty acids in relation to mammary carcmogenesis. *Prog Lipid Res* 20:685-690, 1982.

Carter CA, Milholland RJ, Shea W, et al Effect of the prostaglandin synthetase inhibitor indomethacin on 7, 12-dimethylbenz (a) anthracene-induced mammary tumorigenesis in rats fed different levels of fat. *Cancer Res* 43:3559-3562, 1983.

Chung BH, Mitchell SH, Zhang JS, et al Effects of docosahexaenoic acid and eicosapentaenoic acid on androgen-mediated cell growth and gene expression in LNCaP prostate cancer cells. *Carcinogenesis* 22(8):1201-1206, 2001.

Collett ED, Davidson LA, Fan YY, et al n-6 and n-3 polyunsaturated fatty acids differentially modulate oncogenic Ras activation in colonocytes. *Am J Physiol Cell Physiol* 280(5):C1066-1075, 2001.

Fujino H, Regan JW. Prostannoid receptors and phosphatidylinositol 3-kinase: a pathway to cancer? *Trends Pharmacol Sci* 24(7):335-340, 2003.

Honn KV, Cicone B, Skoff, A. Prostacyclin: A potent antimetastatic agent. *Science* 212:1270-1272, 1981.

Honn KV, Busse WD, Sloane BF. (1983). Prostacyclin and thromboxanes: Implications for their role in tumor cell metastasis. *Biochem Pharmacol* 32, 1-11, 1983.

Huang YC, Jessup JM, Forse RA, et al (1996) n-3 fatty acids decrease colonic epithelial cell proliferation in high-risk bowel mucosa. *Lipids* 31(Suppl):S313-S317, 1996.

Ip C, Carter CA, Ip MM. Requirement of essential fatty acid for mammary tumorigenesis in the rat. *Cancer Res* 45(5):1997-2001, 1985.

Ip C. Review of the effects of trans fatty acids, oleic acid, n-3 polyunsaturated fatty acids, and conjugated linoleic acid on mammary carcinogenesis in animals. *Am J Clin Nutr* 66 (6):S1523-S1529, 1997.

Karmali RA, Welt S, Thaler HT, et al Prostaglandins in breast cancer: Relationship to disease stage and hormone status. Br *J Cancer* 48:689-696, 1983.

Kato T, Hancock RL, Mohammadpour H, et al Influence of omega-3 fatty acids on the growth of human colon carcinoma in nude mice. *Cancer Lett* 187(1-2):169-177, 2002.

Kollmorge GM, King MM, Kosanke SD, et al Influence of dietary fat and indomethacin on the growth of transplantable mammary tumors in rats. *Cancer Res* 43:4714-4719, 1983.

Lands WEM. Dose-response Relationships for n-3/n-6 Effects. In Simopoulos A, Kifer R, Martin R, Barlow SE (eds.) *World Review of Nutrition and Diet*. Karger Press, Inc, 1991, pp. 177-194.

Liu G, Bibus DM, Bode AM, et al Omega 3 but not omega 6 fatty acids inhibit AP-1 activity and cell transformation in JB6 cells. Proc *Natl Acad Sci USA* 98(13):7510-7515, 2001.

Maillard V, Bougnoux P, Ferrari P, et al V. N-3 and N-6 fatty acids in breast adipose tissue and relative risk of breast cancer in a case-control study in Tours, France. *Int J Cancer* 98(1):78-83, 2002.

Narayanan BA, Narayanan NK, Simi B, et al. Modulation of inducible nitric oxide synthase and related proinflammatory genes by the omega-3 fatty acid docosahexaenoic acid in human colon cancer cells. *Cancer Res* 63(5):972-979, 2003.

Narisawa T, Sato M, Tani M, et al. Inhibition of development of methylnitrosourea-induced rat colon tumors by indomethacin treatment. *Cancer Res* 41:1954-1957, 1981.

Nkondjock A, Shatenstein B, Maisonneuve P, et al. Assessment of risk associated with specific fatty acids and colorectal cancer among French-Canadians in Montreal: A case-control study. *Int J Epidemiol* 32(2):200-209; discussion 209-210, 2003a.

Nkondjock A, Shatenstein B, Maisonneuve P, et al. Specific fatty acids and human colorectal cancer: an overview. *Cancer Detect Prev* 27(1):55-66, 2003b.

Plescia OJ, Smith AH, Grinwich K. Subversion of immune system by tumor cells and role of prostaglandins. *Proc Natl Acad Sci* 72, 1848-1851, 1975.

Rawls RL. In search to control cancer, understanding metastasis is crucial. *Chem Eng. News* 10-17, 1985.

Rogers AE. Influence of dietary content of lipids and lipotropic nutrients on chemical carcinogenesis in rats. *Cancer Res* 43:2477s-2484s, 1983.

Rose DP, Connolly JM. Omega-3 fatty acids as cancer chemopreventive agents. *Pharmacol Ther* 83(3):217-244, 1999.

Roynette CE, Calder PC, Dupertuis YM, et al. n-3 polyunsaturated fatty acids and colon cancer prevention. *Clin Nutr* 23(2): 139-151, 2004.

Singh J, Hamid R, Reddy BS. Dietary fat and colon cancer: modulation of cyclooxygenase-2 by types and amount of dietary fat during the postinitiation stage of colon carcinogenesis. *Cancer Res* 57(16):3465-3470, 1997.

Takayama K, Garcia-Cardena G, et al. (2002) Prostaglandin E2 suppresses chemokine production in human macrophages through the EP4 receptor. *J Biol Chem* 277(46):44147-44154, 2002.

Terry P, Lichtenstein P, Feychting M, et al. Fatty fish consumption and risk of prostate cancer. *Lancet.* 2001; 357(9270): 1764-1766. Comment. *Lancet* 358(9290):1367, 2001.

Terry P, Wolk A, Vainio H, et al. Fatty fish consumption lowers the risk of endometrial cancer: a nationwide case-control study in Sweden. *Cancer Epidemiol Biomarkers Prev* 11(1):143-145, 2002.

Yu W, Murray NR, Weems C, et al. Role of cyclooxygenase 2 in protein kinase C beta II-mediated colon carcinogenesis. *J Biol Chem* 278(13):11167-11174, 2003.

2005 National Library of Medicine Search Results:

(http://www.ncbi.nlm.nih.gov/entrez/query.fcgi)

cancer = 1,646,486; cancer eicosanoid = 5,942; cancer fish = 6,502; cancer omega-3 = 800

cell cycle = 243,526; cell cycle eicosanoid = 2,935; cell cycle omega-3 = 23

angiogenesis = 21,602; angiogenesis eicosanoid = 311; angiogenesis omega-3 = 13

Part 2—Metabolic Differences Among Polyunsaturated Fatty Acids

Foods move down
Crowded paths
To life
And death.

12—Maps and the Unknown

In ancient days, navigators and pilots who guided expeditions carried maps, sometimes in carefully guarded chests and sometimes memorized and locked in their minds. People who could go out into frightening and unknown places and return safely had mystery and power associated with them. Maps not only could lead the way to a hidden treasure, they were a treasure of information needed by generals and captains who conquered, kings and other rulers and merchants who wanted new routes to new markets.

Maps can also permit an easier understanding of the terrain to be covered and the distance to be traveled when reaching out to another source of food or water or cultural comfort. With a good map we can decide on a rational course of action and prepare more successfully for what lies ahead. This is true when exploring the links between diet and disease. Knowing what imbalanced events must be treated will also help people plan how to prevent such events. Primary prevention of some diseases is a goal of this book.

Because all maps give some structure to what is known, they also give some structure to what is *not* known. It is possible for a map to indicate where something might occur even if it is not possible to be sure exactly what will occur. Maps often can give an overall pattern to things that can eventually be learned in greater detail. Sometimes knowing the general shape of the territory is enough, but if one is planning to live and farm in a particular place, a detailed map of the soil and water conditions could be essential to a wise choice of a new home site.

The following chapters include some maps that show how essential fatty acids can change as they move along their metabolic pathways and form potent hormones. As we trace each acid in its trip along the pathway, we can learn how different results will occur with different polyunsaturated fatty acids that we eat. We need a chance to learn how some of these nutrients relate to what we call health and disease. How can a pound of grain or meat or fish be a factor in stroke, hypertension, diabetes or cancer?

The land on which our parents lived and bore us may be a good place to stay, and no new place is needed, or desired, or perhaps even possible. There is some wisdom and comfort in continuing to live as our parents and grandparents did, even as our curiosity grows about other ways and other lands. The same holds true with our choice of living conditions and diets. While we continue to live and eat in ways that we learned at the tables of our parents and friends, we may not feel a need for detailed maps of this familiar "territory." Somehow, however, new stories come to us about other ways from other cultures and other places, and the wondering begins again: "What if . . . ?"

Pathways Link Diet and Disease

The following chapters contain crude maps prepared from records of the early researchers of polyunsaturated fatty acids. The maps show hazy outlines of the metabolic relationships among some of these acids with the eicosanoids that affect the body's functions. The different effects that dietary fats can have on human health are the consequences of the invisible processes by which dietary fatty acids are metabolized to form important regulatory autacoids. Polyunsaturated acids of the n-3 and n-6 types are formed originally in plants that convert sunlight and CO_2 into materials that support animal life (Fig. 2-2 [Chapter 2]). Animal tissues depend on the sunlight-supported plants for the vitamin-like fats that must be ingested in the diet. Thus a map of the origins of eicosanoids in our tissues includes a trail that wanders from tissue polyunsaturated fatty acids back through the food chain to its origin in the type of plant that formed it. When we know where the trail begins, the map can help us guess better where the trail may end.

Large amounts of 18:2n-6 occur in the oils of seeds and grains of many land-based plants which are major items of attention in agricultural and nutritional research in Midwestern United States. However, the starting point of the n-3 family, 18:3n-3, is more likely associated with the fatty materials in chloroplasts of the green portion of the plants.

The ocean does not have seeds, grains or cereals of the type found in agriculturally developed land plants. Instead, maritime plants (phytoplankton and seaweeds) contain large amounts of the n-3 fatty acids in highly unsaturated forms (see Table 18-8, Chapter 18). In the ocean, the photosynthetically fixed energy and carbon are stored less in the form of the two common precursor acids (18:2n-6 and 18:3n-3) than in the more highly unsaturated fatty acids (HUFA) of the n-3 type. In this way, plants of the ocean provide to their corresponding animal food chains a pattern of long-chain HUFA rich in the n-3 type. The two different food chains from oceans and continents deliver very different materials to human diets. This difference in foods leads to differences in the body's behavior.

The aim of Chapters 13-16 is to describe the flow of fatty acid material through the many biochemical processes that occur between dietary intake and eicosanoid action. Biochemists have partially described and mapped these routes to show how one compound can be formed from another. From these maps, we can begin a rational evaluation of how the composition of dietary fat alters the availability of arachidonate for formation of n-6 eicosanoids. We now know enough biochemistry to predict some of the complex interactions of the various fatty acids. The information in the following chapters was selected to show how dietary n-3 acids affect the conversion of the dietary n-6 acids to n-6 eicosanoids.

Biochemists generally regard eicosanoids to be formed from nonesterified HUFA that exists momentarily in a "pool" of nonesterified fatty acids (see Fig. 12-1). This pool of raw material is being used continually for various reactions to make cellular components, and it is being continually replaced by the hydrolysis of cell storage components and by the intake of dietary fats. The material in this pool available for eicosanoid formation (and for antagonizing eicosanoid formation) has a transient existence that depends on material flowing in and out along the various pathways involved.

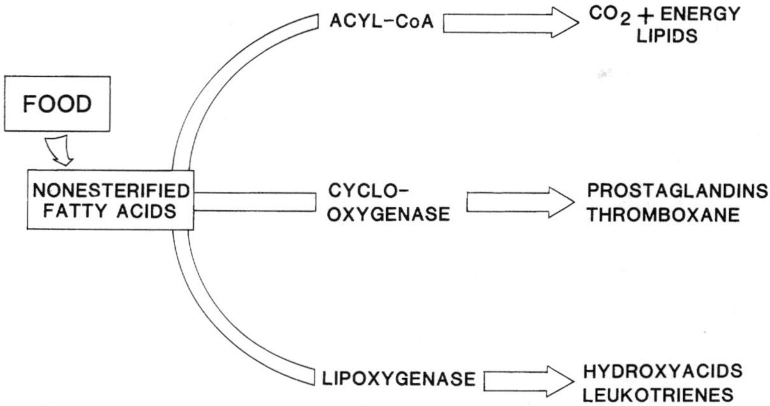

Fig.12-1. HUFA paths.

Animals ingest both n-3 and n-6 types of polyunsaturated acid in the form of fat (triacylglycerols and phospholipids). During digestion, absorption, and transport, the fatty acids are handled as combined esterified forms and as free nonesterified forms. They go into the cells of a tissue mostly as the nonesterified form. From this point, three separate metabolic fates of the nonesterified acid can be described: the acyl-CoA pathways, the cyclooxygenase pathways, and the lipoxygenase pathways.

The degree to which a given fatty acid moves through these three general sets of metabolic processes (Fig. 12-1) depends on the amount of each enzyme in the cell or tissue being studied, the availability of cofactors for the enzymes, the specificity of each enzyme for the individual fatty acids, and the relative abundance of the acid accessible to the enzymes. All four of these factors have important roles in regulating the fate of a dietary polyunsaturated fatty acid in each cell (Fig. 12-2).

The acyl-CoA pathways predominantly regulate the oxidation of fatty acid to CO_2 which provides energy and the cellular lipids that store fatty acids. The cyclooxygenase pathway provides prostaglandins, thromboxanes, and prostacyclin, whereas the lipoxygenase pathway provides leukotrienes and hydroxy fatty acids. Competition among the different fatty acids for the enzymes in these three pathways may provide the underlying basis for the different effects of these acids on the disease mechanisms noted in earlier chapters.

High Rates Driven by Overabundance

The speed and intensity of movement or interaction along the pathways in maps is seldom shown, but is a very important aspect of molecular collisions underlying all of metabolism. Moderate actions of autacoids give reversible healthy responses to stimuli, whereas overly intense actions can create irreversible harm. A large influx of food speeds the movement of acyl-CoA into fat and lipoproteins that circulate in the

- Enzyme Activity
- Enzyme Cofactors
- Enzyme Specificity For Fatty Acids
- Acid Abundance

Fig. 12-2. Factors regulating the speed of each pathway.

blood where the fat (called triglycerides) continues to give more nonesterified fatty acids to tissues than they can oxidize completely in a few hours (see Fig. 12-3).

Expanding on the broad concepts in known maps of metabolism (Figs. 12-1, 13-1, and 13-2 [Chapter 13]) and combining them with some details about inflammation (Fig.5-4 [Chapter 5]) led to a newer overview map discussed at the Third International Conference on Nutrition in Cardio-cerebrovascular Diseases in Japan (now modified as Fig.12-3). The two nutrient imbalances in the upper left of Fig.12-3 are readily modified targets for population-wide primary prevention. Both remain major points for correction in the U.S. diet at the time of this writing.

These could be reduced by more focused primary prevention efforts. This figure was discussed further as 5-3 (Chapter 5).

Excess food energy leads to higher plasma triglycerides and nonesterified fatty acids. It also increases formation of HMG-CoA, mevalonate and prenylated proteins

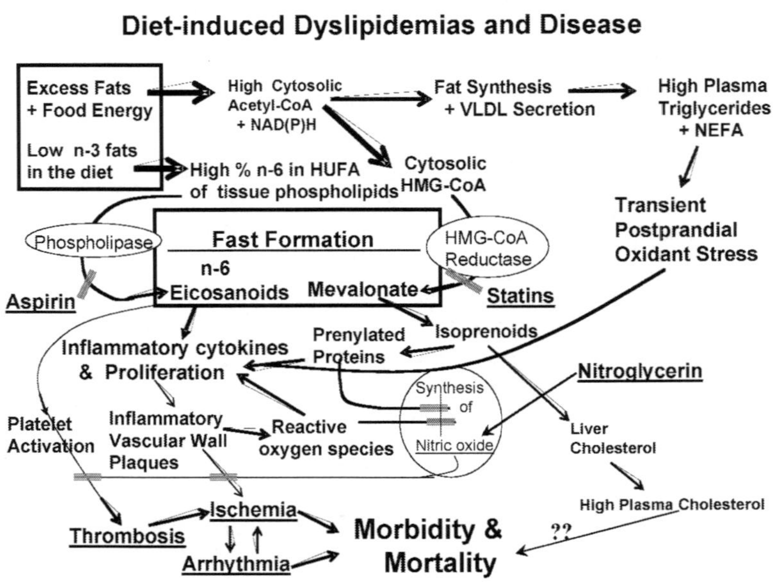

Fig. 12-3. Two chronic dietary imbalances cause serious dyslipidemias and health problems.

in cells. High postprandial transient energy imbalances with their inflammatory tendencies can combine with imbalanced tissue proportions of highly active n-6 (compared to n-3) eicosanoid precursors. When this occurs, tissues can develop amplified immune inflammatory and proliferative events, a condition often seen in U.S. geriatric patients with chronic disease.

The previous 11 chapters noted many diseases with excessive signaling by n-6 eicosanoids. The following chapters discuss how quantitative differences among the competing n-3 and n-6 fatty acids moving along metabolic pathways create such a high proportion of n-6 HUFA in the HUFA of tissues of Americans. Storage and release of HUFA from the 2-position of tissue phospholipids are pivotal steps in the overall diet-disease relationship.

Chapter 13 details how dietary fatty acids and their cellular acyl-CoA intermediates move to and from the tissue reservoirs of precursors for the important autacoids, prostaglandins and leukotrienes. The process of forming these autacoids from tissue HUFA is discussed in chapters 14, 15 and 16. The structures and the maps in those chapters will help readers see more clearly the functional link between EFA in the diet and the disease mechanisms described in the earlier chapters.

The composition of HUFA in tissues fits an empirical quantitative metabolic diet-tissue relationship developed after 1986, with support from the Pfizer Biomedical Research Award. Converting the pathways in the maps into quantitative terms (Chapter 17) now predicts and interprets how deliberate voluntary food choices can provide the EFA nutrients (Chapter 18) that create likely proportions of n-6 HUFA in tissue HUFA at whatever level desired for acceptable risk levels (Fig. 1-3 [Chapter 1]). Values from 15 to 90% n-6 HUFA in tissue HUFA are possible with simple food choices (Chapter 19). People already near the high end of this range (Figs. 1-3 [Chapter 1] and 6-4 [Chapter 6]) may wish to change to a lower value. Each person can easily identify the proportions of tissue HUFA and the risk level that they wish to maintain. Moving toward the left by eating less n-6 and more n-3 fats would be preferred by people averse to risk.

13—Acyl-CoA Pathways

Competition Among Acyl-CoA Actions

The acyl-CoA pathways are initiated by an enzyme that catalyzes the reaction that combines free fatty acid with coenzyme A (CoA) to give an acyl-CoA ester (Fig. 13-1). This reaction proceeds rapidly even with small amounts of nonesterified fatty acid so that it keeps the amount of nonesterified acid very low in healthy tissues. The fatty acid in the acyl-CoA form is the starting point for many metabolic conversions (Fig. 13-1). It may be transferred to an intermediate acylcarnitine that is transported to the part of the cell where it undergoes oxidation to CO_2 with the generation of cellular energy, very similar to the way that burning coal in a locomotive can be transformed into work. The oxidation provides energy that allows humans to move heavy objects, plow fields, and build cities. Throughout our history, human labor has been fueled by this sort of oxidative energy, and the high calorie intake of laborers doing heavy work has been aided by the rich caloric content of fats. So long as a high expenditure of energy balanced the dietary intake, the dietary fat was "burned" and did not accumulate.

We may increase the intensity of forming n-6 eicosanoids, by increasing the proportion of arachidonate in the small pool of nonesterified acids (see Figs. 2-2 [Chapter 2], 14-1 [Chapter 14], and 16-1 [Chapter 16]). Megadoses of linoleate were once proposed to partially displace arachidonate from this pool and interfere with eicosanoid formation. When there are not many other fatty acids competing for the acyl-CoA and acylcarnitine pathways, arachidonate is also oxidized to CO_2.

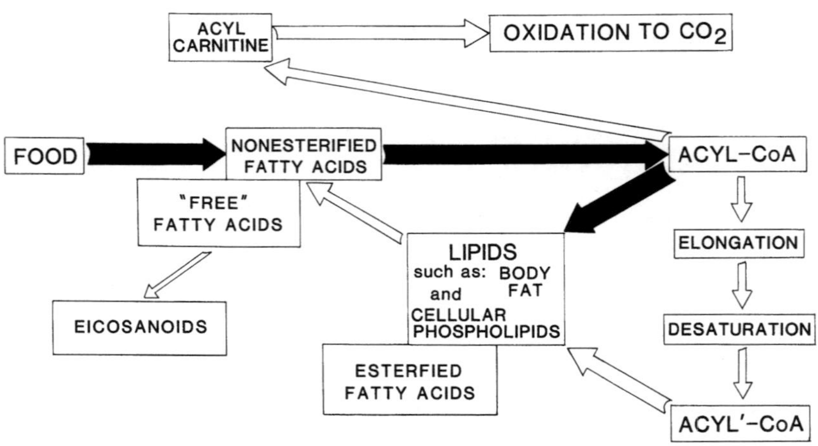

Fig. 13-1. Paths for acyl-CoA derivatives.

High fat diets might make this oxidation less likely and allow arachidonate to move more to other paths.

An important feature of the oxidation process in our tissues is that it operates in close connection with energy expenditure. If we do not expend the energy, the fatty acid is not oxidized. When the oxidation path is not available, the fatty acid of the acyl-CoA transfers to the storage form of the lipid that we call fat. I remember the huge meals we ate as farmhands at harvest time when the work was intense. If I ate such meals now, they would lead to a rapid accumulation of fat and a likely increased risk of bad health (Fig. 12-3 [Chapter 12]). Of course, increased physical labor could move the fatty acid from storage lipids (via nonesterified fatty acids) to form acyl-CoA and acylcarnitine and produce energy by oxidation to CO_2. Each of us must examine his/her choices of energy intake and expenditure to avoid undesired imbalances noted in Fig 12-3 (Chapter 12).

Transient Overabundances

When we eat large meals, the overall balance between energy intake and expenditure causes our tissues to convert the food not burned at the moment to fat and cholesterol. The food fragments (as acetyl-CoA) that would have been oxidized for energy if we needed it are accumulated and recombined by other complex reaction sequences into saturated fatty acids (see Fig. 13-2) and cholesterol.

Although our tissues have ways to control the conversion of food to cholesterol, the unfortunate consequence of overeating can be an overproduction of fat and cholesterol in the blood stream. Both contribute to a higher risk of heart disease and

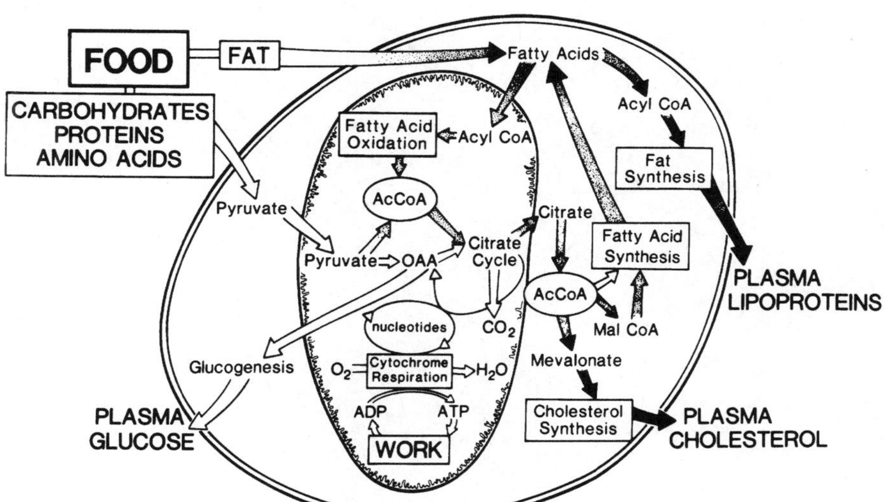

FIG 13-2. Conversion of food to CO_2, fat and cholesterol.

heart attacks. Metabolic maps show us how excess food materials can move from one form to another, claryifying how they cause an effect. The map in Fig. 13-2 reinforces the general advice to exercise caution on the fatty content and total daily calories of food eaten. Some nutritionists advise that the U.S. diet is "ideal," and that 40% calories as fat will be hard to change. However, good health maintained by diets with as little as 10% calories as fat (e.g., the Pritikin diet) indicates that palatable diets can be successfully maintained by motivated individuals.

Rather than forming acylcarnitine, the acyl-CoA may also react with a wide variety of acyltransferases to synthesize lipid esters, some of which function in membranes while others appear to be a storage form, such as fat. Alternatively, the enzymes catalyzing elongation and desaturation (see Figs. 13-1, 13-3) may take the acyl-CoA along paths that provide longer or more highly unsaturated acyl-CoA esters which, in turn, can be also esterified into lipid.

Controlled, quantitative evidence for enzyme selectivity among the various possible reactions of the acyl-CoA esters is very limited. Evidence available at this time suggests that the intermediates in the elongation and desaturation reactions tend to be present in extremely small amounts. Our current understanding of the complex pathways is attributed to the perseverance and ingenuity of investigators such as Rodolfo Brenner and Howard Sprecher who, with their colleagues, extended the pioneering work of Jim Mead and Ralph Holman.

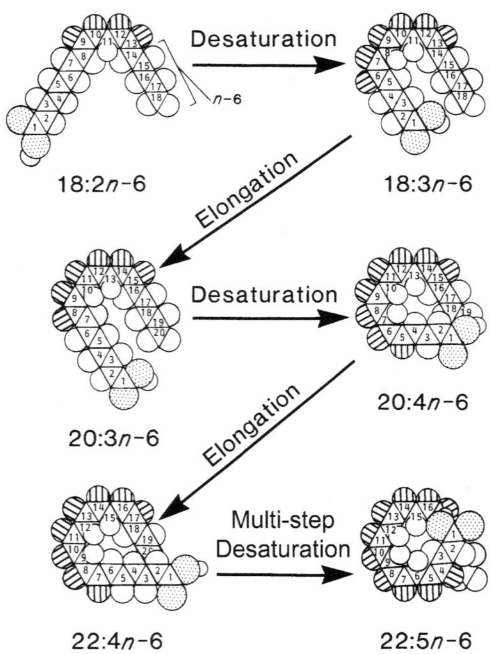

Fig. 13-3. Desaturation and elongation of dietary 18:2n-6.

Four different families of polyunsaturated fatty acid participate in desaturation and elongation reactions in vertebrate tissues (Fig. 13-4). The various members of the four families of unsaturatedfatty acids (n-3, n-6, n-7, and n-9) do not occur in equal amounts, and some are more common than others. Our tissues form 16:0 and 18:0 from the food fragment, acetyl-CoA (AcCoA in Fig.13-2), and a desaturase enzyme converts them to the starting forms of the n-7 and n-9 type of fatty acid (see Fig. 13-5). The starting materials for the n-3 and n-6 acids in humans come from plants. Complex competitions occur among all four types of unsaturated fatty acids as they are handled by the desaturation and elongation enzymes of our tissues. More information on regulating desaturase actions at the 9, 6, 5, and 4 positions of acyl-CoAs is needed before we can predict in detail what to expect from our daily food intake.

Consequences of Competition

Competition occurs when metabolizing nutrient polyunsaturated fatty acids, and increasing the amount of one type can decrease the amount of elongated forms of another. Thus, increasing an n-3 acid, 18:3n-3, caused less 20:4n-6 to be accumulated from dietary 18:2n-6 (Mohrhauer and Holman, 1963a) and increasing 18:2n-6 caused

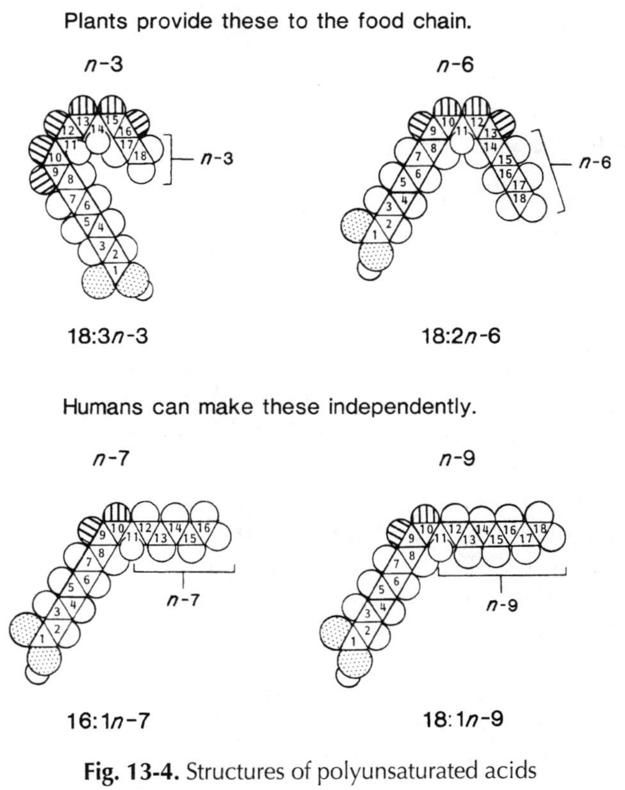

Fig. 13-4. Structures of polyunsaturated acids

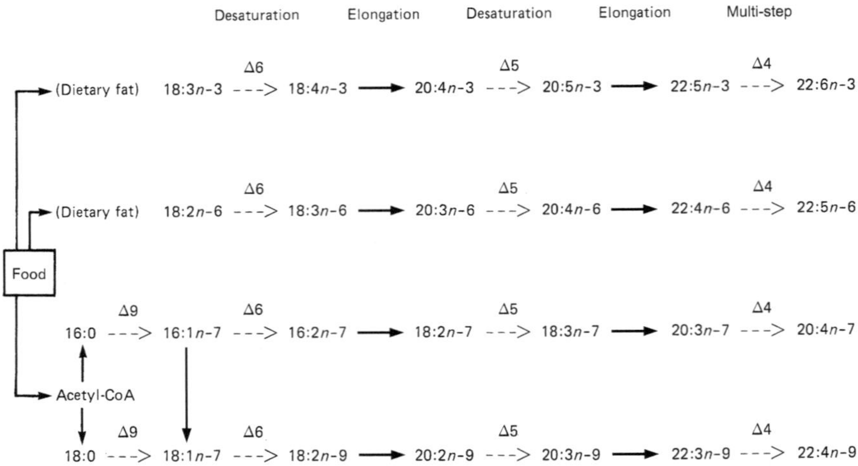

Fig. 13-5. Four families of unsaturated fatty acids. Sequential desaturation and elongation reactions are indicated with bold arrows for elongation reactions and dashed arrows for desaturation reactions catalyzed by the Δ9-, Δ6- and Δ5-desaturase enzymes as indicated. The multistep desaturation that produces Δ4 derivatives is described in the text.

less n-3 HUFA to be accumulated from dietary 18:3n-3 (Rahm and Holman, 1964).

Such metabolic shifts may be due to competition among the structurally similar unsaturated acyl-CoA esters as they compete for the same enzyme site and as they change the induced levels of desaturation/elongation enzymes. In 1963, Mohrhauer and Holman provided a unique series of papers that extensively illustrated dose-dependent effects of EFA interacting with each other as they accumulated in liver (1963a, b), brain (1963c) red blood cells and adipose fat (1963d).

An example of the way that tissue fatty acids can suppress the conversion of a dietary fatty acid to its longer chain derivatives was described by Sanders and Younger (1981). Feeding linseed (flaxseed) oil (containing much 18:3n-3) to people who were ingesting only 1 en% 18:2n-6 led to a significant rise in eicosapentaenoic acid (20:5n-3), although there was no significant rise in docosahexaenoic acid (22:6n-3). In contrast, feeding the same flaxseed oil to people already ingesting appreciable amounts of linoleic acid (18:2n-6) in their diets did not give significant increases in the long chain unsaturated forms 20:5n-3 and 22:6n-3 formed from 18:3n-3.

Competitions during elongation and desaturation processes of 18-carbon acids are circumvented when 20:5n-3 and 22:6n-3 are fed. In this situation, the amounts of both HUFA circulating in the esterified form were increased. When eicosapentaenoic acid was administered to a tissue, most of it was rapidly esterified directly into glycerolipids without change. Only 8% of the material was esterified after forming an elongation product, and only 4% was a desaturation product (Bazan et al., 1982).

These results illustrate a greater tendency for 20:5n-3 to esterify to cellular phospholipids than to move along the steps of elongation and desaturation. More research can determine whether the apparent suppression of certain elongation/desaturation reactions occurs at the level of induced enzyme formation or at competitions among closely related CoA thiolesters. The data provided at the time of this writing are inconclusive.

In adults who maintain healthy weight and physical activity, the usual fate of all food is to be burned (oxidized) to release energy (calories), water (H_20) and carbon dioxide (CO_2). However, each large meal has food that is in excess of immediately needed energy. As a result, the food gives excess acetyl-CoA that is not burned but diverted to form additional fatty acids (stored as fat) and mevalonate-based products (farnesol, geranylgeraniol and cholesterol derivatives) as mapped in Fig. 13-2 (and 12-3 in Chapter 12).

The diverted unburned products, like cholesterol and plasma triglycerides, can be biomarkers of excessive intake of food and saturated fat, and some may be mediators by which food imbalances cause disease and death. When dietary EFA are not burned for energy, they move as acyl-CoA esters along pathways that esterify them into fats and cellular phospholipids as well as pathways of elongation and desaturation (Figs. 13-3, 13-5) forming the 20- and 22-carbon *highly unsaturated fatty acids* (HUFA). The HUFA accumulated in tissue lipids can come only from EFA in the diet, and they serve as biomarkers of EFA intake (Lands, 1995). Because some tissue HUFA act in autacoid-mediated diseases, the acyl-CoA pathways maintaining HUFA in tissue lipids are important.

Many metabolic steps along acyl-CoA pathways are catalyzed by enzymes that discriminate little between n-3 and n-6 types of acid, letting the acids compete against each other in proportion to their abundance. This enzyme promiscuity lets the daily supply of EFA in foods have a strong influence on the resultant composition of tissue HUFA.

The high proportions of n-6 HUFA, reported for tissue HUFA of laboratory animals and many Americans, reflect a high proportion of n-6 EFA in the dietary supply rather than an indication of any inherent mammalian enzyme selectivity favoring n-6 acids. Neither the acyltransferases putting HUFA at the 2 position of phospholipids nor the phospholipases releasing HUFA from the 2-position discriminate much between n-3 and n-6 structures (although some HUFA seem preferred over acids with less unsaturation).

For example, the cytosolic 85-kilodalton phospholipase A2 (85 kDa PLA_2; $cPLA_2$), which is believed to initiate formation of eicosanoids by hydrolyzing membrane phospholipids, has a preference for more unsaturated acids 20:4>20:3>20:2>20:1>20:0 and 20:4>18:3>18:2>18:1>16:1 (Hanel, 1993). However, this $cPLA_2$ released the n-3 and n-6 20-carbon eicosanoid precursors (20:4n-6 and 20:5n-3) similarly, although the release of 22:6n-3 with its double bond at carbon 4 was much slower (Shikano, 1994).

This selectivity contrasts to action of the secretory14 kDa PLA_2 ($sPLA_2$) that hydrolyzed all three HUFA at similar rates. The lack of selectivity between n-3 and n-6 HUFA by the 85 kDa phospholipase in platelets (Weaver and Holub, 1986) causes platelet membranes with a lower proportion of n-6 HUFA in the HUFA to release a lower proportion of the n-6 precursor of thromboxane and thereby provide a lower aggregation response.

New Insights on Desaturase Processes

During elongation and desaturation (see Figs. 13-3, 13-5), the intermediate acyl-CoA esters are present only in very small amounts and are difficult to analyze. As a result, the selectivity at each intermediate step is not known. However, the accumulated lipid esters give clues to possible selectivity at individual steps in desaturation, elongation and esterification. Since 1986, much evidence indicates that the process of inserting a double bond at position 4 of the acyl-CoA chain (see Fig.13-5) is not catalyzed by a distinct "delta-4 desaturase", but involves a coordinated set of multienzyme steps with movement of a 24-carbon acyl-CoA between anabolic enzymes in microsomes and catabolic enzymes in peroxisomes (Luthria, 1996; Sprecher, 2000).

Sprecher summarized (Sprecher, 2002) the metabolic selectivities that regulate accumulation of 22:6n-3 and 22:5n-6 (with their first double bond at position 4) from 24-carbon precursors (with their first double bond at position 6). The slow rate of microsomal acyltransferase action with the very long 24-carbon acyl-CoA esters allows these intermediates to accumulate and move to peroxisomes where oxidation shortens the chains to give a delta-4 structure. Then, slow oxidation of delta-4 derivatives allows these accumulated intermediates to move back to microsomes where the 22-carbon form is esterified into phospholipids by acyltransferases. Complex interactions of this type seem to act during the impaired accumulation of 22-carbon HUFA in tissue lipids of patients with X-linked retinitis pigmentosa (Hoffman, 2001).

At this time, we still do not know the number of enzymes that selectively bind the n-3 or n-6 structure. An abundance of n-6 arachidonate and n-3 docosahexaenoate in tissue HUFA creates the appearance of a preference for the n-3 type of substrate in the overall multistep delta 4 desaturation process, but the exact discriminating catalyst in this process is still not known. As in many cases in lipid metabolism, isolation and characterization of the different individual enzymes will be needed to know how much selectivity occurs at each step.

Two types of desaturase activities in plants allow them to make their own n-6 and n-3 structures that animals must eat in their food. Considering the physiological consequences of the balance between these two types of fatty acid essential for vertebrates, the origins of n-3 acids gain importance. Although plants have several enzymes that place a double bond at the n-3 position, the substrates are glycerolipids rather than acyl-CoA esters.

However, screening the DNA database of the worm, *Caenorhabditis elegans*, produced one n-3 desaturase, fat-1, that was cloned and expressed in a plant causing a 90% increase in the proportion of alpha-linolenic acid,18:3n-3 (Spychalla, 1997).

The worm appears to have all of the desaturase and elongase enzymes to synthesize arachidonate and eicosapentaenoate from simple precursors (Watts and Browse, 2002; Napier and Michelson, 2001).

Transfer of the fat-1 gene reduced the n-6/n-3 ratio and reduced production of n-6 eicosanoids in cardiac myocytes (Kang et al, 2001), rat cortical neurons (Ge, Wang et al, 2002) and human breast cancer cells (Ge, Chen et al, 2002). Interest in inserting the gene into vertebrate tissues led Kang and his colleagues to breed several generations of genetically modified mice that maintain nearly equal amounts of n-3 and n-6 HUFA while eating diets that gave predominantly n-6 HUFA in wild-type mice (Kang et al, 2004).

Dietary adjustments already have allowed rats and mice to produce tissue HUFA with twice the amount of n-3 HUFA compared to n-6 HUFA. Studies of transgenic mice eating such n-3-rich diets may give 10-fold greater proportions of n-3 to n-6 in tissue HUFA and show unique physiology. Ways to introduce expression of such n-3 desaturase activities in genetically modified domestic plants and animals may decrease the large difference between foods supplied from the oceans and foods from the farms. Such steps might provide more n-3- fortified foods for human consumption and reverse the current imbalance in our foods and tissues.

Biomarkers of EFA Availability

Competitive metabolic interactions of n-3, n-6, n-7, and n-9 acids cause different proportions of HUFA to accumulate in tissue phospholipids. Dietary n-3 or n-6 EFA readily displace the n-7 and n-9 HUFA that are made within the body. A useful biomarker for relative intakes of n-3 and n-6 EFA is the proportion of HUFA that is n-6 HUFA (Lands, 1995). That proportion is high in U.S. adults (see Fig.1-3 [Chapter 1]), who eat linoleate-rich foods and carry much more than adequate amounts (2 to 3 kilograms) of 18:2n-6 in their body fat.

However, n-6 supplies may be less in tissues of patients who cannot digest food efficiently and require total parenteral nutrition. In that case, low supplies of either n-3 or n-6 EFA allow the n-9 HUFA, 20:3n-9, to be a higher proportion of tissue HUFA (similar to the competitive relationship shown in Fig. 3-2). The 20:3n-9/20:4n-6 ratio increased during a continuous supply of high glucose fat-free diets as the "feast of glucose calories led to a famine of linoleate" (Wene et al, 1975). Intermittent feeding lets circulating glucose and insulin levels decrease to normal, which then allows mobilization of the still abundant adipose tissue stores of 18:2n-6. Relatively small amounts of circulating EFA are actually needed to keep 20:3n-9 from accumulating in tissue lipids.

The small amount of dietary EFA needed by humans is evident when comparing clinical signs with biomarker levels. The clinical sign (dry scaly rash) of EFA deficiency appeared only after a month of the arachidonate (20:4n-6) in phospholipid being equal to or less than 20:3n-9 (i.e., 20:3n-9/20:4n-6 ratios >1; Collins, 1971). A related report (O'Neill, 1977) also noted that dermatitis appeared only after 20:3n-9 was almost equal to 20:4n-6 for prolonged periods and disappeared after EFA supplementation returned 20:3n-9/20:4n-6 ratios to values below 0.4.

Another parenteral feeding report in 1978 (prior to EFA supplementation) found similar biomarker results when low dietary n-6 supply competed against internal n-9 oleate during elongation/desaturation/ acylation, and only 2 of 32 patients developed physiological symptoms of EFA deficiency (Goodgame, 1978). Confirming this relationship, Mascioli et al (1996) saw that patients on home parenteral nutrition had 20:3n-9/20:4n-6 ratios ranging from 0.06 to 0.64, and none showed clinical signs or symptoms of linoleate deficiency.

Subsequent parenteral nutrition that provided n-6 acids decreased this biochemical marker to less than 0.2. Similarly, detailed results with home parenteral nutrition patients (Jeppeson, 2000) closely paralleled results with rats by Mohrhauer and Holman (1963b), with progressively lower availability of linoleate associated with progressively greater amounts of 20:3n-9 accumulating in phospholipids. In all these patients, the ratio of 20:3n-9/20:4n-6 did not rise above 1, and physiological signs of deficiency were not apparent. Only prolonged proportions of n-9 to n-6 HUFA above 1 in tissue lipids seem to indicate a physiological insufficiency.

Clearly, biomarker values below 1 for 20:3n-9/20:4n-6 indicate adequate EFA intake, and the biomedical community accepts conservative ratios below 0.4 as a surrogate marker for the absence of EFA deficiency. However, the values less than 0.02 commonly seen for many people in the USA reflect a monopolizing of metabolic systems by high amounts of linoleate (18:2n-6) in the diet. Such high linoleate intakes seem more than adequate for good health (see Chapter 3). In fact, the high incidence of diseases with excessive n-6 eicosanoid actions noted in earlier chapters combines with the very low values for the biomarker of 20:3n-9/20:4n-6 to prompt questions about the healthiness of such high linoleate intakes.

Technical Details

Changes in Tissue Acids After Diet Changes

Holman (1964) and Mead (1971) summarized the evidence of the antagonism among the various polyunsaturated fatty acids in terms of competition among their acyl-CoA intermediates for the desaturation and elongation enzymes (Fig. 13-5), The competition among the many different enzymes for an acyl-CoA has made it extremely difficult for researchers to do specific metabolic studies with intact tissues or their homogenates. Also, an acyl-CoA acyl hydrolase can convert the thiolester intermediate back to the nonesterified acid, making it experimentally difficult to detect significant amounts of the acyl-CoA intermediates in cell-free preparations.

Without direct measurements, workers have used indirect techniques to estimate the paths followed by each fatty acid. Analyses of the total fatty acid content in rat liver showed that increasing dietary amount of linolenate decreased the accumulation of 22:5n-6 appreciably when 1 energy percent (en%) 20:4n-6 was fed (as noted by the size of the up arrow in the upper panel of Fig. 13-6). Little competitive effect, however, was seen in the amount of 22:4n-6 accumulated or in the amount of the other nutrient acid (20:4n-6) esterified in the liver lipids. Thus, competition by 18:3n-3

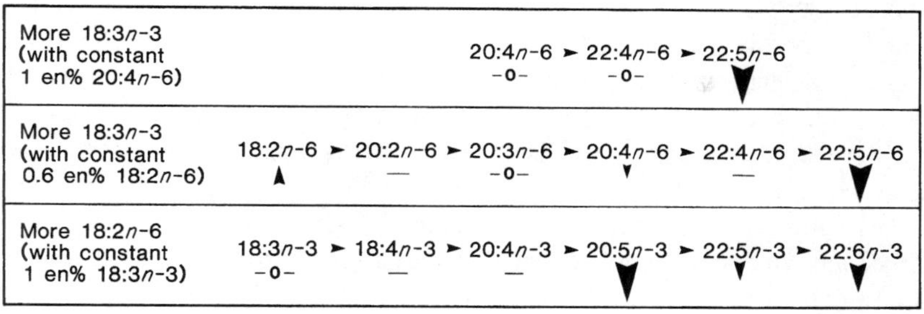

Fig. 13-6. Effects of dietary changes on polyunsaturated fatty acids accumulated in rat liver.

seemed to affect desaturation more than it did elongation or direct esterification. Similarly, the arrows in the second panel show that 18:3n-3 greatly decreased accumulation of 22:5n-6 derived from 0.6 en% dietary 18:2n-6. In this case, however, it had little effect on the amount of esterified 20:3n-6, and actually increased the accumulation of the other nutrient acid (18:2n-6) that accumulated unmodified in liver lipids. When 1 en% 18:3n-3 was antagonized by increasing amounts of 18:2n-6 (lower panel of Fig.13-6), the liver content of 20:5n-3, 22:5n-3, and 22:6n-3 were all decreased while the amount of esterified 18:3n-3 remained unchanged.

These intricate shifts in composition of the liver lipids have parallel, but not identical, counterparts in other tissues. The changes in composition reflect selectivities of the esterifying enzymes as well as of the desaturating and elongating enzymes. It is difficult to characterize all the different processes competing for the small pool of intermediate acyl-CoA esters. When changes in diet shift the relative amounts of the intermediates, the possible numbers of consequences for the acyl-CoAs are too many for interpretations to be more than of limited credibility.

Pioneers in HUFA Metabolism

Each generation of researchers adds stronger insight into the complex metabolic interactions of EFA. Just as Brenner and Sprecher followed Holman and Mead in adding metabolic insights to the pioneering work of Ernst Klenk on the chemical structures of EFA, new methods of studying genetic expression of the enzymes involved now come from Clarke, Jump and Ntambe. This technical section introduces some of those authors and some technical terms describing new measurements of gene expression that complement the earlier studies of HUFA metabolism. Together, the new information helps interpret the impact of diet choices on tissue eicosanoid responses. Further searches in PubMed of terms in the new information will allow readers to update their knowledge as more new reports appear.

Competition among the CoA esters for the 6 desaturase was regarded (Mead, 1971) to favor the n-3 over the n-6 acids (with both types favored over the n-9 acids). Mead (1971) suggested that linolenate (18:3n-3) had about a tenfold greater affinity for the elongation—desaturation system than did linoleate (18:2n-6) which had threefold greater affinity than oleate (18:1n-9). This generalization must be modified with the added concept that the apparent affinity is related to the ratio of unsaturation to chain length. Mead (1971) suggested that the affinity increased with monoenes < dienes < trienes and seemed less for C20 and C22 acids. In this way, he suggested that further elongation and desaturation of the intermediates 18:4n-3, 18:3n-6, and 20:3n-6 might not be prevented by accumulated 20:4, 20:5 and 22:6.

Induction and suppression of enzyme activity represents an alternative concept to direct competitive action by polyunsaturated fatty acids. Brenner (1974) and Brenner et al. (1982) summarized several studies that showed alterations of 6-desaturase activity in response to altered carbohydrate or protein intake and to hormonal influences. Diabetic rats have low activity of 6-desaturase, and added insulin can increase the activity.

Brenner suggested that these changes may be related to a circadian rhythm in hepatic 6-desaturase activity (Actis-Dato et al., 1972). Since dibutyryl-cAMP decreases the 6-desaturase activity in liver microsomes (de Gomez-Dumm et al., 1976), the activity seems regulated by posttranslational kinase modifications. Diet changes can also influence the 5-desaturase activity, and Brenner proposed that this enzyme may be activated only when enough substrate is available to affect the induction.

Placing animals on a diet deficient in essential fatty acids evoked an apparent decrease of the 5-desaturase activity after 4 days and an increase of 6-desaturase on the 11th day (Brenner et al., 1982), Adding linoleate (18:2n-6) or arachidonate (20:4n-6) to a fat-free diet caused a rapid decrease of 6-desaturase activity that was still significant 12 hours after administering 18:2n-6 and 48 hours after 20:4n-6 (Brenner, 1982).

Recognizing Acyltransferase Influences

When Brenner and his colleagues attempted to examine directly the competitions among acyl-CoA esters for the desaturation reaction, they found that many of the thiol esters were so rapidly transferred to phospholipid that the desaturation results were seriously affected and hard to interpret precisely. For example, added arachidonate (20:4n-6) or eicosapentaenoate (20:5n-3) actually enhanced rather than antagonized the action of the 6 desaturase on linoleic acid (18:2n-6) (Brenner and Peluffo, 1966). The apparent activation disappeared when lysolecithin was added (Nervi et al 1968), indicating that the arachidonate spared linoleate by competition between their acyl-CoA intermediates for lipid synthesis and thereby increased the availability of linoleoyl CoA for desaturation (see Fig. 13-3). This competitive "sparing" could not occur when the extra added acceptor allowed all the available acyl-CoA to move quickly to lipid synthesis rather than desaturation.

More than 40 years ago, an uneven entry of added lipid precursors into different glycerolipids indicated that fatty acid was incorporated into phospholipids by both a deacylation/acylation pathway (Lands, 1960) and the phosphatidic acid de novo pathway (Kennedy, 1962). This opened new acyltransferase pathways for producing the various patterns of fatty acid distribution which occur in different cellular lipids. Early studies of fatty acid selectivities for lipid biosynthesis indicated that long-chain HUFA (especially 20:4n-6) tend to incorporate at the 2 position of phospholipids by the reacylation pathway, whereas 18:1n-9 and 18:2n-6 are extensively incorporated by the de novo pathway (for review, see Lands and Crawford, 1976).

De Schrijver and Privett (1982) reported that adding fish (menhaden) oil to diets depressed the 6- and 9-desaturase activities, causing a depressed level of synthesis of the long-chain members of the linoleate family: 20:4n-6, 22:4n-6, and 22:5n-6. This effect was associated with an apparently preferential accumulation of dietary 20:5n-3 and 22:6n-3 in the liver microsomes. The authors hypothesized that dietary 20:5n-3 and 22:6n-3 increased the "minimum requirement" for linoleic acid in the diet.

Unfortunately, the definition of minimum requirement has not been rigorously dealt with in the past or reexamined in light of our current understanding of eicosanoid biochemistry. An example of the difficulty in describing minimum requirements is illustrated by the studies of Galli et al. (1981) in which a diet with 11 en% linoleic acid gave high levels of linoleic acid and low levels of arachidonate in platelet phospholipids. This decreased level of arachidonic acid in certain cellular lipids seemed to depress platelet cyclooxygenase activity and impair platelet function.

Pooviah et al. (1976) concluded that dietary supplements of n-6 acids reduced the activity of 5-desaturase whereas n-3 acids reduced the activity of the elongation enzymes. Kurata and Privett (1980) noted that the 6-desaturase activity in rats was lowest in the liver microsomal fraction from animals that were fed a mixture of corn oil and fish (menhaden) oil. The desaturase activity was regarded to be suppressed by the high levels of eicosapentaenoic and docosahexaenoic which accumulated in the microsomal membrane lipids. The 6-desaturase activity was higher in animals receiving 5 en% EFA than in those receiving 20 en% EFA.

Early studies of the mechanism for the hypolipidemic and hypocholesterolemic response to dietary PUFA were reported by Flick et al. (1977) who showed that the rate of synthesis of the enzyme complex that forms fatty acids in livers of rats fed a PUFA-supplemented diet was one-half that for rats on fat-free diets. The lower induction of fatty acid synthetase activity was attributed to a combined reduced rate of synthesis and increased rate of degradation of the synthetase enzyme. Apparently, PUFA may directly or indirectly regulate the transcription or translation (or both) of the messenger RNA of the fatty acid synthetase. Iritani et al. (1980) showed that eating shellfish fatty acids could reduce the activity of several lipogenic enzymes in rats. The reduced level of these enzymes and decreased formation of lipoproteins might be the basis for the well-recognized lowering of serum lipids generally observed after feeding polyunsaturated fats. The evidence generally indicates that this lowering effect may occur with either the n-6 or n-3 fatty acids, but is greater with n-3 HUFA.

The competitive effectiveness of various polyunsaturated acyl-CoAs in the reacylation reaction catalyzed by isolated rat liver microsomes was described by Lands et al. in 1982. The most effectively transferred acids in this acyl transfer reaction were 20:5n-3 and the two 18:3 isomers (n-3 and n-6), all of which were slightly more efficient with isolated rat liver enzymes than the eicosanoid precursor, 20:4n-6. Such in vitro results contrast with an apparent exclusion of 18:3n-3 from membrane phospholipids in vivo. The contrast suggests that unknown regulatory processes occur in vivo and remain to be discovered (Lands, 2000). Although no acyl transfer discrimination between n-3 and n-6 types of acids seemed apparent, the high efficiency for 20:5n-3 suggests that it might tend to displace 20:4n-6 in situations of competitive turnover. Such competition has a paradoxical consequence in that feeding 20:5n-3 might displace 20:4n-6 from cellular esters into the pool of nonesterified eicosanoid precursors and transiently increase the availability of arachidonate (20:4n-6) for eicosanoid biosynthesis. Such a result contrasts with the direct antagonism by 20:5n-3 of 20:4n-6 conversion to eicosanoids by the cyclooxygenase.

Data of van Gent et al. (1979) suggested that dietary intake of the fully elongated desaturated form, 22:6n-3, may shift arachidonate from the phospholipids and glycerides in the serum lipids to cholesterol esters. Thus, a possible consequence of ingesting a fish oil concentrate might be to make more cholesterol arachidonate available to vascular tissues and to facilitate antithrombotic phenomena by increasing PGI_2 formation. Clearly, more carefully controlled studies are needed to determine details about outcomes in humans.

A very high selectivity for 22-carbon fatty acids (22:4n-6 and 22:6n-3) in the ether-containing ethanolamine phospholipids of tumor cells was due to a unique selectivity of the cytidine-mediated ethanolamine phosphotransferase, rather than to an acyltransferase selectivity (Masuzawa, et al., 1982). In a similar manner, forming phosphatidyl serine (PS) from phosphatidyl choline (PC) in microsomes from cerebral cortex was faster with the 18:0,22:6n-3-PC molecular species, with the order of preference being 18:0,22:6n-3 >18:0,22:5n-6 >18:0,20:4n-6 = 18:0,18:1n-9 (Kim et al, 2004a). Liver microsomes also preferred 18:0,22:6-PC as substrate in PS synthesis, but the 18:0,22:5-PC species was converted to PS at rates the similar to18:0,20:4-PC or 18:0,18:1-PC species. Both brain and liver microsomes preferred 18:0 over 16:0 as the sn-1 fatty acid. The observed selectivity may maintain PS at a lower level in brain when 22:6n-3 is replaced by 22:5n-6 during n-3 fatty acid deficiency.

Comparing DPA (22:5n-6) and DHA (22:6n-3)

Enrichment of cultured neuronal cells with 22:5n-6 protected them against apoptotic death induced by staurosporine, but to a lesser extent than 22:6n-3 enrichment. Also, the in vitro interaction between Raf-1 and membranes was decreased by lower PS contents and also by the fatty acyl composition in PS. Thus, depletion of 22:6n-3 from neuronal tissues may have a compounding effect on Raf-1 translocation in growth factor signaling. The fact that the 22:5n-6 cannot fully support the protective role played by 22:6n-3 may explain the adverse effect of n-3 fatty acid deficiency on neuronal development and function (Kim, et al, 2004b).

Many different reactions participate in the selective movement of polyunsaturated fatty acids among the various cellular lipids. We can anticipate that future research will identify different preferred paths of incorporation for the various elongation and/or desaturation products of dietary fatty acids. More carefully controlled experiments are required before we can fully explain the impact of dietary fatty acids on the fatty acid composition of the many different tissue phospholipids, glycerol and sterol esters.

Another aspect of selectivity that merits attention is the slightly lower rate of lipase-catalyzed hydrolysis of glycerol esters of the highly unsaturated acids that have a double bond at the 3- or 4-position near the carboxy ester group (Brockerhoff, 1965; Bottino et al., 1967). This phenomenon influenced interpretations of fat composition because the analyses depended on a uniform and random rate of cleavage of the ester bonds. The interference should be regarded as due to relative rates and not to inability of pancreatic lipase and other digestive hydrolases to cleave these esters. All fats are normally digested with high efficiency in the small intestine, which apparently has much more lipase available than the minimum needed to cleave dietary fats. Fatty acids of marine origin are readily incorporated into triglycerides and phospholipids of mammals (Brockerhoff et at., 1967).

Ayala et al (1973) reported that docosatetraenoic acid (22:4n-6) was preferentially esterified into triglycerides, with only small amounts into phospholipid. The researchers were unable to measure direct conversion of 22:4n-6 to 22:5n-6 in vitro even though the process does occur in vivo. This result again illustrates the difficulty of studying elongation/desaturation events that tend to occur more slowly than direct acylation. This phenomenon means that many hours or even days may pass before a dietary polyunsaturated fatty acid will be converted fully within an animal to all of the possible elongated desaturated forms. Furthermore, while rearrangement and transformation occurs, there will be a concomitant steady competition for the acyl-CoA intermediates to move into the acylcarnitine-mediated oxidation to CO_2 that eliminates the fatty acid from further considerations.

This phenomenon has particular significance in interpreting the different actions reported for the 18-carbon member of the n-3 family (18:3n-3) relative to the 20-carbon eicosapentaenoic acid (20:5n-3) that is so abundant in the tissues of fish. Dyerberg and his co-workers (1980) reported that dietary linolenic acid (18:3n-3) was esterified in humans predominantly into the plasma triglycerides, and produced only slight increases in the levels of the common elongated and desaturated HUFA, eicosapentaenoic and docosahexaenoic acids. This result in humans appears to contrast sharply with results in rats in which dietary linolenic acid rapidly provided 22-carbon polyunsaturated acids to the cardiac phospholipids (Kramer, 1980). Pooviah et al. (1976) reported that ^{14}C-linolenic acid fed to rats was recovered predominantly in the form of 20:5n-3 and 22:6n-3. Years of research reports still leave unresolved the question of how effective dietary 18:3n-3 is in producing n-3 HUFA in human tissues.

Influencing Gene Expression

Both n-6 and n-3 PUFA suppress transcription of a number of hepatic lipogenic and glycolytic genes, whereas saturated and monounsaturated fatty acids do not (Clarke and

Jump, 1996). Both n-6 and n-3 HUFA suppress the transcription of hepatic genes encoding lipogenic and glycolytic enzymes while concomitantly inducing enzymes for mitochondrial and peroxisomal fatty acid oxidation (Clarke and Jump, 1997). Arachidonic acid (20:4n-6) and eicosapentaenoic acid (20:5n-3) suppressed mRNAs encoding fatty acid synthase, and the effect was blocked by an inhibitor of cyclooxygenase (Mater et al, 1998). Prostaglandins PGE_2 and PGF_2 inhibited expression through a pertussis toxin-sensitive Gi/Go-coupled signalling cascade. Apparently, 20:4n-6 inhibits lipogenic gene expression in 3T3-L1 adipocytes through a prostanoid-related process different from HUFA-mediated suppression of hepatic lipogenic genes.

n-6 PUFA suppress de novo lipogenesis in hepatocytes and adipocytes by inhibiting the transcription of genes encoding key lipogenic proteins, perhaps by prostaglandins PGE_2 and PGF_2 acting through EP3 receptors to suppress fatty acid synthase, l-pyruvate kinase, and the S14 protein mRNA, while having no effect on acyl-CoA oxidase or CYP4A2 mRNA (Mater et al, 1999). Eicosa-5, 8,11,14-tetraynoic acid prevented 18:2n-6 from suppressing hepatic fatty acid synthase mRNA, and it induced hepatic delta-6-desaturase mRNA two-fold (Nakamura et al, 2000). Decreased hepatic 20:4n-6 and increased 18:2n-6 accompanied decreased delta-6 desaturase activity, making delta-6 desaturation appear essential for n-6 and n-3 PUFA to suppress expression of lipogenic genes. Hepatic expression of delta-5-desaturase (D5D) and delta-6-desaturase (D6D) was highly activated in transgenic mice overexpressing nuclear SREBP-1a, -1c, and -2, and expression of both desaturases was downregulated by dietary PUFA (Matsuzaka et al, 2002). Apparently, D5D and D6D expression is dually regulated by SREBP-1c and PPAR(alpha), reciprocal transcription factors for fatty acid metabolism.

The basal fatty acid levels in the NEFA pool coupled with rates of fatty acid esterification, elongation, desaturation, peroxisomal beta-oxidation, and fatty acyl thioesterase activity seem to affect NEFA pool composition and PPAR(alpha) activity (Pawar and Jump, 2003). Changes in NEFA 20:5n-3 and 22:6n-3, but not 22:5n-3, correlated with dynamic changes in the PPARalpha-regulated transcript mRNA for CYP4A. Eicosapentaenoic acid (20:5n-3) suppressed mRNA expression of SREBP-1-regulated lipogenic genes independent of LXR(alpha) (Pawar et al, 2003).

References

Actis Dato SM, Catala A, Brenner RR. Circadian rhythm of fatty acid desaturation, *Lipids* 8:1-6, 1972.

Ayala S, Gaspar G, Brenner RR, et al. Fate of linoleic, arachidonic, and docosa-7, 10, 13, 16-tetraenoic acids in rat testicles. *J Lipid Res* 14:296-305, 1973.

Bazan HEP, Careaga MM, Sprecher H, et al.Chain Elongation and desaturation of eicosapentaenoate to docosahexaenoate and phospholipid labeling in the rat retina in vivo. *Biochim Biophys Acta* 712:123-128, 1982.

Bottino NR, Vandenburg CA, Reiser R. Resistance of certain long-chain polyunsaturated fatty acids of marine oils to pancreatic lipase hydrolysis. *Lipids* 2:489, 1967.

Brenner RR. The oxidative desaturation of unsaturated fatty acids in animals. *Mol Cell Biochem* 3:41-52, 1974.

Brenner RR. Nutritional and hormonal factors influencing desaturation of essential fatty acids. *Prog Lipid Res* 20:41-47, 1982.

Brenner RR, Peluffo RO. Effect of saturated and unsaturated fatty acids on the desaturation in vitro of palmitic, stearic, oleic, linoleic, and linolenic acids. *J Biol Chem* 241:5213-5219, 1966.

Brenner RR, Garda H, Dumm LNT, et al. Early effects of EFA deficiency on the structure and enzymatic activity of rat liver microsomes. *Prog Lipid Res* 20:315-321, 1982.

Brockerhoff H. Stereospecific analysis of triglycerides: An analysis of human depot fat. *Arch Biochem Biophys* 110:586-592, 1965.

Brockerhoff H, Hoyle RJ, Hwang PC. Incorporation of fatty acids of marine origin into triglycerides and phospholipids or mammals. *Biochim Biophys Acta* 144:541-548, 1967.

Clarke SD, Jump DB. Polyunsaturated fatty acid regulation of hepatic gene transcription. *Lipids* 31 Suppl: S7-S11, 1996.

Clarke SD, Jump D. Polyunsaturated fatty acids regulate lipogenic and peroxisomal gene expression by independent mechanisms. *Prostaglandins Leukot Essent Fatty Acids* 57(1): 65-69, 1997.

Collins FD, Sinclair AJ, Royle JP, et al. Plasma lipids in human linoleic acid deficiency. *Nutr Metab* 13(3):150-167, 1971

Consensus conference. Lowering blood cholesterol to prevent heart disease. *JAMA* 253(14):2080-2086, 1985.

de Gomez-Dumm INT, de Alaniz, MJL, Brenner RR. Comparative effect of glucagon, dibutyryl cyclic AMP, and epinephrine on the desaturation and elongation of linoleic acid by rat liver micmsomes. *Lipids* 11:833-836, 1976.

de Schrijver R, Privett OS. Effects of dietary long-chain fatty acids on the biosynthesis of unsaturated fatty acids in the rat. *J Nutr* 112:619-626, 1982.

Dolecek TA, Granditis G. Dietary polyunsaturated fatty acids and mortality in the Multiple Risk Factor Intervention Trial (MRFIT). *World Rev Nutr Diet* 66:205-216, 1991.

Dyerberg J, Bang HO, Aagaard O. Alpha-linolenic acid and eicosapentenoic acid. *Lancet* 1:199, 1980.

Flick PF, Chen J, Vagelos PR. Effect of dietary linoleate on synthesis and degradation of fatty acid synthetase from rat liver. *J Biol Chem* 252:4242-4249, 1977.

Galli C, Agradi E, Petroni A, et al. Differential effects of dietary fatty acids on the accumilation of arachidonic acid and its metabolic conversion through the cyclooxygenase and lipoxygenase in platelets and vascular tissue. *Lipids* 16(3):165-172, 1981.

Ge Y, Chen Z, Kang ZB, et al. Effects of adenoviral gene transfer of C. elegans n-3 fatty acid desaturase on the lipid profile and growth of human breast cancer cells. *Anticancer Res*;22(2A):537-543, 2002.

Ge Y, Wang X, Chen Z, et al. Gene transfer of the Caenorhabditis elegans n-3 fatty acid desaturase inhibits neuronal apoptosis. *J Neurochem* 82(6):1360-1366, 2002.

Goodgame JT, Lowry SF, Brennan MF. Essential fatty acid deficiency in total parenteral nutrition: time course of development and suggestions for therapy. *Surgery* 84:271-277, 1978

Hanel AM, Schuttel S, Gelb MH. Processive interfacial catalysis by mammalian 85-kilodalton phospholipase A2 enzymes on product-containing vesicles: application to the determination of substrate preferences. *Biochemistry* 32(23):5949-5958, 1993.

Hoffman DR, DeMar JC, Heird WC, et al. Impaired synthesis of DHA in patients with X-linked retinitis pigmentosa. *J Lipid Res* 42(9):1395-1401, 2001.

Holman RT. Nutritional and metabolic interrelationships between fatty acids. *Fed Proc* 23:1062, 1964.

Iritani N, Inoguchi K, Endo M, et al. Identification of shellfish fatty acids and their effects on lipogenic enzymes. *Biochim Biophys Acta* 618:378-382, 1980.

Jeppesen PB, Hoy CE, Mortensen PB. Deficiencies of essential fatty acids, vitamin A and E and changes in plasma lipoproteins in patients with reduced fat absorption or intestinal failure. *Eur J Clin Nutr* 54(8):632-642, 2000.

Kang JX, Wang J, Wu L, et al. Transgenic mice: fat-1 mice convert n-6 to n-3 fatty acids. *Nature* 427(6974):504, 2004.

Kang ZB, Ge Y, Chen Z, et al. Adenoviral gene transfer of Caenorhabditis elegans n-3 fatty acid desaturase optimizes fatty acid composition in mammalian cells. *Proc Natl Acad Sci* 98(7):4050-4054, 2001.

Kennedy EP. The metabolism and function of complex lipids. *Harvey Lec Ser* 57:143, 1962.

Kim H-Y, Akbar M, Lau, A. Effects of docosapentaenoic acid on neuronal apoptosis *Lipids* 38:453-457, 2004.

Kim H-Y, Bigelow J, Kevala JH. Substrate preference in phosphatidylserine biosynthesis for docosahexaenoic acid containing species. *Biochemistry* 43:1030-1036, 2004.

Kobayashi M, Sasaki S, Kawabata T, et al. Single measurement of serum phospholipid fatty acid as a biomarker of specific fatty acid intake in middle-aged Japanese men. *Eur J Clin Nutr* 55(8):643650, 2001.

Kobayashi T, Umemura U, Iso H, et al. Differences in dietary habits, serum fatty acid compositions and other coronary risk characteristics between freshmen and fourth-year male university students. *Environ Health Prev Med* 6:143-148, 2001.

Kramer JKG. Comparative studies on composition of cardiac phospholipids in rats fed different vegetable oils. *Lipids* 15(9):651-660, 1980.

Kurata N, Privett OS. Effect of dietary fatty acid composition on the biosynthesis of unsaturated fatty acids in rat liver microsomes. *Lipids* 15:512-518, 1980.

Lands WEM. Metabolism of glycerolipids. II. The enzymatic acylation of lysolecithin. *J Biol Chem* 235:2233-2237, 1960.

Lands WEM. Long-term fat intake and biomarkers. *Am J Clin Nutr* 61(suppl):721S-725S, 1995.

Lands WEM. Stories about acyl chains. *Biochim Biophys Acta* 1483:1-15, 2000.

Lands WEM, Crawford CC. (1976). Enzymes of membrane phospholipid metabolism in animals. In Martonosi A (ed.). *The Enzymes of Biological Membranes*, vol.2. New York: Plenum, 1976, pp 3-85.

Lands WEM, Culp BR, Hirai A, et al. Relationship of thromboxane generation to the aggregation of platelets from humans: effects of eicosapentaenoic acid. *Prostaglandins* 30:819-825, 1985.

Lands WEM., Inoue M, Sugiura Y, et al. Selective incorporation of polyunsaturated fatty acids into phosphatidylcholine by rat liver microsomes. *J Biol Chem* 257:14968-14972, 1982.

Lands WEM, Libelt, B, Morris A. Maintenance of lower proportions of n-6 eicosanoid precursors in phospholipids of human plasma in response to added dietary n-3 fatty acids. *Biochim Biophys Acta* 1180:147-162,m 1992.

Luthria DL, Mohammed BS, Sprecher H. Regulation of the biosynthesis of 4,7,10,13,16,19-docosahexaenoic acid. *J Biol Chem* 271(27):16020-16025, 1996.

Mascioli EA, Lopes SM, Champagne C, et al. Essential fatty acid deficiency and home total parenteral nutrition patients. *Nutrition* 12(4):245249, 1996

Masuzawa Y, Nakagawa Y, Waku K, et al. Distinctive selectivity for docosatetraenoic acid incorporation by Ehriich ascites tumor cells. *Biochim Biophys Acta* 713:185-192, 1982.

Mater MK, Pan D, Bergen WG, et al. Arachidonic acid inhibits lipogenic gene expression in 3T3-L1 adipocytes through a prostanoid pathway. *J Lipid Res* 39(7):1327-1334, 1998.

Mater MK, Thelen AP, Jump DB. Arachidonic acid and PGE2 regulation of hepatic lipogenic gene expression. *J Lipid Res* 40(6):1045-1052, 1999.

Matsuzaka T, Shimano H, Yahagi N, et al. Dual regulation of mouse Delta(5)- and Delta(6)-desaturase gene expression by SREBP-1 and PPARalpha. *J Lipid Res* 43(1):107-114, 2002.

Mead JF. The metabolism of the polyunsaturated fatty acids. *Prog Chem Fats Other Lipids* 9, 159-192, 1971.

Mohrhauer H, Holman RT. Effect of linolenic acid upon the metabolism of linoleic acid. *J Nutr* 81: 67-74, 1963a.

Mohrhauer H, Holman RT. The effect of dose level of essential fatty acids upon fatty acid composition of the rat liver. *J Lipid Res* 58:151-159, 1963b.

Mohrhauer H, Holman RT. Alteration of the fatty acid composition of brain lipids by varying levels of dietary essential fatty acids. *J Neurochem* 10 523-530, 1963c.

Mohrhauer H, Holman RT. The effect of dietary essential fatty acids upon composition of polyunsaturated fatty acids in depot fat and erythrocytes of the rat. *J Lipid Res* 58:346-350, 1963d.

Nakamura MT, Cho HP, Clarke SD. Regulation of hepatic delta-6 desaturase expression and its role in the polyunsaturated fatty acid inhibition of fatty acid synthase gene expression in mice. *J Nutr* 30(6):1561-1565, 2000.

Napier JA, Michaelson LV. Genomic and functional characterization of polyunsaturated fatty acid biosynthesis in Caenorhabditis elegans. *Lipids* 36(8):761-766, 2001.

Nervi AM, Brenner RR, Peluffo RO. Effect of arachidonic acid on the microsomal desaturation of linoleic into γ-Iinolenic acid and their simultaneous incorporation into the phospholipids. *Biochim Biophys Acta* 152:539-551, 1968.

O'Neill JA Jr, Caldwell MD, Meng HC. Essential fatty acid deficiency in surgical patients. *Ann Surg* 185(5):535-542, 1977

Pawar A, Botolin D, Mangelsdorf DJ, et al. The role of liver X receptor-alpha in the fatty acid regulation of hepatic gene expression. *J Biol Chem* 278(42):40736-40743, 2003.

Pawar A, Jump DB. Unsaturated fatty acid regulation of peroxisome proliferator-activated receptor alpha activity in rat primary hepatocytes. *J Biol Chem* 278(38):35931-35939, 2003.

Pooviah BP, Tinoco J, Lyman PL. Influence of diet on conversion of ^{14}C-linolenic acid to docosahexaenoic acid in the rat. *Lipids* 11:194-202, 1976.

Rahm JJ, Holman RT. Effect of linoleic acid upon the metabolism of linolenic acid. *J Nutr* 84:15-19, 1964.

Sanders TAW, Younger KM. The effect of dietary supplements of o3 polyunsaturated fatty acids on the fatty acid composition of platelets and plasma choline phosphoglycerides. *Br J Nutr* 45:613-616, 1981.

Simon JA, Hodgkins ML, Browner WS,et al. Serum fatty acids and the risk of coronary heart disease. *Am J Epidemiol* 142:469-476, 1995.

Shikano M, Masuzawa Y, Yazawa K, et al Complete discrimination of docosahexaenoate from arachidonate by 85 kDa cytosolic phospholipase A2 during the hydrolysis of diacyl- and alkenylacyl glycerophosphoethanolamine. *Biochim Biophys Acta* 1212(2):211-21 1994.

Sprecher H. The roles of anabolic and catabolic reactions in the synthesis and recycling of polyunsaturated fatty acids. *Prostaglandins Leukot Essent Fatty Acids* 67(2-3):79-83, 2002.

Sprecher H. Metabolism of highly unsaturated n-3 and n-6 fatty acids. *Biochim Biophys Acta* 1486(2-3):219-231, 2000.

Spychalla JP, Kinney AJ, Browse J. Identification of an animal omega-3 fatty acid desaturase by heterologous expression in Arabidopsis. *Proc Natl Acad Sci* 94(4):1142-1147, 1997.

van Gent CM, Luten JB, Bronsgeest-Schoute WC, et al. Effect, on serum lipid levels of n-3 fatty acids, of ingesting fish oil concentrate. *Lancet* 2:1249-1250, 1979.

Watts JL, Browse J. A palmitoyl-CoA-specific delta9 fatty acid desaturase from Caenorhabditis elegans. *Biochem Biophys Res Commun* 272(1):263-269, 2000.

Weaver BJ, Holub BJ. The relative degradation of [14C]eicosapentaenoyl and [3H]arachidonoyl species of phosphatidylinositol and phosphatidylcholine in thrombin-stimulated human platelets. *Biochem Cell Biol* 64(12):1256-1261, 1986.

Wene JD, Connor WE, DenBesten L. The development of essential fatty acid deficiency in healthy men fed fatfree diets intravenously and orally. *J Clin Invest* 56(1):127-134, 1975

2005 National Library of Medicine Search Results:

(http://www.ncbi.nlm.nih.gov/entrez/query.fcgi)

fatty acid desaturation = 1,338; fatty acid desaturation omega-3 = 217

fatty acid elongation = 1,246; fatty acid elongation omega-3 = 147

PUFA = 141,592; PUFA elongation = 599; PUFA desaturation = 891;
PUFA desaturation omega-3 = 200; PUFA elongation omega-3 = 143

arachidonic = 32,623; arachidonic elongation = 216

eicosapentaenoic = 3,780; eicosapentaenoic elongation = 92

14—Pathways to Prostaglandins

The discovery in 1964 that arachidonic acid can be converted to prostaglandins gave the polyunsaturated fatty acids a new and powerful role in our interpretations of human physiology and pathophysiology. The biosynthesis of prostaglandins (Bergstrom et al., 1964; van Dorp et al., 1964) involves an oxidative conversion of the polyunsaturated fatty acid to an endoperoxide intermediate (see Fig 14-1) that was first proposed by Hamberg and Samuelsson in 1966 and isolated 7 years later (Hamberg and Samuelsson, 1973). The exciting physiological and clinical discoveries that followed the successful preparation of the intermediate PGH_2 and the understanding of the importance of its derivatives—thromboxane and prostacyclin in heart attacks and strokes—are noted earlier in this book.

In general, our tissues tend to suppress the formation of prostaglandins. Only a small part of the total synthetic potential of a tissue is expressed at a given time. Some estimates indicate that less than 0.01% of the overall synthetic ability is used during a 24-hour period. The factors that control the rate of synthesis are not fully understood, but one important controlling factor is the amount of nonesterified arachidonate accessible to the catalytic enzyme. Another factor is the amount of hydroperoxide activator, which is rapidly amplified by oxygenase action on arachidonate (see Technical details in this chapter).

Pulsatile oscillations occur in the amount of prostaglandin F_2 released from the brain, indicating that there are probably moment-to-moment fluctuations in the rate of synthesis (Roberts et al., 1976). This finding illustrates one of the difficult prob-

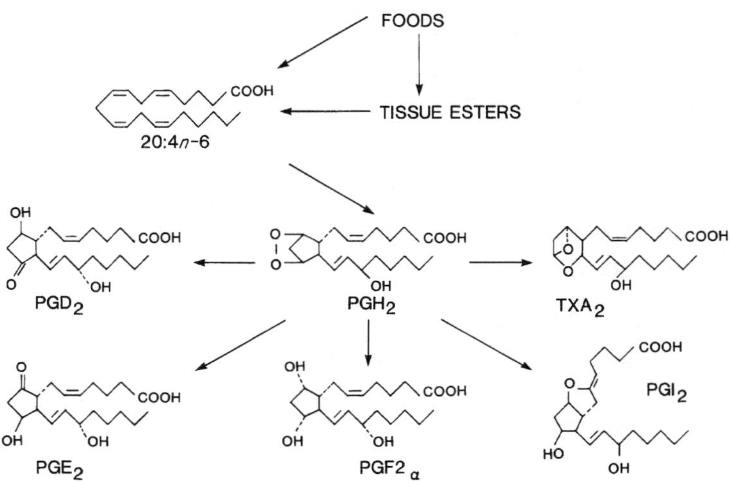

Fig. 14-1. Pathways to prostaglandins.

lems faced by medical researchers trying to study the role of eicosanoids. There is an ever-changing level of these materials as our tissues adapt to varying environmental stimuli and send out a variety of eicosanoid signals in response.

Elisabeth Granström (1978) pointed out that researchers might completely misinterpret the amount of prostaglandin metabolites circulating in the blood if the sampling intervals are infrequent. It has been much easier to discover how the eicosanoids are made than to learn how much is made at a given time by a given tissue. Major analytical efforts are still needed in this area. Nevertheless, researchers have described the pathways involved in converting arachidonate in our tissues to the many recognized prostaglandins, and some preliminary data are available on daily eicosanoid formation.

The principal reactions in cyclooxygenase-initiated pathways are indicated in Fig. 14-1. The enzyme-catalyzed oxidation converts three of the cis double bonds of arachidonate into the five-membered cyclopentane ring with an adjacent trans double bond. Thus the fatty acid with four double bonds, 20:4n-6, produces a prostaglandin, PGH_2, with two double bonds. The subscript "2" indicates the number of double bonds in the eicosanoid. Arachidonic (20:4n-6) and eicosatrienoic acids (20:3n-6) are easily converted to dienoic (two double bond) and monoenoic (one double bond) prostaglandins, respectively, and eicosapentaenoic acid (20:5n-3) is converted into trienoic prostaglandins. Few of the other closely related polyunsaturated acids in our tissues were converted into prostanoids (Struijk et al., 1966; Lands et al., 1973). However, those in vitro studies had low peroxide tone which depressed relative rates of formation of trienoic eicosanoids as noted later in this chapter.

Hydroperoxide Activators Needed

The requirement of the cyclooxygenase for hydroperoxide activator has an interesting relationship to the fact that the initial product of the reaction is a hydroperoxide. Thus, once the enzyme reaction with arachidonate and oxygen is triggered by small amounts of hydroperoxide, it rapidly amplifies the amount of activator available and enhances its own rate of prostaglandin formation. This rapid amplification of cellular hydroperoxide levels when arachidonate (20:4n-6) is the substrate does not occur as readily with the n-3 fatty acids that have a requirement for higher amounts of hydroperoxide activator to maintain the oxygenation reaction. Thus, shifting tissue polyunsaturated fatty acid composition from one rich in n-6 acids to one rich in n-3 acids may suppress the tendency of a tissue to amplify hydroperoxide content (and perhaps diminish carcinogenesis) and lower the tendency to form eicosanoids in general.

A series of isomers of polyunsaturated fatty acids were synthesized (Struijk et al., 1966) to test the selectivity of prostaglandin biosynthesis. Yields obtained with a crude enzyme preparation from sheep are listed in Table 14-1. Polyunsaturated acids that occur in natural mixtures of fatty acids in human tissues are indicated in Table 14.1 by an asterisk. The two HUFA derived from 18:2n-6, 20:3n-6, and 20:4n-6 were excellent substrates. Further studies (Beerthuis et al., 1968), listed in the right-hand

TABLE 14-1
Selectivity for Prostaglandin Formation[a]

Fatty acid	PGE Formed[b]		PG Synthesis relative rate[c]	EFA Assay biopotency[c]
18:3n6*	<5	18:3n-4	0	0
18:4n-6	11	22:3n-8	0	0
19:3n-6	60	19:3n-5	2	22
19:4n-6	41	19:4n-5	43	49
20:3n6*	68	21:3n-7	33	56
20:4n.6*	74	21:4n-7	57	62
21:3n-6	36	20:3n-6*	88	102
21:4n-6	25	20:4n-6*	102	102
22:3n-6	5			
22:4n.6*	24			
20.:5n3*	5			
20:3n-5	<2			
20 :3n-7	18			
20 :3n-8	0			
20 :3n-9	0			

[a]Asterisks indicate a naturally occurring acid.
[b]Data from Struijk et al. (1966).
[c]Data from Beerthuis et al. (1968).

columns of Table 14-1, indicate a close correlation between biological activity as an essential fatty acid and the ability to yield prostaglandin derivatives. Thus we can consider the discovery of essential fatty acids as an early indicator of the importance of n-6 prostaglandins. However, the experiments in Table 14-1 do not acknowledge the earlier demonstrated potency of n-3 EFA (described in Chapter 3).

Various other polyunsaturated fatty acids that resemble 20:4n-6, but differ in small structural details, can bind to cyclooxygenase and serve as competitive inhibitors of the conversion of arachidonate to prostaglandins (Lands et al., 1973; Ziboh et al., 1974). Thus the mixture of nonesterified fatty acids made available to the cyclooxygenase at the time it is stimulated to full activity has an appreciable influence on the degree to which arachidonic acid can be converted into an active prostaglandin. Medical researchers currently have little knowledge of the transient composition of fatty acids in the nonesterified fatty acid pool. It is clear, however, that the pool changes rapidly, and that dietary supply can have both short-term and long-term influences on the composition of the tissue precursors (Ramesha et al., 1985). Also, it is clear that many n-3 fatty acids can antagonize arachidonate (20:4n-6) conversion to eicosanoids while forming alternative eicosanoids.

Results of Culp et al. (1979) confirmed the observation that eicosapentaenoic acid (20:5n-3) was not readily oxidized by cyclooxygenase in some experiments and indicated that the low reactivity was caused by a requirement for greater amounts of lipid hydroperoxide activator when the enzyme reacts with this n-3 fatty acid. The high requirement for activator hydroperoxides with the n-3 acids means that under physiological conditions in which a low level of lipid hydroperoxide is available, the eicosapentaenoate may act more as a competitive inhibitor than a substrate. The in vitro assay conditions commonly used to monitor cyclooxygenase activity in the laboratory often permit sufficiently high levels of peroxide activator to accumulate and thereby allow conversion of eicosapentaenoate to trienoic prostaglandins (with three double bonds). Lands and Byrnes (1982) suggested that if trienoic prostaglandins are eventually found in normal tissues, it may be viewed as an indicator of abnormally elevated levels of tissue peroxides.

For some time, there was some uncertainty among different investigators as to whether trienoic prostaglandins were formed in normal living tissues in vivo. The uncertainty was finally eliminated by the report of a PGI_3 metabolite in the urine of humans who consumed 750 g of mackerel per day (Fischer and Weber, 1984) This evidence finally gave direct support to the hypothesis of Dyerberg et al. (1978) concerning PGI_3 formation in vivo. The transiently elevated lipid hydroperoxides needed to promote oxygenation of the 20:5n-3 may not occur in most tissues, but the vascular endothelial cells that form PGI are in contact with plasma that contains nearly 0.5 picomolar concentrations of peroxide (Warso and Lands, 1985). It will be interesting to learn what amounts of peroxide occur in other tissues and how they influence the rate of prostaglandin formation.

Five Important Aspects

Excessive intensity of n-6 prostaglandin actions described in earlier chapters of this book results from diet choices. To help readers better understand how those harmful effects occur, more details from old and new reports on the pathway to prostaglandin action have been added to this chapter. Autacoid actions of prostaglandins depend on the following five important aspects:

1. How much (and which) HUFA have access to an active cyclooxygenase to make active autacoid at a certain point in time. Access is controlled by activated phospholipase releasing the tissue HUFA that came from eating different foods. A greater speed of oxygenation with 20:3n-6 and 20:4n-6 compared to 20:5n-3 gives more intense formation of n-6 autacoids. This increases with a greater relative abundance of n-6 HUFA in tissue HUFA.
2. How much (and which) active form of the oxygenase is present with the needed level of peroxide activator to form the key intermediate prostaglandin, PGH (see Fig. 14-1). Two separate genes are now known to code three different cyclooxygenases with slightly different catalytic properties. The amount of each variant expressed in a tissue affects the intensity of forming prostaglandins. Also, each catalyst is activated differently by the local ambient peroxide tone in the cell (i.e., the balance between formation and removal of hydroperoxides).
3. How much (and which) active autacoid is formed by the different synthases acting on PGH to give PGD, PGE, PGF, PGI or TXA (see Fig. 14-1) affects subse-

quent actions at different specific cellular receptors. Access to each cellular receptor at a given moment in time depends on the balance between the speed of autacoid being formed near the receptor relative to the speed of its destruction. Most active eicosanoids remain for only a limited number of seconds before they are destroyed.

4. How much (and which) receptor signaling occurs when triggered by n-3 or n-6 types of autacoid. This genetically defined aspect of receptors is very important to predicting when dietary n-3 and n-6 abundance will likely affect disease intensity. Sadly, much of the needed data on eicosanoid receptor specificity for n-3 and n-6 autacoids remain undetermined at this time. Financial support for drug research focuses efforts on making new patented activators and inhibitors of autacoid signaling, neglecting differences among the natural eicosanoids formed from 20:3n-6, 20:4n-6, and 20:5n-3, the abundance of which is affected by people's food choices.
5. How much (and which) signal transduction pathway is altered downstream from the receptor by events that return the overall signaling system back to its original baseline state. This aspect is a generic concern in all transient intracellular signaling events with G-proteins, tyrosine kinases, and protein phosphatases, and it involves details beyond the scope of this book. Clearly, any downstream alterations that involve selective interactions with the n-3 or n-6 structural features of nutrient EFA, may be affected by food choices.

Technical Details

Rate of Cyclooxygenase Action

The pulsatile rates of prostaglandin synthesis described in the first edition depend on a stimulated release of HUFA from tissue lipids with the non-esterified HUFA accessing an active cycloxygenase enzyme with an adequate supply of hydroperoxide activators (Lands, 1979). The phospholipase-catalyzed release seems similar for n-3 and n-6 precursors (Chapter 13), making diet-determined tissue abundance a controlling factor in HUFA competitions for the active site of the cyclooxygenase enzyme. Of course, competing nonsubstrate fatty acids (like DHA) or fatty acid analogs (like many nonsteroidal anti-inflammatory drugs; NSAIDs) can block access of HUFA substrate to the enzyme site.

Some NSAIDs (like ibuprofen or naproxen) are reversible competitors that bind the enzyme site, blocking substrate access until the drug leaves the region. Other NSAIDs (like aspirin or indomethacin) cause a time-dependent inactivation of the enzyme which makes later interactions with substrates unable to form active autacoid. Having active autacoid available for signaling at any given moment depends on access of newly-formed autacoid to the receptor being faster than the rate of autacoid degradation (Lands, 1979). In many tissues, short-lived eicosanoids are inactivated nearly as fast as they are formed. Treatments with NSAIDs succeed by slowing the formation of prostaglandins to a rate below the usual rate of inactivation.

Ex vivo studies have frequently provided evidence that trienoic prostaglandins can be formed outside the body. Hamberg (1980) demonstrated that a suspension of human platelets in vitro could generate thromboxane B_3 (TXB_3) from eicosapentaenoic acid, and Dyerberg et al. (1981) reported the conversion in vitro of added eicosapentaenoic acid to prostaglandin I_3 (PGI_3) by isolated pieces of the umbilical blood vessel. The level of peroxides in these homogenates and slices may be elevated, and the conditions for the successful conduct of these experiments appear to be critical since Needleman et al. (1979) reported that eicosapentaenoate was converted by platelets at one-eighth the efficiency of arachidonate, whereas in 1980 they reported that 20:5n-3 was not detectably metabolized by platelets.

An alternative to in vivo inhibition of cyclooxygenase by eicosapentaenoate was provided by Dyerberg et al. (1978) who suggested that vascular endothelial cells form a trienoic prostacyclin (PGI_3) that antagonizes platelet action. Although the hypothesis does not explain the inhibitory effect observed with eicosapentaenoic acid on isolated platelets, it provides a mechanism whereby fish oil could indirectly decrease thrombotic activity of platelets in vivo.

However, reports by Hamazaki et al. (1980, 1982) and by Hornstra et al. (1981) indicated that feeding fish oil lowered the production of both TXA and PGI, and did not result in the formation of PGI_3. A similar finding was reported by Morita et al. (1983) who saw no detectable conversion of ^{14}C-20:5n-3 to TXB_3 in platelets, and no conversion to PGI_3 by vascular cells in culture. Further, added 20:5n-3 decreased the production of PGI_2 from the endogenous esterified arachidonic acid of these cells. Related results of Ferretti et al. (1981) demonstrated the conversion of tissue 20:5n-3 to a PGI_3 by homogenates of kidney tissue in vitro, even though no PGI_3 was detected in the urinary products from the animals. Such negative results made the report of a PGI_3 metabolite from humans (Fischer and Weber, 1984) more interesting, and subsequent work affirmed in vivo PGI_3 formation (Knapp & Salem, 1989).

Because all fatty acid oxygenases (cyclooxygenases and lipoxygenases) form a hydroperoxide that further activates the oxygenase reaction, the oxygenases are amplifiers of the ambient peroxide tone that supports inflammatory conditions. In contrast, peroxidases act in anti-inflammatory ways. The requirement for maintaining sufficient hydroperoxide activator during oxygenase-catalyzed formation of prostaglandins and leukotrienes is one of the important conditions by which the kinetic balance between prooxidant and antioxidant conditions (Fig. 5-4 [Chapter 5])) affect the intensity of prostaglandin and leukotriene formation and action.

This condition amplifies differences between tissues having different proportions of n-3 and n-6 HUFA. Maintaining a low peroxide tone in cells also allows acetaminophen to slow hydroperoxide amplification of prostaglandin formation rates (Lands and Hanel, 1982) below the prostaglandin inactivation rates so little active autacoid reaches receptors. This illustrates the conditions in which phenolic analgesic agents are effective inhibitors, although they are not when peroxide tone is higher (Hanel and Lands, 1982).

Different Cyclooxygenases

An important aspect of the cyclooxygenase pathway is the inducible nature of that enzyme. Thus, cells in our tissues may not always have a consistent, constitutive amount of cyclooxygenase activity, but rather a level that reflects certain hormonal conditions. This possibility seemed evident in the early report (Tan and Privett, 1973) that the loss of pituitary hormones following hypophysectomy led to a loss of cyclooxygenase activity in rats. The pituitary hormones apparently have an important control over the amount of cyclooxygenase activity in tissues. Since a dietary deficiency of n-6 fatty acids can lead to a loss of pituitary function (see Chapter 3), there may also be a corresponding loss of enzymatic activity for producing prostaglandins. This loss occurs under conditions of EFA deficiency, which gives inadequate synthetic activity to maintain healthy levels of prostaglandins and causes serious imbalances in prostaglandin metabolism and hormone function.

Clues noted earlier for an inducible form of cyclooxygenase became fact by 1990 with cloning of COX-2 that was similar to COX-1 (Herschman, 1994). Immune system signaling induces formation of more molecules of the COX-2 enzyme when amplifying inflammatory pathology, and the development of selective COX-2 inhibitor drugs has been vigorously pursued in recent years (Dewitt et al., 1993; Smith et al., 2000). The two enzymes are now known to occur in different abundances in different cells and tissues. The earlier report of regulating cyclooxygenase activity by pituitary hormone (Privett, 1973) has not been described further, and much remains to be done in understanding the signals that regulate formation of new active cyclooxygenase forms.

A third enzyme form abundant in brain, COX-3, was recently reported to have kinetic features that may make it selectively inhibited by certain phenolic NSAIDs (Chandrasekharan et al., 2002) which antagonize the hydroperoxide activation (Lands and Hanel, 1982). Some kinetic dynamic aspects of the oxygenase enzymes in acting with hydroperoxide activators and NSAID inhibitors is noted below in the context of how diet choices and tissue levels of n-3 and n-6 HUFA may influence diseases. Because of genetic structural differences between COX-1 and COX-2, these enzymes require different ambient peroxide tone and act differently with the carboxyl portion of HUFA substrates.

Carboxylic NSAIDs that are irreversible inhibitors of COX-1 lose that ability when converted to ester or amide forms, but retain irreversible inhibition of COX-2 (Kalgutkar et al., 2000). Similarly, cannabinoid derivatives lacking free carboxylic group are not substrates for COX-1, but are actively oxygenated to prostaglandin esters by COX-2 (Kozak et al., 2002). These differences in the form of cyclooxygenase in a cell give different consequences from the different diet selections that people make. An excellent review describes how differences in the gene-determined structures of the prostaglandin endoperoxide H synthases-1 and 2 (PGHS-1 and PGHS-2), also called cyclooxygenases-1 and 2 (COX-1 and COX-2), relate to mechanisms of cyclooxygenase and peroxidase catalysis and to selective actions of COX-2 inhibitors (Smith et al., 2000).

The large difference between n-3 and n-6 substrates reacting with cyclooxygenase reported in early years of study (see Table 14-1) seems due to assay conditions in which a contaminating peroxidase activity removed the needed hydroperoxide feedback activator, PGG (see Fig. 5-4 [Chapter 5]), and suppressed the self-catalyzed amplification of oxygenase action. We now know that in the absence of other peroxidases, highly purified COX-1 enzyme reacts about 5-fold faster with n-6 substrate than the n-3 substrate (Kulmacz et al., 1993; Malkowski et al., 2001). This faster formation of the activating hydroperoxide PGG gives a more explosively amplified burst of synthesis with n-6 substrates (Chen et al., 1999). The slower formation of the needed hydroperoxide activator by the n-3 substrate with both COX-1 and COX-2 (Laneuville et al., 1995) allows tissue peroxidases to have a greater inhibitory action in slowing formation of n-3 prostaglandins compared to n-6 prostaglandins. This difference causes food choices to affect the intensity of prostaglandin action.

The need for amplifying peroxides is greater with COX-1 (regarded by some as a basic "housekeeping" catalyst), so that a rise above basal peroxide tone is needed to accelerate its action appreciably. In contrast, the COX-2 form that has increased expression during immune responses is activated by low basal levels of hydroperoxides. This sensitivity allows COX-2 to start amplifying peroxide tone from baseline low cellular levels and to create rapid prostaglandin actions. Glutathione peroxidase removal of the needed hydroperoxide feedback activator showed that half-maximal COX activity was maintained with a lower hydroperoxide level with COX-2 (2.3 nM) than with COX-1 (21 nM) (Kulmacz and Wang, 1995).

The ability of COX-2 to proceed at hydroperoxide levels too low to sustain appreciable catalysis by COX-1 gives differential control of the COX isoforms when both are present in the same cell. Thus, low arachidonic acid and low hydroperoxide concentrations cause the observed differences in kinetics and selectivity of COX-1 and COX-2 for substrates and inhibitors (Swinney et al., 1997). The different efficiencies of COX-1 and COX-2 for hydroperoxide feedback activation create a cooperative interdependence between fatty acid and hydroperoxide levels which is not observed when the limitation is removed by added hydroperoxide (Chen et al., 1999).

A third distinct COX isozyme, COX-3, is made from the COX-1 gene but it retains intron 1 in its mRNA (Chandrasekharan et al., 2002). A slow ability to amplify feedback by a slower COX-3 rate of forming hydroperoxide activator may be why acetaminophen inhibits COX-3 under conditions where COX-2 is not inhibited (as noted earlier for COX-1, Lands and Hanel, 1982). In humans, COX-3 mRNA is expressed as an alternative transcript of COX-2, and is most abundant in cerebral cortex and heart.

Comparison of canine COX-3 activity with murine COX-1 and -2 demonstrates that this enzyme is selectively inhibited by analgesic/antipyretic drugs such as acetaminophen, phenacetin, antipyrine, and dipyrone, and is potently inhibited by some nonsteroidal antiinflammatory drugs. The inhibition of COX-3 seems to parallel the inhibition of COX-1 and -2 in low peroxide tone, representing a primary mechanism by which phenolic analgesics like Tylenol decrease pain and possibly fever.

Hopefully, further studies will indicate whether a greater need for peroxide tone also makes n-3 EPA a relatively poor substrate with COX-3, as it is with COX-1.

New knowledge about the enzymes converting HUFA into PGH (see Fig. 14-1) has been accompanied with little new information about the relatively non-specific isomerases forming PGD, PGE, PGF, PGI and TXA. Interestingly, the enzymes may not require a free carboxylic group to form the various isomerized products. They resemble COX-2 by working almost equally well with the endocannabinoids derivatives of PGH (Kozak et al., 2002). The biological significance of the various prostaglandins will continue to be a fertile area of research. Whether or not different signaling occurs with n-3 and n-6 derivatives will be important to nutrition-oriented discussions.

Prostaglandin Receptors

Importance of prostanoid actions is shown using mice that lack the ability to make different prostanoid receptors (Ushikubi et al., 2000). Studies of such "gene knockout" mice show PGI_2 acts at the IP receptor as a mediator of inflammation and as an antithrombotic agent. PGF_2 was found to be an essential inducer of labor via the FP receptor, whereas allergic asthma is affected by PGD_2 with the DP receptor. In different tissues, PGE_2 can act via one of four PGE receptor subtypes: EP1, EP2, EP3 and EP4. PGE_2 acts in colon carcinogenesis via EP1, whereas it acts in ovulation, fertilization and the control of blood pressure via EP2. Febrile responses to both endogenous and exogenous pyrogens and control of bicarbonate secretion in the duodenum are mediated via EP3 (although neurons expressing EP4 receptor are activated during LPS-induced fever, suggesting the involvement of EP4 receptors in the production of fever (Oka et al., 2000)). Closure of ductus arteriosus and bone resorbing action is also regulated by EP4.

Lipopolysaccharide (LPS) enhances expression of EP2/EP4 (but not EP1/EP3), and this was suppressed by a COX-2-selective inhibitor indicating a positive "feed forward" action of the COX-2 product in increasing its receptor (Harizi et al., 2003). PGE_2 and its analogs inhibit immune cell functions through increased EP(2)R actions that lower cellular levels of cyclic AMP (cAMP). The action of PGE_2 in increasing bone mass and bone strength is linked to elevated level of cAMP, implicating the action of EP2 and/or EP4 receptor subtypes (Paralkar et al., 2003). As a result, a selective EP2 agonist can heal canine long bone segmental and fracture model defects without the objectionable side effects that come from using $PGE_{2,}$ which acts also on other EP receptors. PGE_1, PGE_2 and PGE_3 produced from different fatty acid precursors are equipotent in their action to decrease Th1 cytokine production and shifts the Th1/Th2 balance in favor of a The 2 immune response by non-discriminating receptors not yet characterized (Miles et al., 2003).

The protective action of PGE_2 against indomethacin-induced injury of intestine seems mediated by EP3/EP4 receptors, linked to an increase of mucus secretion and enteropooling as well as to inhibition of intestinal hypermotility (Kunikata et al., 2002). The first two processes seem mediated by both EP3 and EP4 receptors, and the third by EP4 receptors. However, a protective action of dimethyl-PGE_2 in the stomach was observed for wild-type and EP3 receptor deficient mice but not for mice lacking EP1 receptors, whereas damage to the intestine was observed in EP1 deficient as well as wild-type mice but not in the animals lacking EP3 receptors (Kunikata et al., 2001).

Apparently, the protection in the stomach is mediated by EP1 receptors, whereas that in the intestine is by EP3/EP4 receptors. EP2 is the major cAMP-generating PGE receptor expressed and regulated in the bovine uterus during the estrous cycle and early pregnancy (Arosh et al., 2003). PGF_2 is an important smooth muscle contractile agent acting on myometrium and implicated in labor, and blocking the PGF receptor (FP) significantly delays preterm delivery (Peri et al., 2002).

Cancer cells implanted in wild-type mice formed a tumor with extensive angiogenesis, which was suppressed by specific inhibitors of cyclooxygenase COX-2 (Amano et al., 2003). Signaling by host tissue PGE_2 acting at EP3 receptors apparently increases expression of vascular endothelial growth factor (VEGF) around the implants and aids tumor development and angiogenesis.

The four different PGE receptors (EP1, EP2, EP3, and EP4) mediate specific functions in different parts of the human kidney (Morath et al., 1999). The human EP1 receptor was mainly in connecting segments, cortical and medullary collecting ducts, and in the media of arteries and afferent and efferent arterioles. The human EP2 receptor was detectable only in the media of arteries and arterioles. The human EP3 receptor subtype protein was strongly expressed in glomeruli, Tamm-Horsfall negative late distal convoluted tubules, connecting segments, cortical and medullary collecting ducts, as well as in the media and the endothelial cells of arteries and arterioles. Human EP4 receptor was in glomeruli and in the media of arteries. However, neither receptor was detected in the thick ascending limb, the macula densa, or in adjacent juxtaglomerular cells.

Receptor Specificities

With diverse receptors mediating prostaglandin actions on different cells, knowledge of their selectivity for n-3 and n-6 autacoids is important to inform us about the likely impact of different food choices. Diet-driven changes in proportions of n-3 and n-6 autacoids may have strong effects with a discriminating receptor but not affect signaling through an indiscriminate one. To study receptor specificity, stable cell lines that individually express the eight known human prostanoid receptors (EP1, EP2, EP3, EP4, DP, FP, IP and TP) were made from human embryonic kidney cells and used in binding assays to determine the affinity and selectivity of known prostanoid receptor ligands with eight individual human prostanoid receptors (Abramovitz et al., 2000). Unfortunately this elegant experimental design was dedicated only to n-6 eicosanoids and pharmaceutical drug development in a way that gave no information on relative actions of n-3 and n-6 ligands to aid in the design of preventive nutrition studies.

References

Abramovitz M, Adam M, Boie Y, et al. The utilization of recombinant prostanoid receptors to determine the affinities and selectivities of prostaglandins and related analogs. *Biochim Biophys Acta* 1483(2):285-293, 2000.

Amano H, Hayashi I, Endo H, et al. Host prostaglandin E(2)-EP3 signaling regulates tumor-associated angiogenesis and tumor growth. *J Exp Med* 197(2):221-232, 2003.

Arosh JA, Banu SK, Chapdelaine P, et al. Molecular cloning and characterization of bovine prostaglandin E2 receptors EP2 and EP4: expression and regulation in endometrium and myometrium during the estrous cycle and early pregnancy. *Endocrinology* 144(7):3076-3091, 2003.

Beerthuis RK, Nugteren DH, Pabon HLJ, et al. Biologically active prostaglandins from some new odd-numbered essential fatty acids. *Red Trav Chim Pays Bas* 87:461-475, 1968.

Bergstrom S, Danielsson H, Samuelsson B. The enzymatic formation of prostaglandin E2 from arachidonic acid prostaglandins and related factors 32. *Biochim Biophys Acta* 90:207-210, 1964.

Chandrasekharan NV, Dai H, Roos KL, et al. COX-3, a cyclooxygenase-1 variant inhibited by acetaminophen and other analgesic/antipyretic drugs: cloning, structure, and expression. *Proc Natl Acad Sci* 99(21):13926-13931. Comment in: *Proc Natl Acad Sci* 99(21):13371-13373, 2002.

Chen W, Pawelek TR, Kulmacz RJ. Hydroperoxide dependence and cooperative cyclooxygenase kinetics in prostaglandin H synthase-1 and -2. *J Biol Chem* 274(29):20301-20306, 1999.

Culp BR, Titus, BG, Lands WEM. Inhibition of prostaglandin biosynthesis by eicosapentaenoic acid. *Prostaglandins Med* 3:269-278, 1979.

Dewitt DL, Meade EA, Smith WL. PGH synthase isoenzyme selectivity: the potential for safer nonsteroidal antiinflammatory drugs. *Am J Med* 95(Suppl. 2A):40S-44S, 1993.

Dyerberg J, Bang HO, Stofferson E, et al. Eicosapentaenoic acid and prevention of thrombosis and atherosclerosis? *Lancet* 2:117-119, 1978.

Dyerberg J, Jorgensen KA, Arnfred T. Human umbilical blood vessel converts all cis-5,8,11,14,17 eicosapentaenoic acid to prostaglandin 13. *Prostaglandins* 22:857-862, 1981.

Ferretti A, Schoene NW, Flanagan VP. Identification and quantification of prostaglandin E3 in renal medullary tissue of three strains of rats fed fish oil. *Lipids* 16:800-804, 1981.

Fischer S, Weber PC. Prostaglandin 13 is formed in vivo in man after dietary eicosapentaenoic acid. *Nature* 307:165-168, 1984.

Granstrom E, Samuelsson, B. Quantitative measurement of prostaglandins and thromboxanes: General considerations. *Adv Prostaglandin Thromboxane Res* 5:1-5, 1978.

Hanel AM, Lands WEM. Modification of antiinflammatory drug effectiveness by ambient lipid peroxides. *Biochem Pharmacology* 31:3307-3311, 1982.

Hamazaki T, Hirai A, Terano T, et al. Oral administration of eicosapentaenoic acid (EPA) stimulates production of prostacyclin .by rat aorta. *Thromb Haemostasis* 46:179, 1980.

Hamberg .M. Transformations of 5,8,11, 14, 17-eicosapentaenoic acid in human platelets. *Bioch Biophys Acta* 618:389-398, 1980.

Hamberg M, Samuelsson B. Novel biological transformation of 8,11,14-eicosatrienoic acid. *J Am Chem Soc* 88:2349, 1996.

Hamberg M, Samuelsson B. Detection and isolation of an endoperoxide intermediate in prostaglandin biosynthesis. *Proc Natl Acad Sci* 70:899-903, 1973.

Harizi H, Grosset C, Gualde N. Prostaglandin E2 modulates dendritic cell function via EP2 and EP4 receptor subtypes. *J Leukoc Biol* 73(6):756-763, 2003.

Hamazaki T, Hirai A, Terano T, et al. Effects of orally administered ethyl ester of eicosapentaenoic acid on PGI_2-like substrate production by rat aorta. *Prostaglandins* 23(4):557-567, 1982.

Herschman HR. Regulation of prostaglandin synthase-1 and prostaglandin synthase-2. *Cancer Metast* 13:241-256, 1994.

Hornstra, G., Christ-Hazelhof E, Haddeman E, et al. (1981). Fish oil feeding lowers thromboxane and prostacyclin production by rat platelets and aorta and does not result in the formation on prostaglandin I_3. *Prostaglandins* 21:727-738, 1981.

Kozak KR, Crews BC, Morrow JD, et al. Metabolism of the endocannabinoids, 2-arachidonylglycerol and anandamide, into prostaglandin, thromboxane, and prostacyclin glycerol esters and ethanolamides. *J Biol Chem* 277(47):44877-44885, 2002.

Knapp HR, Salem N Jr. Formation of PGI_3 in the rat during dietary fish oil supplementation. *Prostaglandins* 38(5):509-521, 1989.

Kulmacz RJ, Wang LH. Comparison of hydroperoxide initiator requirements for the cyclooxygenase activities of prostaglandin H synthase-1 and -2. *J Biol Chem* 270(41):24019-24023, 1995.

Kunikata T, Araki H, Takeeda M, et al. Prostaglandin E prevents indomethacin-induced gastric and intestinal damage through different EP receptor subtypes. *J Physiol Paris* 95(1-6):157-163, 2001.

Kunikata T, Tanaka A, Miyazawa T, et al. 16,16-Dimethyl prostaglandin E2 inhibits indomethacin-induced small intestinal lesions through EP3 and EP4 receptors. *Dig Dis Sci* 47(4):894-904, 2002.

Lands WEM. The biosynthesis and metabolism of prostaglandins. *Ann Rev Physiol* 41:633-652, 1979.

Lands WEM, Byrnes MJ. The influence of ambient peroxides on the conversion of 5,8,ll,14,17-eicosapentaenoic acid to prostaglandins. *Prog Lipid Res* 20:287-290, 1982.

Lands WEM, Hanel AM. Phenolic anti-cyclooxygenase agents and hypotheses of antiinflammatory therapy. *Prostaglandins* 24:271-278, 1982.

Lands WEM, Lettellier PB, Rome LH, et al. Inhibition of prostaglandin biosynthesis. *Adv Biosci* 9:15-28, 1973.

Laneuville O, Breuer DK, Xu N, et al. Fatty acid substrate specificities of human prostaglandin-endoperoxide H synthase-1 and -2. Formation of 12-hydroxy-(9Z, 13E/Z, 15Z)- octadecatrienoic acids from alpha-linolenic acid. *J Biol Chem* 270(33):19330-19336, 1995.

Malkowski MG, Thuresson ED, Lakkides KM, et al. Structure of eicosapentaenoic and linoleic acids in the cyclooxygenase site of prostaglandin endoperoxide H synthase-1. *J Biol Chem* 276(40):37547-37555, 2001.

Miggin SM, Lawler OA, Kinsella BT. Investigation of a functional requirement for isoprenylation by the human prostacyclin receptor. *Eur J Biochem* 269(6):1714-1725, 2002.

Miles EA, Aston L, Calder PC. In vitro effects of eicosanoids derived from different 20-carbon fatty acids on T helper type 1 and T helper type 2 cytokine production in human whole-blood cultures. *Clin Exp Allergy* 33(5):624-632, 2003.

Morath R, Klein T, Seyberth HW, et al. Immunolocalization of the four prostaglandin E2 receptor proteins EP1, EP2, EP3, and EP4 in human kidney. *J Am Soc Nephrol* 10(9):1851-1860, 1999.

Morita I, Saito Y, Chang WC, et al. Effects of purified eicosapentaenoic acid on arachidonic acid metabolism in cultured murine aortic smooth muscle cells, vessel walls and platelets. *Lipids* 18:42-49, 1983.

Needleman P, Raz A, Minkas MS, et al. Triene prostaglandins: Prostacyclin and thromboxane biosynthesis and unique biological properties. *Proc Natl Acad Sci* 76:944-948, 1979.

Needleman P, Sprecher H, Whitaker MO, et al. Mechanism underlying the inhibition of platelet aggregation by Eicosapentaenoic acid and its metabolites. *Adv Prostaglandin Thromboxane Res* 6:61-68, 1980.

Oka T, Oka K, Scammell TE, et al. Relationship of EP(1-4) prostaglandin receptors with rat hypothalamic cell groups involved in lipopolysaccharide fever responses. *J Comp Neurol* 428(1):20-32, 2000.

Paralkar VM, Borovecki F, Ke HZ, et al. An EP2 receptor-selective prostaglandin E2 agonist induces bone healing. *Proc Natl Acad Sci* 100(11):6736-6740, 2003.

Peri KG, Quiniou C, Hou X, et al. THG113: a novel selective FP antagonist that delays preterm labor. *Semin Perinatol* 26(6):389-397, 2002.

Ramesha CS, Gronke RS, Sivarajan M et al. Metabolic products of arachidonic acid in rats. *Prostaglandins* 29:991-1008, 1985.

Roberts IS, Carison IC, McCracken JA. Prostaglandin F. production by the brain and its role in LH secretion. *Adv Prostaglandin Thromboxane Res* 2:609-619, 1976.

Smith WL, DeWitt DL, Garavito RM. Cyclooxygenases: structural, cellular, and molecular biology. *Ann Rev Biochem* 69:145-182, 2000.

Struijk CB, Beerthuis RK, Pabon H, et al. Specificity in the enzymic conversion of polyunsaturated fatty acids into prostaglandins *Rec Trav Chim Pays Bas* 85:1233, 1966.

Swinney DC, Mak AY, Barnett J, et al. Differential allosteric regulation of prostaglandin H synthase 1 and 2 by arachidonic acid. *J Biol Chem* 272(19):12393-12398, 1997.

Tan WC, Privett OS. Studies on the synthesis of prostaglandins in the vesicular glands of essential fatty acid deficient and hypophysectomized rats. *Biohem Biophys Acta* 296:586-592, 1973

Ushikubi F, Sugimoto Y, Ichikawa A, et al. Roles of prostanoids revealed from studies using mice lacking specific prostanoid receptors. *Jpn J Pharmacol* 83(4):279-285, 2000.

Van Dorp DA, Beerthuis RK, Nugteren DH, et al. The biosynthesis of prostaglandins. *Biochim Biophys Acta* 90:204-207, 1964

Warso M,Lands WEM. Presence of lipid hydroperoxide in human plasma. *J Clin Invest* 75:667-671, 1985.

Ziboh VA, Vanderhoek JY, Lands WEM. Inhibition of sheep vesicular gland oxygenase by unsaturated fatty acids from skin of essential fatty acid deficient rats *Prostaglandins* 5:233-241, 1974.

2005 National Library of Medicine Search Results:

(http://www.ncbi.nlm.nih.gov/entrez/query.fcgi)

cyclooxygenase = 24,912; Cyclooxygenase NSAID = 14,254; Cyclooxygenase omega-3 = 260

COX-1 = 2,475 ; COX-2 = 6,886; COX-3 = 41; NSAID = 124,982

prostaglandin synthase= 11,180; Prostaglandin isomerases= 1,675; Prostaglandin receptor= 3,038

isoprostanes = 1023

15—Prostaglandin Formation Following Changes in Diet

An area of research requiring further evaluation is that of determining dynamic time-dependent patterns in the abundance of various eicosanoids that are produced by different tissues during the course of a day. Such studies might permit a more careful description of the influence of diet on the physiology of eicosanoids formed from essential fatty acids. Individuals with different diets will have different proportions of arachidonate in tissue HUFA that affect the intensities in eicosanoid signaling. Exaggerated n-6 eicosanoid responses in some individuals who overreact to stimuli could cause development of a disease state that does not occur in people with lower proportions of arachidonate in their HUFA.

Wide variations seem to occur in the minute-to-minute production of eicosanoids as our tissues respond to stimuli, and the various eicosanoids formed are rapidly inactivated and excreted in the urine. Because of rapid degradation and inactivation, the autacoids act only over short distances and short times with only metabolites left to record their transient presence. As a result, medical researchers have analyzed the metabolites in urine as an index of the total daily eicosanoid production. Unfortunately, such results give little insight into the diverse moment-by-moment intensities of the transient events in different tissues of the body.

Attempts to characterize the production of prostaglandins in living animals or in people by measuring metabolites in the blood or urine are frustrating because the distant and delayed measurements can not indicate the transient intensity of autacoid signaling at local tissue receptors. The time required for collecting and analyzing prostaglandin metabolites prevents knowing the variable intensity of formation that may occur transiently at specific tissue sites at any given time during the day. The analytical results with metabolites allow only a crude index of overall "throughput" of arachidonate to prostaglandin. Also, a slow rate of synthesis could allow all newly formed autacoids to be inactivated to metabolites without ever reaching a receptor and providing a physiological signal.

This slow ineffective state might have a cumulative overall daily formation of eicosanoid metabolites similar to that resulting from states with multiple sharp pulsatile formation events that give active intermittent signaling that markedly affects tissue physiology. Difficulty in interpreting the results of prostaglandin formation from monitoring blood or urine metabolites led to diminished efforts over the years. Nevertheless, such measures remain in use for global measures of overall daily eicosanoid mobilization.

Because of the limitations described previously, this chapter has not been expanded for 2005. In contrast to the decreased interest in monitoring metabolites, the obvious influence of diet on the precursors in tissue HUFA raises interest in reliably monitoring diet-tissue changes with gas chromatographic analyses. The proportions of n-6 HUFA eicosanoid precursors that are likely to be released during a response also predict the likely relative intensity of an eicosanoid response.

Monitoring newly recognized HUFA metabolites, the 20-carbon *isoprostanes* and 22-carbon *neuroprostanes* gives useful monitoring of the overall body burden of oxidant stress rather than monitoring physiological self-healing responses (Roberts and Morrow, 2002; Youssef et al., 2003; Fam and Morrow, 2003). These two new types of biomarker are just some of a large number of different prostaglandin-like oxidized products that are now known. However at the present time, little evidence suggests whether these biomarkers of oxidant stress directly mediate disease processes or whether their observed relative abundance indicates any metabolic selectivity for either n-3 or n-6 forms that may help interpret diet-disease links.

An early study by Seyberth et al. (1975) demonstrated that administering ethyl arachidonate to healthy male volunteers at a level of 6 g daily during a 2 to 3 week period caused a 47% increase in the major urinary metabolite of PGE. Because of a corresponding increased thrombotic tendency indicated by a decrease in the threshold dose of ADP required for platelet aggregation, 2 of the 4 volunteers were removed from the study to preclude any misfortune. The very dramatic increase in the sensitivity of the platelets to aggregation observed 12-14 days after starting the diet returned to control levels 2 weeks after the arachidonate supplementation was discontinued. The study showed that some important eicosanoid responses to diet occur much more rapidly to diet changes than the slow adaptation of adipose tissue to dietary linoleate.

Using an analytical procedure developed by Nugteren in 1975, Adam et al. (1982) demonstrated that increasing amounts of dietary linoleic acid led to increased amounts in the urine of the major metabolites, tetranorprostanedioic acid derivatives. Individuals on a conventional diet produced 300 micrograms (μg) per day whereas those temporarily eating a diet with no linoleate produced only 123 μg per day (however, adipose tissue was likely unchanged). Supplementation at 4 and 20 en% linoleate led to 175 μg per day and 350 μg per day, respectively. These results illustrate what a small fraction of the total daily EFA appears to be converted to prostaglandins; only 380 μg were detected as the tetranorprostanedioic acid derivatives of the 68,000,000 μg of linoleate that were consumed. In general, the results suggest that a higher intake of n-6 polyunsaturated fatty acids leads to greater prostaglandin biosynthesis. The results are inadequate in helping us determine whether dietary arachidonate is 100 or 1000 times more effective than linoleate in influencing our daily eicosanoid output. The difference between eating 18-carbon EFA or 20-carbon HUFA could have an important influence on our responses to stimuli.

A somewhat different analytical result was reported by Friedman (1982) who noted that 20% of daily calories (20 en%) as linoleate fed to infants decreased the amount of prostaglandin E metabolite to a level comparable to that observed in EFA-deficient infants. A recovery period in which the infants received 5-10 calorie percent of linoleate returned the daily PG metabolite levels to the control value. The decreased formation of the PG metabolite in infants receiving very high levels of linoleate (megadoses) may also diminish the arachidonate available for prostaglandin biosynthesis. However, withdrawal from the "megadose" regimen led rapidly to higher production of prostaglandins. The physiological impact of these changes remains undefined.

Brongeest-Schoute et al. (1981) reported that when either cod liver oil or corn oil in the diet decreased the aggregation of platelets and their production of thromboxane, the levels of total urinary prostaglandin metabolites were still unchanged. Similarly, Hansen and Jensen (1982) saw no significant effect of eicosapentaenoic acid administration on urinary excretion of PGE. In the latter case, it is important to note that the measurement in the urine of PGE itself (rather than its metabolites) does not reflect the many other prostanoic metabolites formed in nonrenal tissues and excreted in the urine. The data at present provide clear evidence that diet can alter prostaglandin production in humans, but leave unanswered the question of whether diets rich in n-3 fats that diminish platelet aggregation will alter significantly the total daily urinary metabolites.

References

Adam O, Wolfram G, Zollner N. Prostaglandin formation in man during intake of different amounts of linoleic acid in formula diets. *Ann Nutr Metab* 26:315-323, 1982.

Brongeest-Schoute HC, van Gent CM, et al. The effect of various intakes of n-3 fatty acids on the blood lipid composition in healthy human subjects. *Am J Clin Nutr* 34:1752-1757, 1981.

Brox JH, Killie J-E, Gunnes S, et al. The effect of cod liver oil and corn oil on platelets and vessel wall in man. *Thromb Haemostasis* 46(3):604-611, 1981.

Fam SS, Morrow JD. The isoprostanes: unique products of arachidonic acid oxidation - a review. *Curr Med Chem* 10(17):1623-1740, 2003.

Friedman Z. Effects of dietary variation in linoleic acid Content on prostaglandin synthesis in infants. *Prog Lipid Res* 20:59-66, 1982.

Friedman Z, Oates L. Effects of dietary variation in linoleic acid content on platelet aggregation and the major urinary metabolites of the E prostaglandins (PGE-M) in infants. *Atheroscler Rev* 8:69-86, 1981.

Hansen HS, Jensen B. Urinary PGE excretion in essential fatty acid-deficient (EFA-D), and in ethyl linolenate-fed rats. In. *Prostaglandins-Vth International Conference*. Florence, Italy 1982, p 699.

Roberts LJ 2nd, Morrow JD. Products of the isoprostane pathway: unique bioactive compounds and markers of lipid peroxidation. *Cell Mol Life Sci* 59(5):808-820, 2002.

Seyberth HW, Oelz O, Kennedy T, et al. Increased arachidonate in lipids after administration to man: Effects on prostaglandin biosynthesis. *Clin Pharmacol Ther* 18:521-529, 1975.

Youssef JA, Birnbaum LS, Swift LL, et al. Age-independent, gray matter-localized, brain-enhanced oxidative stress in male Fischer 344 rats: brain levels of F(2)-isoprostanes and F(4)-neuroprostanes. *Free Radic Biol Med* 34(12):1631-1635, 2003.

2005 National Library of Medicine Search Results:

(http://www.ncbi.nlm.nih.gov/entrez/query.fcgi)
prostaglandin metabolites = 4,091; prostaglandin metabolites diet = 132

16—Pathways to Leukotrienes

Leukotrienes are potent eicosanoids that cause smooth muscle contraction, bronchoconstriction, increased vascular permeability and edema. Their discovery has greatly aided our understanding of the mechanisms underlying the immune immediate hypersensitivity reactions and asthma (Dahlen et al., 1983).

The lipoxygenase pathway which converts polyunsaturated fatty acids into leukotrienes (LTB, LTC, LTD, etc.) represents an alternate set of reactions for interpreting the potent autacoid actions of polyunsaturated fatty acids (Murphy et al., 1979; Samuelsson et al., 1980). In these conversions, the double bonds of the substrate fatty acid are retained in the molecule (see Fig. 16-1), but they are rearranged into a conjugated triene pattern which absorbs ultraviolet light strongly at 280 nm. Thus, the leukotrienes derived from arachidonate (20:4n-6) contain four double bonds and those from eicosapentaenoic (20:5n-3), five double bonds. Formation of leukotriene A (LTA) from the 5-hydroperoxide intermediate may be catalyzed by the lipoxygenase (Shimizu et al., 1984).

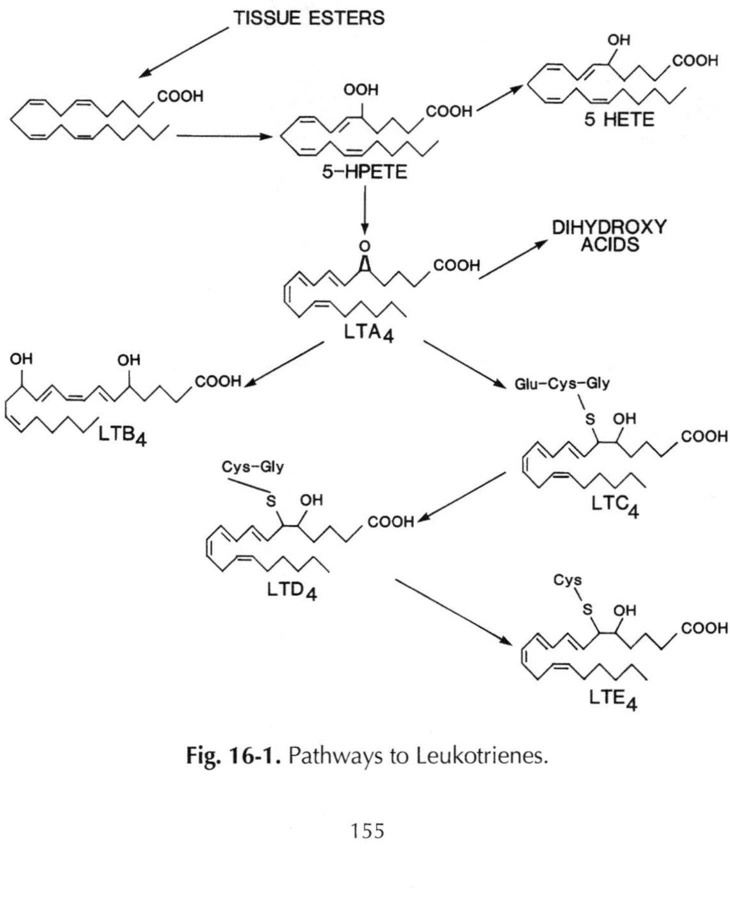

Fig. 16-1. Pathways to Leukotrienes.

The specificity for 5-lipoxygenase catalyzed formation of biologically active leukotrienes from a variety of fatty acids depends on the presence of the 5,6 double bond as described by Jakschik et al. (1980) (see Table 16-1). The hydroxy derivative HETE, is frequently the most abundant product being formed in vitro from the 5 hydroperoxy intermediate by reduction catalyzed by cellular peroxidases. The other products, LTC and LTD, are responsible for most of the slow reacting substance (SRS) activity observed. Smooth muscle contracting activity was reported to be high with products formed from 20:3n-9, 20:4n-6, and 20:5n-3 although several workers indicated that there is significantly lower activity for LTC_5 derived from 20:5n-3 relative to that for LTC_4 derived from 20:4n-6. Further studies should clarify whether the discrimination observed is due to CysLT1 or CysLT2 receptors (see later discussion).

Incubation of mastocytoma cells with 80 nmoles of eicosapentaenoic acid (20:5n-3) yielded 6.4 nmoles of the leukotriene C_5 (Hammarström, 1980; 1981). At the same time, 200 nmoles of leukotriene C_4 were formed from the endogenous arachidonate (20:4n-6) of the cells. Apparently the endogenous n-6 fatty acid was much more effectively utilized than the exogenous n-3 acid. The results of Murphy et al. (1981) gave a more direct comparison of the relative efficiencies of leukotriene biosynthesis with these two fatty acids when they come simultaneously from the endogenous phospholipids of mastocytoma cells. Cells were grown either in mice eating standard chow diets or mice raised from birth on a diet enriched with fish oil fatty acids, containing low proportions of arachidonate in the HUFA.

Similar proportions of two HUFA in mastocytoma phospholipids (3.9% 20:4n-6 and 4.5% 20:5n-3) led to similar amounts of LTB_4 and LTB_5. This result suggests

TABLE 16-1
Selectivities for Fatty Acid in Leukotriene Synthesis by RBL-1 Cell Homogenates[a,b]

	HETE Formed	SRS Activity
18:4n-4	37	moderate
19:4n-5	43	moderate
20:3n-9	31	high
20:4n-6	26	high
20:5n-3	34	high
19:4n-6	9	low
19:5n-3	10	very low
20:3n-6	7	low
20:4n-3	10	low
21:4n-6	7	very low
21:5n-6	7	very low
22:4n-6	7	low

[a]Data from Jakschik et al. (1980).
[b]The first five acids listed have 5, 8, 11 double bonds.

that both acids are mobilized and converted with similar efficiencies to the leukotriene epoxide derivative, LTA, when the cells were activated. However, in contrast to the similar amounts of LTB derivatives, the amount of LTC_4 was ten-fold greater than LTC_5. This indicated that LTC synthase action on LTA may be selective and depend on the structure of the unsaturated fatty acid. This apparent ten-fold greater tendency of the n-6 LTA to react with LTC synthase rather than the expoxide hydrolase may lead to different degrees of edema and inflammatory responses in ischemic tissues when eicosapentaenoic acid is abundant.

The formation of similar amounts of LTB_4 and LTB_5 merits further interpretation since the pentaenoic compound (LTB_5) was only about 5-10% as active as LTB_4 in stimulating neutrophils (Lee et al. 1984, Goldman et al. 1983) and 500-fold less able to bind to the high affinity receptor on neutrophils (Goldman et al., 1983) Thus, the effect of the n-3 HUFA in tissues is to decrease the amount of leukotriene B formed and to also give a less potent leukotriene (Prescott, 1984). At the present time, relatively little is known about the selectivity for the different unsaturated acyl chains of the lipoxygenase or the other synthase enzymes. Also, competition of n-3 with n-6 acids, which was clearly evident for the cyclooxygenase activity (Lands, 1973; Corey 1983), still remains to be demonstrated for mammalian lipoxygenase activity. Present evidence suggests that dietary fish oil can diminish the in situ biosynthesis of leukotrienes (Terano et al., 1984). This may have an important consequence in modifying some leukocyte responses in our immune system.

Other Lipoxygenase Products

Another lipoxygenase activity found in platelets converts either arachidonate or eicosapentaenoate to a 12-hydroxy derivative, presumably by way of the 12-hydroperoxide (Hamberg, 1980). This enzyme appears to act in platelets separately from TXA_2 formation, and its physiological significance is not well defined. Many different lipoxygenases form oxidized products that are somewhat related to leukotrienes and different from 5-lipoxygenase products of AA, 20:4n-6, shown in Fig. 16-1. However, the physiological significance of these oxidized materials (HETE, HODE, lipoxins, hepoxylin, resolvins, etc.) remains an active area of research (e.g., Serhan and Chiang, 2004).

The five aspects that control prostaglandin formation and action described in Chapter 14 parallel those that control leukotriene formation and action, and they are not repeated here. However, one important difference that relates to food choices is the fact that 5-lipoxygenase does not discriminate between n-3 and n-6 substrates like the cyclooxygenase does. Rather, leukotriene A of both n-3 and n-6 types seem provided at comparable speeds to tissue synthases, leaving synthase and receptor specificity as the most likely sites where diet choices may impact with leukotriene effects on health.

The dramatically greater signaling through the LTB receptor, BLT, by LTB_4 over LTB_5 gives strong motivation for studying further effects of dietary n-3 and n-6 intakes on the immune inflammatory events noted earlier in this book. Unfortunately, specificities in different tissues for n-3 and n-6 ligands of the leukotriene synthases and receptors (like those for the prostaglandin synthases) are still not yet characterized sufficiently to interpret their importance in human health. Some of what we have learned recently is shown below to illustrate what further answers we need to understand the impact of dietary EFA on health.

The n-6 leukotrienes, LTB_3 and LTB_4, cause similar dose- and time-dependent pro-inflammatory enhancement of complement receptors and release of lysozyme, whereas the n-3 LTB_5 was approximately 100 times less potent than LTB_4 in enhancing complement receptors and 10,000 times less potent than LTB_4 in releasing lysozyme from human neutrophils (Lee et al., 1988). In chemotactic attraction of human neutrophils, LTB_5 was 100-fold less potent than LTB_4 (and LTB_3 was only 5-fold weaker). The high affinity of leukotriene B_4 for the leukotriene B (BLT) receptor (Kd approx. 0.4 nM) is very similar in human, mouse and guinea pig (Boie et al., 1999). The guinea pig and human BLT receptors couple to the signaling pathway that inhibits cAMP formation and the one mobilizing intracellular Ca^{2+}. The relative potency in competition for [^{3}H]-LTB_4 binding is leukotriene B_4 >20-OH-leukotriene B_4 >12(R)-HETE ((5Z,8Z,10E,12(R)14Z)- 12-hydroxyeicosatetraen-1-oic acid) > 12(S)-HETE ((5Z,8Z,10E,12(S)14Z)- 12-hydroxyeicosatetraen-1-oic acid) >>> leukotriene C_4 = leukotriene D_4 = leukotriene E_4.

The cysteinyl leukotrienes, derived from eicosapentaenoic acid (LTC_5 and LTD_5) seem five times less damaging than those derived from arachidonic acid (LTC_4 and LTD_4), in terms of susceptibility of gastric mucosa to damage and reducing gastric blood flow (Wallace and McKnight, 1990). Contractile and inflammatory actions of the cysteinyl leukotrienes, LTC_4, LTD_4, and LTE_4, are mediated by at least two distinct G protein-coupled receptors, CysLT1 and CysLT2, which elevate intracellular calcium when activated. The human CysLT1-receptor gene maps to the X chromosome, and CysLT1 messenger RNA was found in spleen, peripheral blood leukocytes and in smooth muscle cells and tissue macrophages of lung (Lynch et al., 1999). The CysLT2 gene maps to chromosome 13q14, a region linked to atopic asthma, and CysLT2 receptor mRNA was detected in lung macrophages and airway smooth muscle, cardiac Purkinje cells, adrenal medulla cells, peripheral blood leukocytes, and brain (Heise et al., 2000).

Competition for [^{3}H]LTC_4 binding in lung tissue followed LTC_2 > LTC_3 > LTC_4 > LTC_5 >>> LTD_4 and LTB_4 (Metters et al., 1994), suggesting a possible stronger signaling by the n-6 autacoid. The mouse cysteinyl-leukotriene D(4) receptor (mCysLT(1)R) has 87% amino acid identity with the human CysLT(1) receptor (hCysLT(1)R) and binds leukotriene D_4 (LTD_4, K(d) = 0.25 nM), 100-fold more tightly than LTE_4 and LTC_4 and 6,000-fold more than LTB_4 (Martin et al., 2001).

References

Boie Y, Stocco R, Sawyer N, et al. Characterization of the cloned guinea pig leukotriene B4 receptor: comparison to its human orthologue. *Eur J Pharmacol* 380(2-3):203-213, 1999.

Corey EJ., Shih C, Cashman JR. Docosahexaenoic acid is a strong inhibitor of prostaglandin but not leukotriene biosynthesis. *Proc Natl Acad Sci* 80:3581-3584, 1983.

Dahlen S.-E, Hansson G, Hedqvist P, et al. Allergen challenge of lung tissue from asthmatics elicits bronchial contraction that correlates with the release of leukotrienes C4, D4, and E4. *Proc Natl Acad Sci* 80:1712-1716, 1983.

Goldman DW, Pickett WC, Goetzl EL. Human neutrophil chemotactic and degranulating activities of leukotriene B5 (LTB5) derived from eicosapentaenoic acid. *Biochem Biophys Res Commun* 117:282-288, 1983.

Hamberg M. Transformations of 5,8,11,14,17-eicosapentaenoic acid in human platelets. *Biochim Biophys Acta* 618:389-398, 1980.

Hammarström S. Leukotriene C5: A slow reacting substance derived from eicosa pentaenoic acid. *J Biol Chem* 255:7093-7094, 1980.

Hammarström S. Conversion of 14C-labeled eicosapentaenoic acid (n-3) to leukotriene C5. *Biochim Biophys Acta* 663:575-577, 1981.

Heise CE, O'Dowd BF, Figueroa DJ, et al. Characterization of the human cysteinyl leukotriene 2 receptor. *J Biol Chem* 275(39):30531-30536, 2000.

Jakschik BA, Sams AR, Sprecher H, et al. Fatty acid structural requirements for leukotriene biosynthesis. *Prostaglandins* 20:401-410, 1980.

Lands WEM, Letellier PE, Rome LH, et al. Inhibition of prostaglandin biosynthesis. *Adv Biosci* 9:15-28, 1973.

Lee TF, Mencia-Huerta J-M, et al. Characterization and biologic properties of 5,12-dihydroxy derivatives of eicosapentaenoic acid, including leukotriene B5 and the double lipoxygenase product. *J Biol Chem* 259: 2383-2389, 1984.

Lee TH, Sethi T, Crea AE, et al. Characterization of leukotriene B3: comparison of its biological activities with leukotriene B4 and leukotriene B5 in complement receptor enhancement, lysozyme release and chemotaxis of human neutrophils. *Clin Sci* 74(5):467-475, 1988.

Lynch KR, O'Neill GP, Liu Q, et al. Characterization of the human cysteinyl leukotriene CysLT1 receptor. *Nature* 24:789-793, 1999.

Martin V, Sawyer N, Stocco R. Molecular cloning and functional characterization of murine cysteinyl-leukotriene 1 (CysLT(1)) receptors. *Biochem Pharmacol* 62(9):1193-2000, 2001.

Metters KM, Gareau Y, Lord A, et al. Characterization of specific binding sites for cysteinyl leukotrienes in sheep lung. *J Pharmacol Exp Ther* 270(1):399-406, 1994.

Murphy RC, Hammarström S, Samuelsson B. Leukotriene C: A slow-reacting substance from murine mastocytoma cells. *Proc Natl Acad Sci.* 76:4275-4279, 1979.

Murphy RC, Pickett WC, Culp BR, et al. Tetraene and pentaene leukotrienes: Selective production from murine mastocytonia cells after dietary manipulation. *Prostaglandins* 22:613-622, 1981.

Prescott SM. The effect of eicosapentaenoic acid on leukotriene B production by human neutrophils. *J Biol Chem* 259:7615-7621, 1984.

Samuelsson B, Borgeat P, Hammarstrom S, et al. Leukotrienes: A new group of biologically active compounds. In Samuelsson B, Ramwell PW, Paoletti R (eds.). *Advances in Prostaglandin and Thromboxane Research*, vol. 6. New York: Raven Press, 1980, pp 1-18.

Serhan CN, Chiang N. Novel endogenous small molecules as the checkpoint controllers in inflammation and resolution: entree for resoleomics. *Rheum Dis Clin North Am* 30(1):69-95, 2004.

Shimizu T, Radmark O, Samuelsson B. Enzyme with dual lipoxygenase activities catalyzes leukotriene A4 synthesis from arachidonic acid. *Proc Natl Acad Sci* 81:689-693, 1984.

Terano T, Salmon JA, Moncada S. Effect of orally administered eicosapentaenoic acid (EPA) on the formation of leukotreine B4 and leukotriene B5 by rat leukocytes. *Biochem Pharmacol* 33:3071-3076, 1984.

Wallace JL, McKnight GW. Comparison of the damage-promoting effects of leukotrienes derived from eicosapentaenoic acid and arachidonic acid on the rat stomach. *J Exp Med* 171(5):1827-1832, 1990.

2005 National Library of Medicine Search Results:

(http://www.ncbi.nlm.nih.gov/entrez/query.fcgi)
leukotriene = 15,177; leukotriene receptor = 1,584; leukotriene omega-3 = 306;
lipoxygenase = 11,290; lipoxygenase omega-3 = 287
lipoxin = 465; lipoxin omega-3 = 21

Part 3—Choosing Diets

In crowds,
Each person
Makes
A choice
Alone.

17—Polyunsaturated Acids in Tissues and Foods

Each of us may choose very different foods when we are free to select what we want to eat. And the foods may vary greatly from day to day. If eicosanoids are formed from the small tissue pools of rapidly changing nonesterified acids, then even day-to-day changes in diet can affect the amount and type of eicosanoid formed by our tissues. Researchers do not yet know what influence short-term changes in diet have on eicosanoid actions.

Since diseases involving eicosanoids are long-term and short-term, we can start understanding them by interpreting evidence available on long-term diet choices. Much long-term evidence averages many variables involved in day-to-day changes and gives results "averaged over time." These resemble some of the general epidemiologic clues in Chapter 1 that gave averages of many individual food choices. General information available on human diets consists of many different specific observations grouped as a whole; however, these often may ignore possible metabolic differences among individuals and day-to-day differences in foods eaten.

Even as Eskimos, Danes, Japanese and North Americans have many similar traits, certain differences among these groups (and of individuals among a given group) must be recognized and interpreted. Some Americans, Danes, or Japanese might consume foods similar to those of average Eskimos, but most do not. People need a way to estimate whether their personal dietary intakes, tissue HUFA, and eicosanoid responses meet the goals they want to achieve. Ways to predict what eicosanoid responses are likely for a given dietary balance of polyunsaturated fatty acids also need to be developed. Other questions that need to be addressed include:

- How to confirm the balance of n-3 and n-6 acids consumed by an individual during the past months?
- Can researchers recommend some proportions of n-3 and n-6 acids in the diet that would have a desirable potential for making the "right" amount of eicosanoids?
- Considering the nutritional factors involved in complex diseases, we need more definitive information on how dietary habits affected the tissue HUFA of those with the disease—not just the average dietary and disease data for the general population of the individual's native country.

Bang et al. (1976, 1980) indicated that the amounts of individual fatty acids (expressed as average percent of all fatty acids) measured in food consumed by village Eskimos relative to those in the food of urbanized Danes, were as follows: 18:2n-6, 4.7/10.0; 18:3n-3, 0.4/2.0; 20:4n-6, 0.1/0; 20:5n-3, 2.3/0.4; and 22:6n-3,

2.2/0.3. These values show that the average total intake of n-6 acids (linoleate and arachidonate) by Eskimos was about one half that of the Danes although total fat intake was similar. Eskimos consumed about equal amounts of n-3 relative to n-6 fatty acids, whereas people in the Western nations tended to consume much less n-3 relative to n-6 fatty acids.

Diverse Daily Intakes

The average consumption of fats by a given population reflects the combined effects of the average supply and demand. For example, when vegetable foods are scarce, Australian Aborigines tend to ingest tropical sea foods which contain 4.8-14.3% 20:4n-6, 13-30% n-3 fatty acids in the fat and almost no 18:2n-6 (O'Dea and Sinclair, 1982). This shift might lead to seasonal changes in the daily eicosanoid production. When the annual fish harvest was poor in a Japanese fishing village, the villagers had a lower average intake of n-3 fatty acids in their diet that year as their livelihood depends on selling whatever fish they caught. This need resulted in their diets being much more similar to that of the farming villagers that year.

The amount of body fat that accumulates in the human body provides a reservoir of fatty acids that continually mixes with the daily intake of fat. The amount of stored fat is often so great that more than a year is needed for it to respond to a diet-induced change (Hirsch et al., 1960). In fact, progressive increases in the linoleate content of adipose tissue were observed over several years for patients on a diet containing 9-11% of their calories as linoleate (Christakis et al., 1965). Apparently, even three years did not fully equilibrate body fat with the diet. Individuals adhering to the diet for three years did have about 19% of the body fat as linoleate. This corresponds to daily intakes of fat, of which 28.8% is linoleate or 22 g of linoleate per day based on the equations of Beynen et al. (1980). A similar study in California showed that serum triglycerides (of people on a three-year diet) contained about 33% linoleate, higher than the content in body fat, but closely resembling that for dietary fat (Dayton et al., 1966).

To estimate the relative amount of ingested polyunsaturated fatty acids, medical scientists analyzed adipose tissue biopsies. The percentage of linoleate in adipose fat related to the amount of linoleate eaten per day: % 18:2 in fat=7.44 + 0.52 x [g 18:2/day]. This relationship allows medical researchers to estimate the average daily amount consumed by measuring a biopsy sample of the body fat (Beynen et al., 1980). Also, the relative percentage of linoleate in the body fat relates to its average relative percentage in the foods eaten: % 18:2 in body fat=3.43 + 0.54 x [% 18:2 in dietary fats].

In one study (Albutt and Chance, 1969), only half the patients on a long-term (four to seven years) prescribed diet rich in linoleate had tissue linoleate significantly higher than those on a standard diet. However, a check of the compliance confirmed that most of the patients did not adhere to the prescribed diet; some objected to the food restrictions; and others found it unpalatable.

The situation seems common when special diets are recommended. People do not generally follow diets that are either too restricted or too different from their customary ones. Whatever food choices you make based on the information in this book, your revised diet will be easier to maintain if you have selected a variety of foods—many of us humans find it difficult to be regimented for long periods unless by personal choice.

Large-scale shifts in the average consumer demand for different compositions of food oils occurred over the years. Taylor et al. (1979) noted that the British diet shifted over a 40 year period (1935-1975). It went from an annual per capita consumption of 2.6 kg 18:2n-6 plus 0.41 kg of 18:3n-3 to one of 4.3 kg 18:2n-6 and 0.43 kg 18:3n-3. Note that a seven-fold increase in deaths from coronary heart disease accompanied that increase in dietary linoleate.

Another retrospective view of national average British dietary trends (Katan and Beynen, 1981) reported that during the 15 year-period of 1960-1975 linoleate (8% 18:2n6) in the body fat of the British population was unchanged. However, it seemed to increase in the adipose tissue of Americans from 8% to 16%. One might infer from that result that there was a higher intake of linoleate-rich fats and oils in America than in Britain. From the equation of Beynen et a1. (1980), we can estimate that the American diet may have shifted from 8.5 g per day to 23 g per day during those decades. The apparent lack of change in the average linoleate content of dietary fats in Britain parallels the unchanged mortality rate for heart disease during that period, and suggests that the increased linoleate consumption noted by Taylor et al. (1979) had occurred between 1935 and 1960.

The linoleate intakes in Britain were appreciably greater than the 1% of daily calories needed in the form of n-6 fatty acids (see Chapter 3), and they may have led to exaggerated eicosanoid responses. Of course, many other factors related to changes in lifestyle or medical procedures influence mortality rates. Dietary factors alone cannot explain all the differences. Nevertheless, industrialized nations are now at a point where it seems both necessary and possible to develop a clearer view of a desirable nutritional balance of n-3 and n-6 fatty acids. If we wish to lower risk factors for the diseases noted in earlier chapters, can we agree on the proportions of tissue HUFA that achieve such lowering? If some agreement develops, we then will have to find a variety of suitable food sources to provide the desired proportions of dietary n-3 and n-6 EFA.

Diverse Tissue HUFA

Health and disease depend on eicosanoid-mediated events that reflect the proportions of HUFA available in tissue membranes. Since tissue HUFA come only from the consumption of EFA, the proportions of the essential n-3 and n-6 acids in food determine the proportions stored in tissues. Voluntary food choices give human tissue HUFA proportions of n-6 HUFA ranging from 15% to 90% (Fig. 1-3 [Chapter 1]). Fig. 17-1 shows how the n-6 HUFA compete with the n-3 HUFA for placement in tissue lipids. Knowing the quantitative competitions in the diet-tissue relationship for essential fatty acids is very important for health professionals to design effective credible programs of primary prevention with nutrition education for the public. Experiments funded by the 1985 Pfizer Biomedical Research Award allowed me to develop an empirical quantitative metabolic relationship (Lands et al., 1992) that gives new ways to educate professionals and the public for primary prevention of diseases caused by excessive n-6 eicosanoid actions.

The first edition of this book (1986) noted the problem of using only average (mean) values for a population in which there is considerable variance among the individuals (see Fig. 17-1) and their likely risk of disease (e.g., Fig 1-3 [Chapter 1] or 19-5 [Chapter 19]). Each of us needs personal advice about steps we can take in daily life to prevent nutrient and tissue imbalances. We will want to tailor our choices to fit our personal tastes and lifestyle. This helps ensure a comfortable and successful life-long adoption of healthy eating habits.

When we started quantitative metabolic measurements with the Pfizer Award in 1986, we rediscovered that a very low level (less than 0.1 energy percent) of n-6 linoleate gave a half-optimal status for laboratory animals and humans (see Chapters

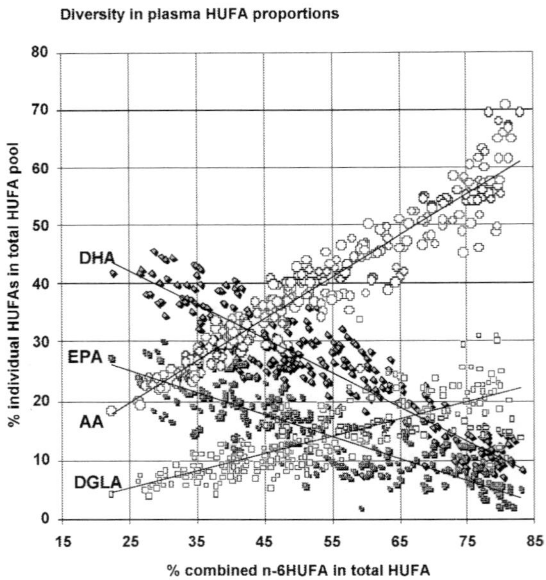

Fig. 17-1. Human diversity in HUFA proportions: Gas chromatographic analyses of HUFA in plasma phospholipids. Values are from individual Japanese and Americans (380 samples) eating their customary voluntary personal food choices without and with omega 3 supplements. Docosahexaenoic acid (DHA; 22:6n-3) and eicosapentaenoic acid (EPA; 20:5n-3) are lower proportions when arachidonic acid (AA; 20:4n-6) and dihomo-gamma-linolenic acid (DGLA; 20:3n-6) are higher.

3 and 13). Apparently, 0.5 energy percent of the n-6 linoleate is more than adequate to meet human needs for essential fatty acid with an ample margin of safety (Cuthbertson, 1976). We thus realized how the food habits in the United States had gone far beyond what was needed. It made us reexamine the concepts of what is normal and what is a megadose level of dietary linoleic acid.

Our research results developed an empirical quantitative metabolic relationship for the hyperbolic competitive interactions of n-3 and n-6 acids in maintaining tissue HUFA. The equation and constants developed for laboratory rats (Lands et al., 1990) gave a surprisingly good fit to data from humans in Chicago (Lands et al., 1992). The relationship between the amounts of EFA ingested and the amounts of EFA in plasma phospholipids was developed with limited data from U.S. patients who were taking dietary supplements of fish oil capsules. We used gas chromatographic analyses of plasma lipids to fit constants to the empirical relationship shown in the following equation.

The equation expresses as percent of daily food energy (en%) the intake of four types of dietary essential fatty acid, the 18-carbon n-3 and n-6 PUFA (P3 and P6) and the 20- and 22-carbon n-3 and n-6 HUFA (H3 and H6) to predict the proportion of n-6 HUFA accumulated in tissue HUFA. The proportion reflects competitive interactions among dietary EFA and it also predicts the likely intensity of forming n-6 eicosanoids.

$$\text{20:3+20:4n-6 in HUFA} = \frac{100}{1 + \frac{HC_6}{\text{en\%H6}}\left(1 + \frac{\text{en\%H3}}{HC_3}\right)} + \frac{100}{1 + \frac{PC_6}{\text{en\%P6}}\left(1 + \frac{\text{en\%P3}}{PC_3} + \frac{\text{en\%H3}}{HI_3} + \frac{\text{en\%O}}{C_O} + \frac{\text{en\%P6}}{Ks}\right)}$$

Analyses from a recent detailed study of 87 subjects (Kobayashi et al., 2001) with diverse voluntary food choices were added to the small data set for humans in Chicago (Lands et al., 1992) to cover a wider range of values (20 to 80% n-6 HUFA in total HUFA). To fit the new combined data set, only three constants needed to be revised: HC_3 = 3.0 (from 8.8); HC_6 = 0.7 (from 0.5); HI_3 = 0.005 (from 0.008), and the other four remain.

The relative values for HC6 and HC3 (0.7 and 3.0) reflect a more effective competitive influence of dietary n-6 over n-3 HUFA during storage of dietary HUFA into tissue lipids. In contrast, the similar values for PC_6 and PC_3 (0.0555 and 0.0441) reflect a similar competitive interaction of dietary 18-carbon n-6 and n-3 PUFA during conversion of dietary PUFA to tissue HUFA. Further, the contribution of dietary fatty acids other than essential fatty acids was inversely related to a constant, Co, whose magnitude was about 100-fold greater than that for essential fatty acids (5 vs. 0.05). Such a result suggests little influence of overall total dietary fat upon the competitions among EFA maintaining the proportions of n-3 and n-6 HUFA in tissue HUFA. The equation with the new revised constants also fits closely with results from a recent detailed diet-tissue study of 94 middle-aged Japanese dietitians (Kuriki et al., 2002).

Individualized Diet Planning on Web

For easy use of the empirical equation and new constants, they were embedded in a handy "calculator" placed on this website: http://efaeducation.nih.gov/sig/dietbalance.html. We also developed an interactive database for planning personalized daily menus to fit an individual's personal taste preferences, lifestyle, and level of risk aversion. The software, which can be downloaded free from the distance learning websites: http://ods.od.nih.gov/eicosanoids/ and http://efaeducation.nih.gov/, easily converts combinations of food servings (with their dietary EFA) into estimates of the probable resulting %n-6 HUFA in total HUFA of plasma phospholipids. The final two chapters of this book show how to choose foods to ensure that personal consumption of EFA meets personal goals for an acceptable level of risk.

Technical Details

A detailed analysis of the fatty acids in the average British household food supply (Bull et al., 1983) noted that the daily intake of 103 g of fat per person was divided among milk and non-butter milk products (19%), butter (12%), other visible fats (25%), meats and meat products (27%), cereal products (10%), and all other foods (7%). Of the fatty acids in the fats, 45% were saturated; 9.8% linoleate (l8:2n-6); 1.6% linolenate (18:3n-3); 0.5% arachidonate (20:4n-6); 0.1% eicosapentaenoate (20:5n-3), and 0.4% 22:5n-3 plus 22:6n-3.

The values are for food brought into the home; no one can be certain what parts were eaten and what discarded. This is a common problem in estimating the food intake of a large population. National data keep us informed on the food being sold, but different ways of preparing food can set aside or discard appreciable amounts of fat as people try to curtail the amount of fat in their daily caloric intake. We can only guess at what is actually consumed.

Only small differences in the fatty acid patterns of body fat were noted for several groups of people: East Africans (with a low incidence of myocardial infarction), North American whites (with a high incidence of infarction), and North American blacks (with an intermediate rate of infarctions). The linoleate content of all adipose samples was reported to be about 11-13 mole percent (Lee et al., 1962). No evidence was presented for the presence of l8:3n-3, no values were reported for other n-3 acids, and no linoleate contents were higher than those reported by Hegsted for Bostonians (Hegsted et al., 1962). The latter report claimed "rather similar" mean values for most fatty acids in adipose biopsies of different populations. Values for the linoleate content of adipose were from Japanese (9.4), Bostonians (7.9), and Nigerian (7.9-8.7). Jamaicans (5.8) and Columbians (5.5). Only samples from Japanese had a significant amount of 20-carbon polyunsaturated fatty acid reported to be in the adipose tissue. All values obtained for linoleate were lower than that reported by Lee et al. (1962), although they agree with the 8% reported by Katan and Beynen (1981).

Analysis of the fatty acids in adipose tissue and plasma free fatty acids for citizens of Oslo, Norway, had good agreement between the two types of data for linoleate

(Albutt and Chance, 1969). However, another report described arachidonate as 0.5% of the body fat and it was not detected at all in the plasma free fatty acids (Jacobsen et al., 1983). In contrast, a study of Koreans and Americans detected arachidonate (20:4n-6) in serum triglycerides, but not in adipose tissue (Scott et al., 1964). In these analyses, a significant amount of 18:3n-3 was found in the adipose tissue of Koreans, but not of Americans. The different values probably reflect long-term effects of voluntary diet preferences. The difficulties in securing consistent values and sufficient information on 18:3n-3 or other n-3 fatty acids make it hard to use the data to assess in a scientific manner the trends among dietary polyunsaturated acids with different groups of people. Also, the wide diversity in diet preferences for n-3 intake noted for different sets of individuals indicates that we must expect that many individuals within a general group will have fatty acid patterns appreciably different from the group average.

The average fatty acids in adipose tissue reported for patients in Sweden (Walldius, 1976) contained 9-14% linoleate (18:2n-6) and detectable amounts of both 18:3n-3 (1-2%) and 20:4n-6 (0.2-0.7%). Similar amounts of these acids might be present in other populations, but inadequate analytical procedures have prevented researchers from detecting them. Some ideas that now need testing cannot be evaluated with data gathered in the past. Newer data indicate that plasma triglycerides of fasting individuals have EFA compositions similar to those in adipose tissue. The proportion of any EFA in the fasting plasma or adipose triglycerides seems linearly related to its en% in the diet.

References

Albutt EC, Chance GW. Plasma and adipose tissue fatty acids of diabetic children on long-term corn oil diets. *J. Clin Invest* 48:139-145, 1969.

Bang HO, Dyerberg I, Hjorne N. Composition of food consumed by Greenland Eskimos. *Acta Med Scand* 200:69-73, 1976.

Bang HO, Dyerberg J, Sinclair HM, et al. The composition of the Eskimo food in northwestern Greenland. *Am J Clin Nutr* 33:2657-266, 1980.

Beynen AC, Hermus RJJ, Hautvast JGAJ, et al. A mathematical relationship between the fatty acid composition of the diet and that of the adipose tissue in man. *Am J Clin Nutr* 33:81-85, 1980.

Bull NL, Day MJL, Burt R, et al. Individual fatty acids in the British household food supply. *Hum Nutr Appl Nutr* 37A:373-377, 1983.

Christakis GJ, Rinzler SH, Archer M, et al. Effect of a serum cholesterol-lowering diet on composition of depot fat in man. *Am J Clin Nutr* 16:243-251, 1965.

Cuthbertson WFJ. (1976) Essential fatty acid requirements in infancy. *Am J Clin Nutr* 20:559-568, 1976.

Dayton S, Hashimoto S, Dixon W, et al. Composition of lipids, in human serum and adipose tissue during prolonged feeding of a diet high in unsaturated fat. *J Lipid Res* 7:103-111, 1966.

Hegsted DM, Jack CW, Stare FJ. The composition of human adipose tissue from several parts of the world. *Am J Clin Nutr* 10:11-18, 1962,

Hirsch J, Farquhar JW, Ahrens EH Jr, et al. Studies of adipose tissue in man: A microtechnic for sampling and analysis. *Am J Clin Nutr* 8:499-511, 1960.

Jacobsen BK, Trygg K, Hjermann I. Acyl pattern of adipose tissue triglycerides, plasma free fatty acids, and diet of a group of men participating in a primary coronary prevention program (The Oslo Study). *Am J Clin Nutr* 38:906-913, 1983.

Katan MB, Beynen AC. Linoleic acid consumption and coronary heart disease in USA and U. K. *Lancet* 2:371, 1981.

Kobayashi M., Sasaki S, Kawabata T, et al. Single measurement of serum phospholipid fatty acid as a biomarker of specific fatty acid intake in middle-aged Japanese men. *Eur J Clin Nutr* 55:643-650, 2001.

Kuriki K, Nagaya T, Imaeda N, et al. Discrepancies in dietary intakes and plasma concentrations of fatty acids according to age among Japanese female dietitians. *Eur J Clin Nutr* 56:524-531, 2002.

Lands WEM, Morris AJ, Libelt B. Quantitative effects of dietary polyunsaturated fats on the composition of fatty acids in rat tissues. *Lipids* 25:505-516, 1990.

Lands WEM, Libelt B, Morris A, et al. Maintenance of lower proportions of n-6 eicosanoid precursors in phospholipids of human plasma in response to added dietary n-3 fatty acids. *Biochim Biophys Acta* 1180:147-162, 1992.

Lands WEM. Functional foods in primary prevention or nutraceuticals in secondary prevention? *Current Topics Nutraceutical Research* 1(2):113-120, 2003.

Lee KT, Shaper AG, Scott HRF. Geographic studies pertaining to arteriosclerosis. *Arch Pathol* 74:481-488, 1962.

O'Dea K, Sinclair AJ. Increased proportion of arachidonic acid in plasma lipids after 2 weeks on a diet of tropical seafood. *Am J Clin Nutr* 36:868-872, 1982.

Scott RF, Lee KT, Kim ON, et al. Fatty acids of serum and adipose tissue in six groups eating natural diets containing 7 to 40 per cent fat. *Am J Clin Nutr* 14:280-290, 1964.

Taylor TG, Gibney MJ, Morgan JB. Haemostatic function and polyunsaturated fatty acids. *Lancet* 2:1378, 1979.

Walldius G. Serum triglycerides and fatty acid incorporation into human adipose tissue (FIAT). *Acta Med Scand* 200:409-421, 1976.

18—Overall Supply of n-3 Fatty Acids

Many of our foods contain fat distributed within the plant or animal tissue in ways that are not visible, and thus its presence is hard to recognize. Considerable fat also may be added during the cooking process. Some concentrated forms of fat such as butter, margarine, or salad oil are also added to our foods. Use of these more visible forms of fat allows us to supplement our daily food intake with the particular fatty acids we wish.

How much supplement and what type we use are often a personal choice. Visible fats are available from many sources, and nearly 60 million tons of such fats were produced and marketed worldwide in 1980. These fats contain mixtures of saturated fatty acids with n-3, n-6, and n-9 unsaturated fatty acids. Table 18-1 shows that large-scale sources of n-3 fatty acids are rapeseed (canola), soybean and linseed (flaxseed) oil (all containing 18:3n-3) and fish oil (containing long-chain n-3 HUFA). Tables of fatty acid composition can help people choose visible fats that would give the dietary balance desired among the various fatty acids. Until now, the composition of available oils seemed driven more by producers' priorities than by public health rationales or priorities.

Because the n-3 HUFA abundant in seafoods are more effective than 18:3n-3 in moderating the formation of eicosanoids from arachidonate, their availability is the first feature we will examine. The fish most often consumed by Americans tend to have low contents of fat in their tissues, and one of the attractions of replacing meat with fish has been the opportunity to decrease the total fat and saturated fatty acids in the diet.

TABLE 18-1
Fats and Oils Produced Worldwide

	Kilotons produced[a]	n-3/n-6 Content[b]
Fish	1,015	13–35/1–4
Linseed	961	26–58/5–23
Soybean	14,570	2–10/49–52
Rapeseed	3,542	1–10/10–22
Sunflower	5,425	—/44–68
Cottonseed	3,291	—/50
Peanut	3,492	—/13–34
Olive	1,374	—/4–15
Coconut	3,275	—/1–3
Palm	4,300	—/6–12
Butter	5,100	—/3
Lard	3,800	—/4–9
Tallow	5,865	—/1–3
Total overall	58,918	

[a]Data from Young (1982) for 1979–1980.
[b]Data from Applewhite (1980).

There are many fish sources of n-3 HUFA that have not been directly used as food materials in Western nations. Most fish oils produced in the United States are derived from small oily fish like the Atlantic menhaden that are harvested principally for their oil and not generally used for food (Stansby, 1978). Fish oils account for only 2% of the fats and oils that are marketed in the world (Table 18-1), but they are an economically important product in several countries. Because the U.S. Food and Drug Administration had not included fish oil with other edible oils in preparing the list of materials generally regarded as safe (GRAS), the U.S. population was for a while the only major country not consuming fish oil as an edible oil. As a result, the U.S. production of 95.6 kilotons of fish oil in 2002 was disbursed by selling 96.5 kilotons to Japan, Chile, Canada, Netherlands, Norway, and other countries. Now purified grades of fish oil have U.S. FDA GRAS status and a long list of foods has FDA approval for being fortified with n-3 HUFA.

Using Hydrogenated or HUFA Forms?

The 1986 edition stated the annual worldwide production of oils and fats was approximately 59 million metric tons in 1979-1980. However, worldwide use of fat rose from 52 million metric tons (MMT) in 1976-1980 to 104 MMT in 1996-2000. It is expected to rise to 184 MMT in 2016–2020, corresponding to 12.1, 17.7, and 24.8 kg/yr/person or 33, 48 and 68 g/d/person, respectively (Gunstone, 2003).

The worldwide average intake of fat per person is approaching the mean intake of 75g/d/person seen in the United States (Food and Nutrition Board, 2002). The tons of fats and oils produced overall, worldwide, are a major source of EFA in human diets, and they generally contain more n-6 than n-3. As a result, finding ways to balance the EFA in people's diets and in their tissues remains a worldwide health challenge.

Vegetable oil consumption in the United States steadily increased during the past 50 years, to become the major source of the current high intake of n-6 fatty acids in the typical U.S. diet. Soybean oil is now the major component in the 72 g/d/person of food oils and fats currently used by Americans (Gunstone, 2003). As a result, dietary fat available now in the United States (71 g/d; about 33% of overall food energy) has nearly 50% in the form of n-6 linoleate (31 g/d). Intake of n-3 linolenate (4 g/d) is appreciably less. Even if all of the consumed soybean oil was in the partially hydrogenated form, n-6 linoleate intake would still be about 10% of daily food energy and n-3 linolenate would be about 0.8 en%. The values for overall supply of fats and oils in the United States (Table 18-2) should be considered in the context of current information about what is a biologically adequate dietary supply of n-3 and n-6 fats.

Fish oil has been used in many countries for many years as hydrogenated edible oil and incorporated into margarine and shortening. Hydrogenation changes the chemical nature of the fat, making it more saturated and destroying the n-3 polyunsaturated acids that could moderate eicosanoid formation. In this way, hydrogenation of either fish or vegetable oil greatly changes the way in which its fatty acids partici-

TABLE 18-2
Fats and Oils Consumed in U.S.

Oils & fats	MMT/y	g/d/person	g LA/d	g LNA/d
Soybean	5.73	56.55	28.03	3.76
cottonseed	0.18	1.78	0.64	0.00
groundnut	0.06	0.59	0.18	0.00
canola	0.22	2.17	0.44	0.20
corn	0.23	2.27	1.28	0.02
coconut	0.07	0.69	0.01	0.00
butter	0.41	4.05	0.08	0.05
lard	0.13	1.28	0.12	0.01
tallow	0.12	1.18	0.03	0.01
total =	7.15	70.57	30.83	4.05
% food energy =		31.64%	13.82%	1.81%

pate in eicosanoid-related health and disease processes. Sometimes we may want that change and sometimes we may wish to avoid it. The balance of n-3 and n-6 EFA that will be recommended for the coming years is yet to be determined.

Chemical Composition of Fish Oils

Generally speaking, ocean fish oils are complex mixtures containing many fatty acids, some with as many as six double bonds. Nevertheless, for practical purposes, eight fatty acids can describe the composition of fish oil reasonably well. These fatty acids fall into four pairs of particular structure and origin, namely, 14:0 and 16:0, 16:1 and 18:1 (n-7 and n-9), 20:1 and 22:1 (n-9 and n-11), and 20:5 and 22:6 (n-3). These eight fatty acids make up 80-85% of the total fatty acids in fish oil, and normally can be used to determine the type of oil and its value in different markets.

We will focus on the n-3 HUFA of fish oil. The nonessential 14:0, 16:0, 16:1n-7, 18:1n-7, and 18:1n-9 are of nutritional interest here only as substrates for the acyl-CoA pathway to CO_2 and energy (Figure 13-1 [Chapter 13]). All of the nonessential fatty acids can be formed by vertebrate tissues from simple amino acid or carbohydrate precursors, and the acids have no recognized role in modifying the metabolism of eicosanoids.

Overall, the world production of 1 million tons of fish oil contains an annual combined total of about 100,000-250,000 tons of 20:5n-3 plus 22:6n-3. This represents a significant amount of material capable of antagonizing the conversion of arachidonate to eicosanoids. If 50% of the average U.S. annual fish oil production of about100,000 metric tons (which has been primarily exported until recently) were converted to a concentrated form of n-3 fatty acid, it would represent about $1.2\text{-}2.8 \times 10^{10}$ g of n-3 HUFA. This amount could provide a daily supplement of about 1 g per day of n-3 HUFA for about 40 million people (less than 14% of the U.S. population). Making this dietary supplement available to all U.S. citizens seems desirable; and added sources of n-3 fats will be sought.

General information suggests that 14% of the U.S. population might be a realistic and significant market for 20:5n-3 and 22:6n-3. At 1 g per day and five cents per gram, annual sales for this market could represent almost $1,000,000,000 that would be derived from raw materials costing far less. Millions of dollars of profit could be obtained in marketing the oil and fortified foods for health purposes.

Since 1986, millions have been spent in understanding how the n-3 HUFA influence our health. Medical researchers have added thousands of reports, and we still need to know more about reducing the causes of diseases that are driven by dietary EFA imbalances. Questions still to be addressed and answered include:

- Who will carry out the public education needed for primary prevention?
- Who will fund the education about what is already known about the health benefits of increasing n-3 fats and decreasing n-6 fats?

The average values for the polyunsaturated fatty acid composition in fish oils listed in Table 18-3 indicate that much more 20:5n-3 relative to 22:6n-3 occurs in Atlantic menhaden than in most other species. This fish provides a major portion of the fish oil produced in the United States. Canadian tuna, however, has relatively more 22:6n-3. Because each source of oil has important financial consequences for the community marketing the product, information on its potential health benefits will be needed.

Sources of Fish Fatty Acids

Consumers need to know whether the seafood being considered for consumption has been fed from a food chain from the land or the sea. Since the fish cannot make either n-3 or n-6 fatty acids, its tissues will have polyunsaturated acids of the type that it eats. Some commercial fish farms may use feeds derived from soybean or other seeds or grains in which the major polyunsaturated fats are of the n-6 type. This may explain why the composition of catfish shown in Table 18-3 is so similar to that commonly found in chicken meat.

Not all fish in the market will have the n-3 fats of seafoods. Also, not all meat is rich in the n-6 fatty acids. If the food chain of the chicken or pig were changed to resemble the food of the seal or whale, the meat of the chicken or pig might have the large abundance of n-3 acids found in seals and whales. In this respect our tissues can only reflect the pattern of the mix of food chains that feeds us.

Eskimos consume large quantities of meat, but it is a meat derived from the maritime food chain rich in n-3 fats. The meat Americans eat is derived from a continental food chain rich in n-6 fats. Thus, the terms “meat” and “fish” do not always adequately inform us of what we need to know in balancing our own dietary n-3 and n-6 polyunsaturated fatty acids. The food chain that supplies the meat or fish plays a major role in determining the fatty acids that will eventually influence the production of eicosanoids in our tissues.

TABLE 18-3
Polyunsaturated Fatty Acids in Fish Oils

Fatty acid	Atlantic menhaden[b]	Maine sardine[b]	Canadian tuna[b]	Atlantic herring[b]	Atlantic mackeral[c]	Mexican anchovy[b,c]		Michigan salmon[d]	Mississippi catfish[b]	S. African mackerel[c]	Redfish[c]	Iceland cod liver[e]	Iceland capelin[e]
16:2n-7	0.8	0.3	—	1.1	—	0.9	—	1.5	0.1	—	—	—	—
16:3n-4	1.7	—	—	1.1	—	1.0	—	2.0	—	—	—	—	—
16:4n-4	2.9	0.7	1.0	1.0	0.4	0.9	1.3	—	—	1.3	0.4	—	—
18:2n-6	1.0	1.6	1.6	3.8	1.2	1.2	1.1	5.0	13.6	1.6	1.2	1.4	1.4
18:3n-6	1.1	1.3	0.8	1.2	—	0.9	—	4.3	0.9	—	—	0.5	0.6
18:4n-3	2.1	4.7	0.8	3.0	1.3	2.0	1.5	1.4	0.1	3.1	1.3	0.4	0.4
20:3n-3	0.2	—	—	—	—	0.2	—	2.0	0.4	—	—	—	—
20:4n-3/n-6	1.7	0.5	2.0	0.7	4.0	0.9	4.5	2.0	0.4	2.9	4.0	0.6	0.4
20:5n-3	16.7	7.4	6.9	9.0	11.5	16.7	14.3	3.2	0.4	16.1	11.5	7.9	8.9
22:5n-3	0.9	0.6	2.2	0.6	1.8	1.1	1.8	5.1	0.4	0.8	1.8	1.2	1.2
22:6n-3	7.0	5.2	19.7	4.0	15.1	15.6	13.1	5.2	0.6	11.4	15.1	8.7	10.5

[a]Expressed as percentage of total fat.
[b]Unpublished data from Zapata Haynie Corp., United States.
[c]Unpublished data from Fishing Industries Research Institute, Republic of South Africa.
[d]Data from Braddock and Dugan (1969).
[e]Unpublished data from Pall Olafsson, Icelandic Fisheries Laboratories, Iceland.

Consequences of Choices

With each species of fish selected as a source of EFA for our diet, some community will experience some financial and social consequences. Will we know enough to choose wisely and fairly? If we want to deliberately alter our intake of n-3 and n-6 acids, we will need more agreement among medical researchers on the impact of this intake. It would be helpful to have more advice on the impact that the present levels of both n-3 and n-6 acids in our normal diets have on our normal responses.

Current "normal" U.S. diets reflect adaptation to life in an industrial nation in which soybean products are more economically handled and more vigorously marketed than seafood. The relative lack of 18:3n-3 and other n-3 acids in our dietary EFA may reflect marketer's convenience more than our deliberate food choices. The food shifts noted in Chapter 17 reflect a major marketing effort by organizations that provide large amounts of linoleate (18:2n-6) to our diets. Wouldn't more dietary n-3 fats and less 18:2n-6 help us achieve a healthier balance of polyunsaturated acids in our tissues like that observed in seafoods and in people who eat them?

Considering Alternatives to Fish

The supply of long-chain n-3 fatty acids in seafoods may be too limited to provide adequate supplementation to all who wish to balance the n-3 and n-6 acids in their diet. For this reason, my curiosity about the Eskimo way of life and their foods from the sea led to examining other ways to provide a similar balance that the sea provides.

For that balance, we must study the types of plants that could enter our food chain. In contrast to the algae of the ocean, our farmed land plants do not form 20:5n-3 and 22:6n-3. Instead, they tend to accumulate n-6 fatty acids in their seeds, and only three species have significant amounts of 18:3n-3: *Linum usitatissimum*, linseed or flaxseed; *Brassica spp.*, rapeseed; and *Glycine max*, soybean.

A brief review of the data in Table 18-4 indicates that only flaxseed has higher amounts of n-3 than n-6 fatty acids. Most previous production of linseed oil has been for the paint industry, which took no precautions to prevent oxidation that produces toxic materials and unpleasant odors and flavors. Commercial procedures used to harvest and prepare the oil need to be modified to let us use the oil for supplementing

TABLE 18-4
Polyunsaturated Fatty Acids in Plant Oils[a]

Fatty acid	Linseed	Rapeseed	Soybean	Sunflower	Corn	Peanut	Olive	Butter	Margarine[b]
18:3n-3	53	11	7	0.2	0.7	0	0.6	0.3	0.3
18:2n-6	13	22	51	66	58	32	8	1.8	25
kcals	884	884	884	884	884	884	884	717	714

[a]The values are grams or kilocalories per 100 g of oil.
[b]Values for margarines can vary widely (from 11% to 48% 18:2n-6).

our diets. An unusual plant used to provide herbal flavorings in Japan (Perilla, or "beefsteak" plant) also has a high percent of 18:3n-3 in its seed oil. Professor Okuyama, a distinguished lipid scientist, informed me that the content can be as high as 64% (with 12% as linoleate) and it has a range of uses. Presumably other seed oils with high n-3/n-6 ratios not commonly used at this time can be identified.

The polyunsaturated fatty acid 18:3n-3 tends to oxidize more easily than does linoleate, 18:2n-6. For that reason, many producers of soybean oil consider ways of decreasing the content of the n-3 fatty acid (*JAOCS* 59:34, 1982). If the oil is "lightly" hydrogenated, the content of 18:3n-3 can be decreased from 7.6 to 3.3% and of 18:2n-6 from 53 to 37%.

As expected, such a product is more stable on storage, etc., but its lower content of polyunsaturated fatty acids and higher content of *trans* acids may make it less able to lower the levels of plasma lipoproteins (Lame et al., 1982). Different priorities work in the marketplace for food. What people need is balanced with what they want and what can be economically provided. The purpose of this book is to provide insights for readers to better appreciate whether what they think they want is truly what they and their children need for good health.

The anwers to these questions can shed light on this topic.

- What happens to people if they turn away from the simple food from coastal regions and develop an industrialized way of life?
- What happens to the balance of polyunsaturated acids in mothers who do not have enough n-3 fatty acids in their food chain?
- How much does the early food provided to Eskimo babies differ from what babies are fed in industrialized nations?
- Does the early balance of eicosanoids affect the development of our immune responses?
- How will we learn if small genetic differences are amplified by early environmental influence?
- In comparing our disease pattern with that of Eskimos, is there more importance in the differences in our mother's genes or in our mother's milk?
- A mother's milk can provide only the fatty acids that are in her food chain. How does she choose what to eat?
- Will we be able to choose diets that differ from those on which we were raised?
- Will the knowledge we need on nutrition and the mechanisms of diseases be available?

Knowing the EFA in our present food chain is an important first step in making wise future food choices.

As we began to use the empirical equation described in Chapter 17 to predict the likely intensity of n-6 eicosanoid responses of people who eat different foods, we saw more clearly the dietary sources of tissue HUFA imbalance. Changing food oils can make a big difference in the relative tissue balance. However, managing information on EFA in all of the daily foods is needed for effective preventive nutrition education. To help readers sense the different amounts of EFA in different types of food, this book gives specific examples of the EFA content in some servings listed by the USDA Nutrient Database, which is the primary database for estimating nutrient intakes in the United States (http://www.nal.usda.gov/fnic/cgi-bin/nut_search.pl).

Inadequacies are evident in the analytical values provided for individual essential fatty acids (e.g., Taber et al., 2001), but the database remains the best overall comprehensive source of information. Readers are advised to use the quantitative analytical data on EFA nutrients as a first approximation to the likely content in food. The values should be used with an expectation that precise details can be clouded by questions of time and place of harvest, nutrients provided to the plant or animal BEFORE food was harvested, as well as differences in food preparation. Nevertheless, this is a "first step."

The database values from USDA version 15 were put into an interactive personalized computer program that uses the equation described in Chapter 17 to help people estimate the likely impact of a person's overall daily food choices. The software called KIM (Keep It Managed) sorts foods in arrays that make the relative proportions of EFA more evident. After four years of use, KIM was replaced recently by KIM-2, which has improved software and updated USDA nutrient data. It can be downloaded free from the distance learning sites http://ods.od.nih.gov/eicosanoids/ and http://efaeducation.nih.gov/.

The next chapter illustrates how the different food items (and their EFA) combine in an overall daily meal plan to fit each individual's personal tastes, preferences and life-styles. The amounts of EFA that are in typical, readily available food servings are discussed below to help people begin to see how rational choices of foods will give EFA intakes that can balance the proportions of n-3 and n-6 HUFA in their tissue HUFA at almost any level they desire.

Cereals, grains and bread make up the base of the current USDA food pyramid, and 1,652 different servings of these foods are listed in the USDA Nutrient Database (Version 15). These foods, with their polymeric carbohydrates, are an important source of energy. One cup of wild rice (166 kcals) has 195 mg n-6 and 158 mg of n-3 EFA, whereas 1 cup of regular boiled rice (242 kcals) contains only 76 mg of n-6 and 17 mg n-3 EFA. The balance of EFA shifts even more toward n-6 with one slice of rye bread (81 kcal) that has 236 mg n-6 and only 19 mg of n-3, and a regular cracker (20 kcals) containing 355 mg of n-6 and 26 mg of n-3. Less helpful in maintaining a balance among EFA would be one cup of brown rice (218 kcals) with 552 mg of n-6 and only 25 mg of n-3 or a regular hamburger roll (123 kcals) with 1,065 mg of n-6 and only 15 mg of n-3. The n-6 EFA predominate over the n-3 throughout this whole food group, and the n-6 proportions become even greater when vegetable oils or margarine spreads are included with these foods.

Vegetables, of which 1,385 servings are listed, include some foods with more n-3 than n-6 EFA. Thus the top of the sorted list has a canned grape leaf (3 kcal) with 6 mg of n-6 and 34 mg of n-3, and 1 cup of cooked spinach (41 kcals) has 29 mg of n-6 with 153 mg of n-3. Cauliflower, broccoli, turnips and lettuce all have more n-3 than n-6, but the total amount of EFA in a serving is not very high. Further down the list, 1 cup of chopped kale (34 kcals) has 92 mg of n-6 and 121 mg of n-3 and 1 cup of shredded cabbage (18 kcals) has a balance of 36 mg of n-6 with 48 mg of n-3. Near the bottom of the list, vegetables like red ripe tomatoes, onions, sliced beets, and sweet green peppers have more than 10 times the amount of n-6 compared to n-3 EFA. For example, 1/2 cup of asparagus (18 kcals) has 98 mg of n-6 and only 5 mg of n-3 and 1/2 cup of sweet corn (76 kcals) has 277 mg of n-6 with only 8 mg of n-3. Overall, vegetables contribute vitamins, minerals and fiber to the diet with only modest amounts of calories, and many vegetables have balanced amounts of n-3 and n-6 EFA.

Fruits, (532 entries) have little fat, and only a few items have more n-3 than n-6 EFA. One cup of papaya (55 kcals) has 8 mg of n-6 with 35 mg of n-3 and 1 cup of cantaloupe (56 kcals) has 75 mg of n-6 and 101 mg of n-3. Somewhat balanced proportions of EFA are found in cherries, pineapple, strawberries and blueberries, but almost no n-3 fatty acid is reported for watermelon, prunes, pears, grapes or apricots. Avocado is one fruit that stands out from all the others in having lots of fat energy (242 kcals per cup); it contains 2,760 mg of n-6 and 167 mg of n-3 EFA.

Dairy and egg products (454 entries) necessarily reflect the balance of EFA supplied by farmers to the animals producing the milk or eggs. As a result, U.S. dairy products tend to have a balance that reflects the green pasturage eaten by cows. Thus, 1 oz of Parmesan cheese (129 kcals) has 90 mg of n-6 and 98 mg of n-3, and 1 oz of fontina cheese (110 kcals) has 245 mg of n-6 and 224 mg of n-3 EFA. Similarly 1 pat of butter (36 kcals) has 92 mg of n-6 and 59 mg of n-3, whereas a cup of 2% milk (122 kcals) has 105 mg of n-6 and 68 mg of n-3. When cows have limited pastures and are fed supplemental grain, the milk, cheese and butter inevitably have higher levels of n-6 fats. Because chickens are customarily fed grains with relatively high proportions of n-6 EFA, one large hard boiled egg (78 kcals) has 594 mg of n-6 with only 18 mg of n-3 EFA. Finally, 1/4 oz. of liquid egg substitute (96 kcals) has 3,706 mg of n-6 with only 38 mg of in-3 EFA, reflecting the fats added in formulating the product. Obviously, the producers could have used other fats to give much healthier outcomes. Readers can readily sense how easily a large number of formulated food products could be made "functional foods" suited to help in primary prevention of diseases in the general public.

Meat, fish, and legumes (4,538 entries) provide an important source of protein; legumes (peas and beans) are especially important to vegetarians and vegans. Wide differences in the EFA balance of legumes are illustrated by the amounts of 43 mg n-6 and 603 mg n-3 in 1 cup of boiled mungo (Urd or matpe) beans (189 kcals). This contrasts greatly with the content in 1 cup of boiled mung beans (212 kcals) with 240 mg of n-6 and only 18 mg of n-3 EFA. Alternatively, 1 cup of boiled kidney beans or pinto beans has balanced proportions with 133 mg of n-6 and 186 mg of n-3 or 217 mg and 181 mg, respectively. The high proportion of n-3 EFA in mungo beans is matched by that in ground flaxseed, which has 518 mg of n-6 with 2,175 mg of n-3 in 1 tbsp. (59 kcals). Unfortunately, many other legumes, such as lentils and chick-peas resemble mung beans with n-6 EFA dominating their relative EFA proportions. As a result, people could not gain balanced EFA in their tissues from the typical legumes eaten in the United States.

Pork, turkey, and chicken also have a predominance of n-6 fatty acids in accord with the grain and soybean feeds used by the farmers. For example 3 oz. of roasted turkey dark meat (222 kcals) contains 2,534 mg of n-6 but only 134 mg of n-3. This contrasts with the composition in beef and lamb, which come from animals that have eaten a lot of green pasturage during their growth. Three ounces of New Zealand lamb (259 kcals) has 519 mg n-6 and 340 mg of n-3, whereas U.S. domestic lamb has 1,165 mg of n-6 with 357 mg of n-3. Domesticated farm animals can only accumulate in their tissues the proportions of EFA permitted by the foods fed by the farmers. Again, farmers, producers and marketers (when they wish to do so) can deliberately provide meats that give humans more n-3 and less n-6.

Fish and seafood are the focus of this book because their algal-based food chain lets their tissues accumulate rich supplies of n-3 fats that can correct an imbalance toward n-6 EFA from a grain-rich food chain for humans. It is this n-3 rich food chain in the oceans that needs no human farmers' wisdom to yield food that helps human health. In addition, seafoods have relatively high amounts of 20- and 22-carbon n-3 HUFA accompanying the 18-carbon n-3 EFA. The combination ensures a greater dietary impact on tissue HUFA compositions. As people choose and eat their daily foods, they give to their tissues diverse mixtures of EFA that reflect the land-based food chain rich in the n-6 fats of grains and cereals and the foods rich in n-3 fats from the algae-based food chain. These voluntary food choices provide people with plasma phospholipid HUFA that range from 15-90% n-6 HUFA (Figure 17-1 [Chapter 17]).

The commercial feed for domestic farm animals is controlled by the farmer, who currently tends to make domestic animal tissues richer in n-6. This trend occurs also with farmed seafoods. For example, 3 oz. of wild Atlantic salmon (155 kcal) has 291 mg of n-6 HUFA and 1,877 mg of n-3 HUFA accompanying 187 mg of n-6 and 411 mg of n-3 18-carbon EFA. In contrast, farmed Atlantic salmon has a higher fat and n-6 content with 1,082 mg n-6 HUFA and 1,825 mg n-3 HUFA that accompany 566 mg n-6 and 252 mg n-3 18-carbon EFA. Similarly, farmed coho salmon had n-3 HUFA similar to wild salmon, but had more n-6 EFA per serving than the wild fish. Nuts and seeds are popular items for snacks, and they provide protein and lots of energy in the form of fat. However, they usually add much more n-6 than n-3 EFA. For example, 1 oz. of pistachios (161 kcals) has 3,866 mg of n-6 but only 74 mg of n-3, and 1 oz. of pecans (201 kcals) have 5550 n-6 compared to 282 n-3 EFA. English walnuts are popularly described as being rich in n-3 fats, but 1 oz. has 10,799 mg of n-6 and only 2,574 mg of n-3. Thus, the relative proportions closely resemble those of soybeans, a less expensive source of protein and energy. It was a personal disappointment to learn that a corresponding serving of 2 tbsp. of the very popular peanut butter brings 4,387 mg of n-6 with only 25 mg of n-3. Adding nuts and seeds to the typical diet will not help balance the already high proportions of n-6 EFA in Americans.

Daily consumption of various fats in the United States may average 70-100 g per person with a great proportion being from soybean oil, which may provide 80-90% of linoleate (18:2n-6) that Americans eat. The preceding information alerts readers to the challenge that must be overcome in reaching safer personal goals for the balance of tissue HUFA. Chapter 19 shows how personalized computer-aided menu planning can ease the challenge.

Technical Details

Production of fish body oil in 1980 was greater than 100,000 tons in each of five countries: Chile, Denmark Japan, Norway and the United States. It would be interesting to know how much additional fish oil is discarded during processing of the fish that we do eat. Excellent authoritative summaries of the technical aspects of fish oil composition and production were provided by Ackman (1982) and Young (1982) in the book, *Nutritional Evaluation of Long Chain Fatty Acids in Fish Oil* (see References).

All fish oils from the ocean contain 20:5n-3 and 22:6n-3, and Table 18-3 lists some reported compositions of various marine oils to help the reader recognize oils that are rich in certain polyunsaturated fatty acids. Because different procedures of preparing food tend to discard varied amounts of the fat in the food, it will be difficult to predict how much of a particular polyunsaturated fatty acid is actually eaten when a selected species of fish is consumed.

Each person will choose the way that n-3 HUFA are consumed: as a food, a fortified food, or a food supplement. Herring, mackerel, salmon, and sprat may have 12-16% fat containing large amounts of 20:5n-3 and 22:6n-3. The fillets of these fish usually contain less fat (see Table 18-5), and the composition changes from season to season as the food supply changes. The values listed in Table 18-5 may be useful to individuals selecting fish alternatives for their diets.

We do not know at this time whether our health is affected more by eating 20:5n-3, 22:5n-3 or 22:6n-3 forms. Many vertebrates living on land contain more 22:6n-3 than 20:5n-3. Many fish (and the animals that eat them) tend to accumulate appreciable 20:5n-3 relative to 22:6n-3 in their muscle (meat). It would be interesting to know the details of the food chain that supports each species of fish and how the EFA supply causes body oil of one species to differ from that of another.

The high levels of 20:5n-3 and 22:6n-3 in the crustaceae of the northern oceans may undergo some further elongation or desaturation as the fatty acids pass along the food chain so that 22:6n-3 becomes more abundant than 20:5n-3 in herring, cod, salmon and tuna. The absence of any appreciable amount of polyunsaturated fatty acid other than 18:2n-6 in cultured catfish (see Table 18-3) probably reflects a diet rich in linoleate (perhaps based on soybean and cottonseed meal). These results raise the question of whether the elongation/desaturation reactions in fish are of much sig-

TABLE 18-5
Polyunsaturated Fatty Acids in Fish[a,b]

Fish	n-3 acids	(Total fat)	18:2n-6	20:4n-6	20:5n-3	22:6n-3
Tuna (albacore)	2.33	(6.8)	0.15	0.14	0.63	1.7
Anchovy	1.89	(6.4)	0.12	0.02	0.69	1.2
Herring	0.91	(6.2)	0.29	0.03	0.33	0.58
Mackerel	1.76	(9.8)	0.14	0.12	0.65	1.1
Salmon (Chinook)	1.72	(13.2)	0.13	0.06	1.0	0.72
Tuna (bluefin)	1.16	(4.7)	0.05	0.02	0.28	0.88
Halibut (Pacific)	0.31	(2.0)	0.02	0.08	0.11	0.20
Flounder	0.22	(1.2)	0.01	0.04	0.11	0.11
Cod	0.23	(0.73)	—	0.02	0.08	0.15
Haddock	0.15	(0.66)	0.01	0.01	0.05	0.10

[a]Expressed as grams per 100 grams of food.
[b]Data from Kifer and Miller (1969).

nificance in influencing the composition of the tissue lipids. Little evidence is available at this time on where the polyunsaturated compositions of fish tissues originate. How can we find foods with the n-3 HUFA content that we want?

Does the pattern of polyunsaturated fatty acids in fish merely reflect the pattern of the dietary sources rather than any selectivity of elongation—desaturation enzymes of the fish tissues? Perhaps fish function more as a concentrative system that accumulates and concentrates fat from a widely dispersed variety of sources in the sea and pass it on to the whales and seals in the food chain of the Eskimos.

More concentrated study of the exact origins of the n-3 HUFA in seafood would help us better understand ways of providing more of it to our tissues. High levels of 20:5n-3 occur in some species of phytoplankters and seaweeds (Table 18-6), and the ratio of 20:5n3/22:6n-3 in *M. luthen* resembles that found in *T. longicons* , menhaden, and pilchard. More research on algae might give us new information on useful new sources of these fatty acids.

Isolation and Stability of Fish Oils

Purified fish oil now has many applications as a source of dietary n-3 fatty acids for humans and farmed animals, in contrast with its earlier role as a component in industrial coatings (e.g., paints) and printing inks. Most fish oils are produced via the "wet reduction" process. With good production and storage procedures, crude fish oil will keep for some time with little or no deterioration. The natural antioxidants are lost when the crude oil is refined and bleached, and the oil needs adequate protection by antioxidants, inert gases and closed containers. The oil is chilled and filtered to remove the high-melting fraction which is high in saturated and monounsaturated fatty acids.

This process increases the percentage of unsaturated acids in the oil and provides a product that will not cloud or form a precipitate when stored in cold areas for long periods of time. Subsequent chilling to refrigeration temperatures will not affect

TABLE 18-6
Polyunsaturated Fatty Acids in the Maritime Food Chain[a]

	Phytoplankters		Seaweeds		Copepod
Fatty acid	Phaeodactylum tricornutum	Monochrysis lutheri	Fucus vesicalons	Chondrus crispus	Temora longicons
16:poly	4	4	<1	1	1
18:2n-6	1	1	9	2	1
18:3n-6	<1	<1	1	1	<1
18:3n-3	<1	<1	10	10	<1
18:4n-3	0	5	13	3	1
20:4n-3/n-6	<1	1	13	24	<1
20:5n-3	9	22	14	25	14
22:6n-3	1	10	—	—	7

[a]Data from Ackman (1982).

the clarity (or brilliance) of properly treated oils. The oil may be alkali-refined to remove contaminating nonesterified fatty acids and then, finally, clay-bleached to remove most of the color and any traces of soap or moisture.

A deodorization step can remove any traces of fish flavor, as well as free fatty acids and chlorinated hydrocarbons, and thus make the oil suitable for human consumption. The deodorization step also removes remaining natural antioxidants, making it again necessary to add an antioxidant to protect the oil. TBHQ (tertiary butylhydroquinone) is a very effective antioxidant (and the one of choice in the United States). It was approved for food use after many years of careful testing. Haagsma et al. (1982) used the antioxidant, octylgallate, when the use of TBHQ in fats was not allowed for human consumption in the Netherlands.

Fish oil treated and stabilized as noted above can last for a very long time if adequately protected from light and air. Years ago, Gauglitz and Gruger (1965) described how commercial menhaden oil can be refined by clay bleaching and molecular distillation to a point where it is odorless and taste free. In this form, it remained palatable after months of storage in airtight containers. The tendency of highly unsaturated oils to develop unpleasant "fishy" odors or flavors has often led marketers of food oils to either obtain materials from sources with low polyunsaturated contents or to process the oil in a way that decreases the polyunsaturated content. Neither of these tactics is compatible with providing a food oil that has a high content of the n-3 HUFA that will antagonize the formation of potent eicosanoids from arachidonate.

Thus, there has been little n-3-rich material available from either plants or marine products at the present time that can be marketed in a form suitable for human use. Ironically, a major effort has been made to obtain certain strains of soybean that will produce less than 3% 18:3n-3 rather than the 7-9% currently obtained (*JAOCS* 59:34, 1982). At the present time, nutritional research indicates that a higher level in the diet of n-3 relative to n-6 EFA can have beneficial effects. Clearly, better information on the impact of the n-3 and n-6 fatty acids on human health could appreciably influence the future demand for these fatty acids.

To facilitate evaluations of the role of omega-3 fatty acids in health and disease, the National Marine Fisheries Service of the Department of Commerce joined the National Institutes of Health in 1986 to provide a long-term, consistent supply of quality-assured/quality-controlled test materials to all qualified applicants conducting research studies. This joint program greatly increased the quantity and quality of research on n-3 HUFA. The research-grade, deodorized menhaden oil was prepared from commercial oil that had been winterized and alkali refined. It was processed through a two stage wiped-film evaporator to remove cholesterol, volatile oxidation products and any traces of organic contaminants. The oil contained 0.2 mg/g TBHQ as antioxidant plus 2 mg/g tocopherols and it had approximately 30% n-3 fatty acids in the triglyceride form; 14% EPA, 8% DHA, 8% other n-3 acids. The oil was available in 1 g soft-gel capsules or packaged in bulk quantities depending on investigators' needs. In addition, there were 1 gm soft gelatin capsules of purified (approx. 90 %) EPA ethyl ester (containing 1-2 mg/g tocopherols and 0.02% TBHQ) and purified (approx. 90%) DHA ethyl ester (containing 1-2 mg/g tocopherols and 0.02% TBHQ). Publications of some of the resulting research are cited in the preceding chapters of this book.

Most research on the beneficial effects of seafoods has been directed at the effects of the n-3 HUFA (20:5n-3, 22:5n-3 and 22:6n-3) in fish oil. Earlier researchers noted that beneficial effects seemed due to a combination of fatty acids and/or to some component present in trace amounts. However, Peifer et al. (1962) demonstrated that the hypolipidemic effects of fish were due to the oils and not to other "factors".

Unfortunately, some past publications, without much accompanying rigorous logic, cast doubt on the efficacy of isolated forms of the individual fatty acids and esters and claimed that the oil must be in its "natural" state. Whether the claim is true or just an attempt to sway attitudes of those interested in "natural" or "health" food remained unknown in 1986. By now, large enough quantities of individual purified 20:5n-3 and 22:6n-3 fatty acids have been isolated and fed. Nevertheless, debate continues about whether a particular beneficial health effect being studied is or is not due to a particular fatty acid. The preceding chapters of this book describe results with both purified oils and individual acids.

Fractionation techniques are available to isolate individual fatty acids and their ethyl esters. Haagsma et al. (1982) described the preparation of 265 g of a concentrate of 85% n-3 fatty acids from 1000 g of cod liver oil using urea inclusion complexes of the saponified, acidified fatty acids. The technology to produce concentrated individual n-3 fatty acids exists and can be employed when a suitable market for them has been demonstrated and the right material or product for diet supplementation has been described. The peroxide value of these oils normally remains low throughout the processing and the final deodorization step will drop the value further. Some people regard the peroxide value and the anisidine number as measures of rancidity or oxidation in fish oil as described in *Nutritional Evaluation of Long Chain Fatty Acids in Fish Oil* (Young, 1982).

References

Ackman RG. Fatty acid composition of fish oils. In Barlow SM, Stansby ME (eds.). *Nutritional Evaluation Of Long-Chain Fatty Acids In Fish Oil.* New York: Academic Press, 1982, pp 25-88.

Applewhite TH. Fats and fatty oils. *Kirk-Othmer Encyc Chem Technol* 9:795-831, 1980.

Braddock RJ, Dugan LR Jr. Fatty acids of Lake Michigan coho salmon. *JAOCS* 46:428, 1969.

Exler J, Weihrauch JL. Comprehensive evaluation of fatty acids in foods. VIII. Finfish. *J Am Diet Assoc* 69:243-247, 1976.

Exier J, Weihrauch JL. Comprehensive evaluation of fatty acids in foods. XII. Shellfish. *J Am Diet Assoc* 71:518-521, 1977.

Food and Nutrition Board (FNB)of the Institute of Medicine (IOM), 2002, Dietary Reference Intakes for Energy, Carbohydrate, Fiber, Fat, Fatty Acids, Cholesterol, Protein, and Amino Acids (Macronutrients)-Appendix E- www.nap.edu/books/0309085373/html/

Gauglitz EJ Jr, Gruger EH Jr. Adsorptive bleaching and molecular distillation of menhaden oil. *JAOCS* 42, 561-563, 1965.

Gunstone F. (2003) Prices need to rise if production to meet demand (discussing the book, *The Revised Oil World 2020). INFORM* 13:688-689, 2003.

Haagsma NC, van Gent CM, Luten, JB, et al. Preparation of an w3 fatty acid concentrate from cod liver oil. *JAOCS* 59:117-118, 1982.

Kifer RR, Miller D. Fish oils-fatty acid composition energy values, metabolism, and vitamin content. *Fish Ind* 5:25, 1969.

Peifer JJ, Janssen F, Muesing R, et al. The lipid depressant activities of whole fish and their component oils. *JAOCS* 39:292-296, 1962.

Stansby ME. Development of fish oil industry in the United States. *JAOCS* 55:238–243, 1978.

Taber L, Chiu C-H, Whelan J. 2001 Assessment of the arachidonic acid content in foods commonly consumed in the American diet. *Lipids* 33(12):1151-1157, 1998.

Young FVK. The production and use of fish oils. In In Barlow SM, Stansby ME (eds). *Nutritional Evaluation Of Long-Chain Fatty Acids In Fish Oil.* New York: Academic Press, 1982, pp 1-23.

19—Alternative Diets

One well-established nutritional concept for average Americans in 2005 **is** the desirability of lowering total caloric daily intakes to balance the calories expended. Most people in Western industrialized countries are urged to consume less calories and expend more energy to balance daily energy and avoid the extra calories accumulating as fat and cholesterol associated with inflammatory vascular disease. Another important concept developed in this book is the desirability of raising n-3 intakes and lowering n-6 intakes to balance tissue HUFA and avoid overproduction of n-6 eicosanoids that mediate serious chronic diseases. Important primary prevention should include both of these simple diet alternatives. A reexamination of Fig. I-3 (Introduction) may help us decide what diets can help us achieve these goals as we evaluate the four suggested approaches in the Overview.

Suggestion 1

The earlier suggestion (1965–1985) of consuming very high "megadose" amounts of linoleate 18:2n-6 to elevate tissue 18:2n-6 and decrease the availability of arachidonate 20:4n-6 for eicosanoid formation (Fig. 19-1) has failed to meet expectations from experimental studies. There are three major concerns associated with this approach.

Increased Caloric Intake

First is the concern over the total caloric intake likely to occur when adding to the daily diet the large amounts (40-50 g; about 60 ml) of linoleate-rich oil proposed to suppress the availability of arachidonate for eicosanoid formation. The desire to keep total calories minimal would likely favor vegetable oils richest in 18:2n-6: safflower oil (80%) > sunflower oil (66%) > corn oil (58%) soybean oil (51%). This priority, however, is in the reverse order to the relative abundance of these oils in commerce, and thus would likely meet marketing resistance. Each product will have its marketing advocates, and various rationales for the use of each oil seem certain to evolve.

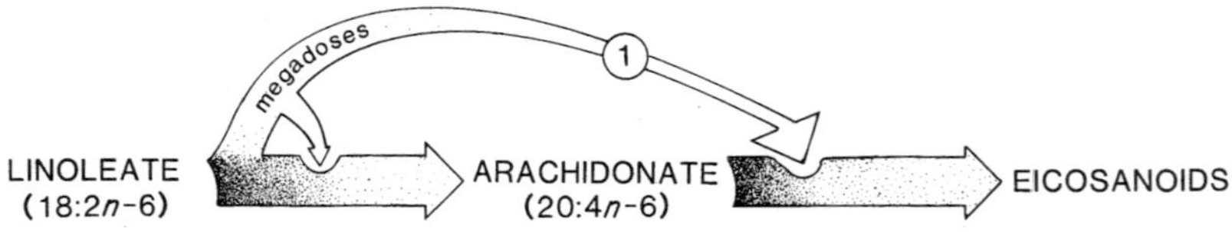

Fig. 19-1. The megadose approach.

Arachidonate from Meat

A second concern is about the amount of arachidonate consumed in the diet from meat, since additional intake of arachidonate can directly form eicosanoids. Fortunately, the content of arachidonate in most foods is generally not very high: approximately 70-150 mg per 100 g of chicken, pork, or beef. Most dietary studies use linoleate, and the seventy years of EFA research still gives no clear answer for the daily dietary intake of arachidonate needed for essential fatty acids. It seems as though most quantitative nutritional studies of EFA ended just prior to recognizing that they form eicosanoids and that different disease states are related to eicosanoids. We can only assume and hope that a moderate intake of meat will avoid "pushing" n-6 eicosanoid formation excessively. Nutrition research still has little controlled evidence to assign suitable or desirable combinations of arachidonate and linoleate intake.

Loss of Control

A third concern for the "megadoses" of Suggestion 1 is even more vexing because it relates to the consequences of dietary noncompliance, a common occurrence in human dietary experience. Suggestion 1 presumes a continued intake of large amounts (megadoses) of 18:2n-6 that may suppress the conversion of arachidonate to eicosanoids. However, it seems likely that every time a daily "megadose" of linoleate is neglected, the pools of precursor acids might progress to lower contents of 18:2n-6 that would then permit tissue arachidonate to support eicosanoid biosynthesis at a greater rate and thus defeat the intended strategy. Would we ever be able to turn away from 18:2n-6 megadoses once we started them?

Suggestion 2

Moderating eicosanoid formation by dietary means might cut the intake of n-6 fatty acids to meet only the optimal level required (Fig. 19-2). Past research has indicated an adequate level of 1 en% linoleate, although the studies failed to consider the amount of arachidonate eaten daily. One concern of this possible approach is whether decreasing the overall content of polyunsaturated fatty acids in the diet might lead to increased saturated fat intakes. Much public attention already has been placed on including polyunsaturated fatty acids in the diet, and there is bound to be confusion and uncertainty regarding the benefits of decreasing the overall amount now. The ubiquitous presence of linoleate in nearly all foods makes even rigorous attempts to cut intake of n-6 fats unlikely to reach 1 en% linoleate. Laboratory studies of adult animals clearly showed how difficult it is to create a deficiency of n-6 fatty acids after tissue levels have been high. The empirical diet-tissue relationship described in Chapter 17 indicates that without added competition by n-3 fats only lowering intakes of n-6 acids is likely inadequate for maintaining balanced tissue HUFA.

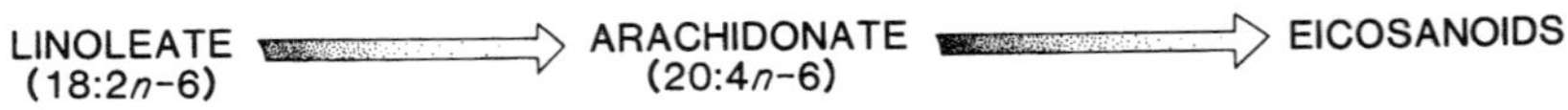

Fig. 19-2. The stringency approach.

Suggestion 3

This approach seems better than the previous alternatives. It would decrease dietary linoleate (18:2n-6) in the current diet and increase linolenate (18:3n-3) to decrease the formation of 20:4n-6 from 18:2n-6 (Fig. 19-3). The dietary n-3 linolenate would also be expected to gradually increase tissue levels of the longer n-3 HUFA, 20:5n-3, 22:5n-3 and 22:6n-3, and give more effective inhibition of arachidonate conversion to eicosanoids.

This dietary alternative favors dietary oils particularly rich in 18:3n-3: flaxseed (53%) >> rapeseed (11%) >> soybean (7%). The ratio of the two acids (18:3/18:2) in flaxseed oil is 53/13, whereas in low-erucic rapeseed oil (e.g., canola) it is 11/22 (see Table 18-4 [Chapter 18]). Soybean has only 7/51, and it is already a major cause of the high proportion of n-6 HUFA in tissue HUFA in the United States.

Some concerns associated with this alternative include keeping a sufficiently low total caloric intake, although this concern could be eliminated by people carefully monitoring their food. A second concern linked to this approach is for inclusion of sufficient antioxidant in food oils for a safe shelf life and including added vitamin E in the diet to protect the tissues from the easily oxidized PUFA.

The old-fashioned mode of preparing and marketing linseed oil for the paint industry favors partial oxidation and polymerization in ways that are unsuited for human consumption. It is necessary to have the oil processors change their methods when producing flaxseed oil for human consumption. If sufficient amounts of flaxseed oil become available for human diet supplements, there might be a restructuring of the basis of financing the flax crop. It would be interesting to see if a new interest in flaxseed oil would result in broader availability of flax fiber and of linen production. The situation would be reminiscent of the slow shift in the financing and

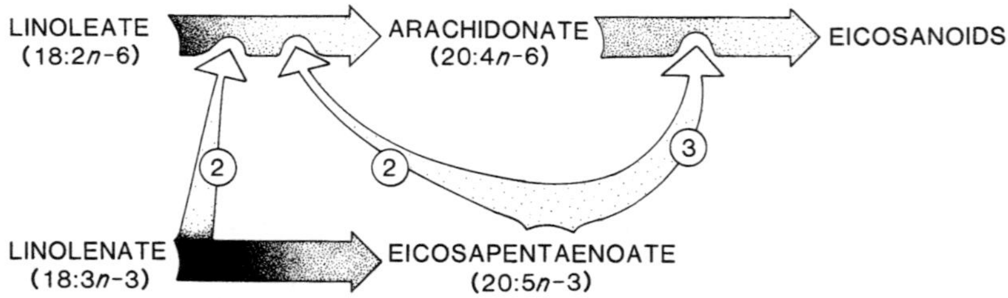

Fig. 19-3. Use of n-3 fats from plants.

marketing of dairy products from a butterfat basis to one more oriented to protein and milk solids.

Suggestion 4

This alternative includes sufficient dietary long-chain n-3 HUFA to suppress the tendency for tissues to overproduce n-6 eicosanoids (Fig. 19-4). The availability of these effective competitors in fish and fish oils permits the metabolic regulations discussed in this book. However, a limited supply of fish and fish oils with high contents of n-3 fatty acids might limit the number of people who could use this approach (as noted in Chapter 18). Another approach would be to fortify foods with n-3 HUFA from unwanted species, limiting the added calories while still moderating eicosanoid formation.

Perhaps alternates for food fortification would be using microbial production or total chemical synthesis of the n-3 HUFA to provide large amounts of the acids. Although the cost of the acids would likely be higher in this approach, the supply would not be limited by natural harvesting factors. Cost of fortification may limit the market, but the health impairments that might be prevented seem much more costly. Finally, the introduction of genetically modified domestic farm animals noted in Chapter 13 might revolutionize the supply of foods for the population to gain desired amounts of n-3 HUFA irrespective of food from the sea.

It seems likely that fish, fish oil supplements, and fish oil fortified foods will be a convenient and economical approach in the near future. Lowering the ingested competing n-6 fats to levels closer to those adequate for optimal nutrition (1-2% of daily calories) will permit even moderate amounts of fish or fish oils to alter our tissue HUFA in a beneficial manner.

A Course for Action

A combination of choices may well provide the best solution. Perhaps a blend of the second, third, and fourth suggestions noted previously can provide a convenient and reasonable compromise for the billions of people who want primary prevention of

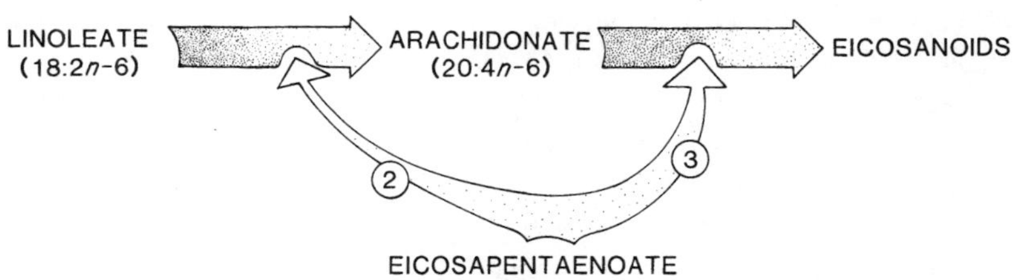

Fig. 19.4. The seafood approach.

the many diet-based chronic diseases noted in earlier chapters. A possible approach could include a significant drop in the total dietary calories in the form of fat with a shift in the balance of dietary polyunsaturated fatty acids to decrease 18:2n-6 and include more 18:3n-3 from selected vegetable oils plus the longer n-3 HUFA from fish and fish oils. Flexible choices still seem best.

The long trail of questions that started with an introduction to the pattern of diseases in Eskimos led to a deeper understanding of how nutrition and genetics influence our health. It seems likely that as we understand more clearly how polyunsaturated acids act, a wide range of new combinations of food can be selected with satisfaction and pleasure to achieve good health.

The data in this book were arranged to help develop an understanding of how certain human diseases are influenced by eicosanoid production and how eicosanoid production is influenced by diet. In following the clues from the lives of Eskimo families, we found new unexpected ways to link the mechanisms of many thrombotic and immune diseases to the n-6 fatty acids in our daily food intake.

There is evidence that the n-3 fatty acids from the sea can modify and prevent some of these disease mechanisms. There is not enough evidence for medical scientists to determine how many of the different aspects in disease prevention are due to diet habits or to genetics. Both aspects are transmitted from parent to child during family life. We have much more to learn of the interactions of these two influences on human health and primary prevention.

We have learned some ways in which n-3 and n-6 polyunsaturated fatty acids in our diets affect our health in general. The oceans of the earth can continue to play important roles in the lives of people. We can see how the food chain of the oceans produces materials that help people balance their lives on land. Understanding that balance may lead to important preventive steps that were neglected for too long. Reviewing the food chain that provides our necessities of life may help us appreciate again what the seas mean to us. Some part of us may reflect early human needs once met by the balanced life found along shores where the tides mark a constantly changing dialog between the land and the sea.

This edition reaffirms the general advice of the 1986 edition. We realized then that any diet alternative to decrease excessive n-6 eicosanoid actions should be in a context of trying at the same time to cut the total caloric intake and the percentage of calories in the form of fat. What we knew then is even truer today.

At that time, I assumed that ongoing nutritional advice to cut overall daily caloric intake and the percentage of daily calories in the form of saturated fat would be implemented soon. However, the imbalance between energy intake and energy expenditure became worse and caused more pathology among Americans in the past decades. An epidemic rise of obesity occurred while billions of dollars were focused on blocking cholesterol formation rather than preventing the dietary energy imbalances that cause high blood cholesterol. Vague and inadequate preventive nutrition information was given to Americans while specific pharmaceutical treatments were extensively marketed.

Prevention of HUFA Imbalances

We now know the diet-tissue relationships for essential fats that are needed for designing effective primary prevention education. Unfortunately, recognizing a public need for effective primary prevention interventions still does not identify the professionals and agencies willing and able to design and deliver effective educational solutions. Obsessive attention to blocking formation of plasma cholesterol with pharmaceutical treatments neglected to acknowledge it as a biomarker for the underlying causal problem of excessive energy intake over expenditure (see Fig.5-3 [Chapter 5] or Fig. 12-3 [Chapter 12]). Primary prevention of energy imbalance needs more definite explicit nutrition advice from public health professionals, just as primary prevention of imbalanced n-3 and n-6 intakes needs more definite and explicit nutrition advice.

This chapter includes insights added since 1986 to show how personalized diet plans can be designed and evaluated by individuals to fit their own life-styles and preferences. The previous chapters noted much published evidence of benefits from raising n-3 intakes while decreasing the competing (and much more than adequate) n-6 intakes. Figure 19-5 reminds readers of the strong link between CHD risk and the balance of tissue and dietary n-3 and n-6 EFA (Lands, 2003). Each reader may have their own level of risk aversion that will point to a personal goal for the proportion of n-6 HUFA in total HUFA.

The 1986 edition suggested general choices for diet plans that met the mood of those times by first considering (but declining to recommend) the common use of megadose levels (11 en%) of the n-6 linoleate which had been claimed to decrease platelet arachidonate. Now, many published results show little merit and some risk in

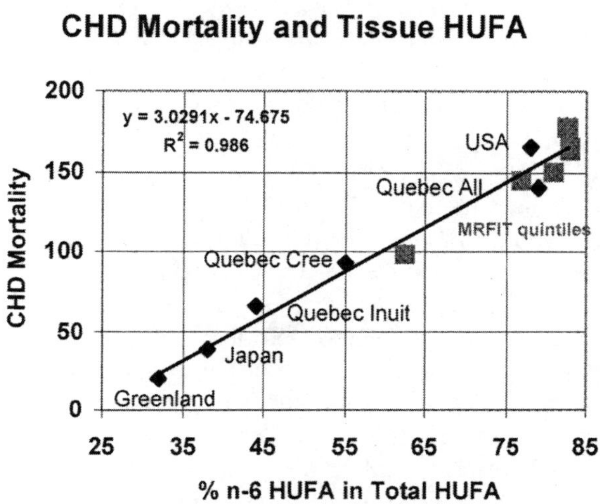

Fig. 19-5. Imbalanced HUFA is a diet-induced dyslipidemia related to CHD risk of death.

having n-6 intakes so much higher than n-3 intakes that tissue HUFA have very high proportions of n-6 HUFA.

The second suggestion of only decreasing n-6 intakes can now also be seen as unlikely to give adequate benefit. The empirical relationship in Chapter 17 predicts that even low linoleate intakes near 1 en% will give high % n-6 HUFA in tissue HUFA when there is inadequate dietary n-3 fats in foods to compete and displace n-6 HUFA from tissue lipids.

The third suggested choice of replacing 18:2n-6 with competing dietary 18:3n-3 is reported to have health benefit, and the fourth suggestion of eating more dietary n-3 HUFA is now recommended by the American Heart Association (2000, 2002). Now, as in 1986, the sound and simple advice to increase n-3 intakes and decrease n-6 linoleate intakes seems desirable. Details about which forms of n-3 and n-6 EFA to eat and how much of each to eat are discussed below.

Making Personal Menu Plans

Daily menu plans in Tables 19-1 to19-7 were developed with the interactive computer program, KIM-2, to illustrate how explicit food choices can meet personal food preferences and personal levels of aversion to risk (see Fig. 19-5). The plans show combinations of foods that create tissue HUFA balances from 15-90% n-6 HUFA in the overall HUFA. The software program combines information on a person's daily food choices and predicts the likely resultant tissue HUFA proportions, and thus a likely risk.

The software is downloadable free from two distant learning websites: http://ods.od.nih.gov/eicosanoids/ and http://efaeducation.nih.gov/ . It manages quantitative information from the USDA about essential fatty acids and calories in nearly twelve thousand different servings of food. The process of discovering suitable foods that fit individual preferences and life-styles is made easier by computerized "find" and "sort" commands. Alternative diets become feasible in the context of the very wide range of EFA intakes that are seen to occur voluntarily in free-living populations. Fig. 19-5 repeats Fig. 1-3 [Chapter 1] to remind readers how tissue HUFA proportions relate to cardiovascular mortality. Choose your foods wisely!

The interactive menu planning software system, KIM (Keep It Managed), displays daily menu plans with the different servings arranged either by mealtimes or by the food group types discussed in Chapter 18. The milligrams of each of four types of EFA in a serving are listed, summed and expressed as a percent of total daily calories (en%).

The en% values are then combined into the empirical predictive relationship described in Chapter 17 to estimate a likely value for the percent of n-6 HUFA in plasma phospholipid HUFA, a biomarker for EFA intakes and a surrogate index of cardiovascular risk as shown in Fig. 19-5. The seven sample plans provided at the end of this chapter have food combinations predicted to give estimated biomarker values ranging from 13% to 93% n-6 HUFA in the phospholipid HUFA. Many other combinations are possible.

TABLE 19-1
Meal Times For 91% Plan That Likely Gives 91% n-6 HUFA in Overall HUFA

Breakfast	Serving Size	grams	kcals	Servings	Short 6	Short 3	Long 6	Long 3
Fast foods, biscuit, with egg and ham	1 biscuit	192	442	1	7087	467	117	35
Milk, reduced fat, fluid, 2% milkfat	1 cup	245	125	1	105	69	0	0
Vegetable juice cocktail, canned	1 cup	242	46	1	87	2	0	0
Lunch	Serving Size	grams	kcals	Servings	Short 6	Short 3	Long 6	Long 3
Egg, whole, cooked, hard-boiled	1 large	50	78	1	594	18	75	22
Mushrooms, canned, drained pieces	0.5 cup	78	19	1	87	1	0	0
Tomatoes, red, ripe, raw,	1 large whole	182	38	1	237	9	0	0
Oil, vegetable corn, salad or cooking	1 tbsp	14	120	1	7888	95	0	0
Onions, raw	1 slice, thin	9	10	3	16	1	0	0
Dinner	Serving Size	grams	kcals	Servings	Short 6	Short 3	Long 6	Long 3
Applesauce, canned, unsweetened	1 cup	244	105	1	29	7	0	0
Cheese, gruyere	1 oz	28	117	1	369	123	0	0
Tofu, soft, with calcium sulfate	1 piece (2-1/2″)	120	73	1	2202	295	0	0
Chicken, broilers, thigh, meat and skin,	1 thigh	68	473	3	5794	265	245	143
Corn, sweet, yellow, kernels, cooked,	0.5 cup kernels	82	76	1	277	8	0	0
Okra, cooked, boiled, drained	8 pods (3″ long)	85	27	1	38	1	0	0
Potatoes, frozen, french fried, extruded,	10 strips	50	333	2	1405	0	0	0
Snacks	Serving Size	grams	kcals	Servings	Short 6	Short 3	Long 6	Long 3
Apple juice, bottled, unsweetened,	1 cup	248	117	1	69	15	0	0
Snacks, pork skins, barbecue-flavor	1 oz	28	153	1	967	0	11	0
				total mg =	**27250**	**1375**	**448**	**199**
Total Energy Choice = 2351 kcals				**%Cal =**	**10.43%**	**0.53%**	**0.17%**	**0.08%**

TABLE 19-2
Meal Times For 71% Plan That Likely Gives 71% n-6 HUFA in Overall HUFA

Breakfast	Serving Size	grams	kcals	Servings	Short 6	Short 3	Long 6	Long 3
Blueberries, raw	50 berries	68	38	1	67	46	0	0
Cereals ready-to-eat, KELLOGG'S	0.75 cup	29	92	1	297	21	1	0
Bread, mixed-grain, toasted (whole-grain)	1 slice	24	131	2	451	30	0	0
Butter, with salt	1 pat	5	72	2	183	118	0	0
Milk, reduced fat, fluid, 2% milkfat	1 cup	244	244	2	210	137	0	0
Lunch	Serving Size	grams	kcals	Servings	Short 6	Short 3	Long 6	Long 3
Strawberries, raw	1 cup, whole	144	43	1	156	112	0	0
Spinach, raw	1 cup	30	13	2	13	69	0	0
Tomatoes, red, ripe, raw, year round average	1 medium	123	26	1	160	6	0	0
Peppers, sweet, red, raw	1 cup, sliced	92	25	1	86	8	0	0
Vegetable oil, canola	1 tbsp	14	124	1	2842	1302	0	0
Chicken, broilers or fryers, meat only, roasted	1 unit	146	277	1	2000	102	161	102
Cheese, cottage, nonfat, large curd	4 oz	113	192	2	25	9	0	0
Dinner	Serving Size	grams	kcals	Servings	Short 6	Short 3	Long 6	Long 3
Lettuce, looseleaf, raw, shredded	0.5 cup	28	5	1	13	32	0	0
Mushrooms, cooked, boiled, drained, pieces	0.5 cup	78	21	1	140	1	0	0
Asparagus, cooked, boiled, drained	4 spears (1/2"	60	29	2	155	8	0	0
Salad dressing, mayonnaise, soybean oil	1 tbsp	14	99	1	5120	580	0	0
Ice creams, chocolate	0.5 cup	66	285	2	330	198	0	0
Crustaceans, shrimp, mixed species	3 oz	85	90	1	24	17	74	447
Pork, fresh, loin, tenderloin, separable lean	3 oz	85	159	1	417	9	34	0
Chickpeas (garbanzo beans, bengal gram)	1 cup	164	269	1	1825	71	0	0
Cheese, gruyere	1 slice (1 oz)	28	116	1	364	121	0	0
Snacks	Serving Size	grams	kcals	Servings	Short 6	Short 3	Long 6	Long 3
Apples, raw, with skin	1 medium (2-3/4"	138	81	1	120	25	0	0
Alcoholic beverage, beer, regular	1 bottle (12 fl.oz.)	356	292	2	0	0	0	0
Snacks, potato chips, plain, salted	1 oz	28	304	2	6793	108	0	0
				total mg =	**21789**	**3129**	**270**	**549**
Total Energy Choice = 3027 kcals				**%Cal=**	**6.48%**	**0.93%**	**0.08%**	**0.16%**

TABLE 19-3
Meal Times For 63% Plan That Likely Gives 63% n-6 HUFA in Overall HUFA

Breakfast	Serving Size	grams	kcals	Servings	Short 6	Short 3	Long 6	Long 3
Blueberries, raw	50 berries	68	38	1	67	46	0	0
Cereals ready-to-eat, CHEERIOS	1 cup	30	221	2	405	19	0	0
Bananas, raw	1 medium (7″)	118	109	1	66	39	0	0
Egg, whole, cooked, scrambled	1 large	61	101	1	1169	51	71	2
Milk, nonfat, fluid, (fat free or	1 cup	245	172	2	25	10	0	0
Lunch	Serving Size	grams	kcals	Servings	Short 6	Short 3	Long 6	Long 3
Cheese, gouda	1 oz	28	101	1	75	112	0	0
Cheese, cottage, nonfat, dry,	1 cup	145	123	1	16	6	0	0
Cabbage, raw	1 cup, shredded	70	18	1	36	48	1	0
Carrots, raw	1 large (7-1/4″ to	72	31	1	48	7	0	0
Bread, cracked-wheat	1 slice	25	195	3	486	25	0	0
Dinner	Serving Size	grams	kcals	Servings	Short 6	Short 3	Long 6	Long 3
Beans, kidney, royal red, boiled	1 cup	177	218	1	64	101	0	0
Apples, raw, with skin	1 medium (2-3/4″	138	81	1	120	25	0	0
New Zealand spinach, raw	1 cup chopped	56	8	1	7	37	0	0
Potatoes, baked, flesh	1 potato (2″)	156	145	1	50	16	0	0
Lima beans, canned, no salt	0.5 cup	124	44	0.5	58	28	0	0
Peas and onions, boiled,	1 cup	180	81	1	140	29	0	0
Snacks	Serving Size	grams	kcals	Servings	Short 6	Short 3	Long 6	Long 3
Candies, fudge, chocolate	1 piece	17	70	1	50	13	0	0
Frozen yogurts, chocolate,	0.5 cup (4 fl oz)	72	115	1	101	50	0	0
				total mg =	**2983**	**659**	**71**	**21**
Total Energy Choice = 1871 kcals				**%Cal =**	**1.44%**	**0.32%**	**0.03%**	**0.01%**

TABLE 19-4
Meal Times For 50% Plan That Likely Gives 50% n-6 HUFA in Overall HUFA

Breakfast	Serving Size	grams	kcals	Servings	Short 6	Short 3	Long 6	Long 3
Bananas, raw	1 medium 7″	118	109	1	66	39	0	0
Bread, cracked-wheat	1 slice, regular	25	130	2	324	17	0	0
Cereal HONEY NUT	1 cup	30	112	1	429	31	0	0
Butter, with salt	1 pat (1″ sq, 1/3″	5	36	1	92	59	0	0
Milk, nonfat, fat free	1 cup	245	172	2	25	10	0	0
Lunch	Serving Size	grams	kcals	Servings	Short 6	Short 3	Long 6	Long 3
Nectarines, raw	1 fruit (2-1/2″)	136	67	1	306	7	0	0
Cabbage, raw	1 cup, shredded	70	18	1	36	48	1	0
Cheese, cottage, nonfat,	1 cup	145	123	1	16	6	0	0
Pork, fresh, top loin (roasts)	1 oz	28	40	1	130	6	17	0
Dinner	Serving Size	grams	kcals	Servings	Short 6	Short 3	Long 6	Long 3
Vegetable oil, canola	1 tbsp	14	124	1	2842	1302	0	0
Corn, sweet, yellow, boiled	0.5 cup cut	82	89	1	481	15	0	0
Lima beans, canned,	0.5 cup	124	88	1	117	56	0	0
\New Zealand spinach, raw	1 cup, chopped	56	8	1	7	37	0	0
Potatoes, baked, flesh	1 potato 2-1/3″	156	145	1	50	16	0	0
Carrots, raw	1 large (7-1/4″	72	31	1	48	7	0	0
Finfish, snapper, grilled	1 fillet	170	218	1	43	0	75	58
Chickpeas (garbanzo)	1 cup	164	269	1	1825	71	0	0
Snacks	Serving Size	grams	kcals	Servings	Short 6	Short 3	Long 6	Long 3
Blueberries, raw	50 berries	68	38	1	67	46	0	0
Apples, raw, with skin	1 medium 2-3/4″	138	163	2	240	50	0	0
Snacks, pretzels, hard	1 oz	28	130	1	564	45	0	0
Candies, fudge, chocolate	1 piece	17	140	2	100	26	0	0
				total mg =	**7808**	**1840**	**93**	**583**
Total Energy Choice = 2247 kcals				**%Cal=**	**3.13%**	**0.76%**	**0.04%**	**0.23%**

TABLE 19-5
Meal Times For 35% Plan That Gives 35% n-6 HUFA in Overall HUFA

Breakfast	Serving Size	grams	kcals	Servings	Short 6	Short 3	Long 6	Long 3
Oil, olive, salad or cooking	1 1tsp	5	80	2	711	54	0	0
Orange juice, raw	1 cup	248	112	1	72	27	0	0
Squash, winter, hubbard, baked	1 cup	205	103	1	199	332	0	0
Mungo beans, mature boiled	1 cup	180	189	1	43	603	0	0
Lunch	Servinq Size	grams	kcals	Servings	Short 6	Short 3	Long 6	Long3
Potatoes, russet, flesh and skin	1 potato small	170	134	1	43	17	0	0
Grape leaves, canned	1 leaf	4	3	1	6	34	0	0
Seeds, flaxseed	1 tbsp	12	59	1	518	2175	0	0
Rice, white, long-grain, regular	1 cup	158	411	2	196	41	0	0
Dinner	Serving Size	grams	kcals	Servings	Short6	Short3	Long6	Long3
Artichokes, boiled, drained	0.5 cup	84	42	1	41	15	0	0
Spinach, boiled, drained	1 cup	180	41	1	29	153	0	0
Cauliflower, cooked	0.5 cup	62	20	1	19	66	0	0
Beans, kidney, royal red, boiled	1 cup	177	218	1	64	101	0	0
Wild rice, cooked	1 cup	164	166	1	195	156	0	0
Snacks	Servinq Size	grams	kcals	Servings	Short 6	Short 3	Long6	Long3
Bananas, raw	1 large 8″	136	125	1	76	45	0	0
				total mg =	**2211**	**3819**	**0**	**0**
Total Energy Choice = 1701 kcals				**%Cal=**	**1.17%**	**2.02%**	**0.00%**	**0.00%**

TABLE 19-6
Meal Times For 26% Plan That Gives 26% n-6 HUFA in Overall HUFA

Breakfast	Serving Size	grams	kcals	Servings	Short 6	Short 3	Long 6	Long 3
Cereals, QUAKER, oatmeal, instant	1 packet	37	135	1	689	65	0	0
Milk, reduced fat, fluid, 2% milkfat,	1 cup	244	122	1	105	68	0	0
Blueberries, raw	50 berries	68	38	1	67	46	0	0
Orange juice, raw	1 cup	248	56	0.5	36	14	0	0
Lunch	Serving Size	grams	kcals	Servings	Short 6	Short 3	Long 6	Long 3
Potatoes, flesh skin, baked	1 medium	173	168	1	55	17	0	0
Cheese, gruyere	1 slice (1 oz)	28	116	1	364	121	0	0
Oil, olive, salad or cooking	1 tbsp	14	60	0.5	533	41	0	0
Pork, fresh, loin, tenderloin,	3 oz	85	139	1	298	9	26	0
Dinner	Serving Size	grams	kcals	Servings	Short 6	Short 3	Long 6	Long 3
Rice, white, long-grain,	1 cup	95	360	1	60	13	0	0
New Zealand spinach, cooked	1 cup, chopped	180	22	1	20	101	0	0
Cauliflower, cooked, boiled,	0.5 cup (1″ pcs)	62	14	1	31	104	0	0
Finfish, salmon, coho, wild	0.5 fillet	155	143	0.5	202	270	131	1293
Ice creams, chocolate	0.5 cup (4 fl oz)	66	143	1	165	99	0	0
Broccoli, cooked, boiled	1 stalk, large	280	78	1	106	361	0	0
Snacks	Serving Size	grams	kcals	Servings	Short 6	Short 3	Long 6	Long 3
Bananas, raw	1 large (8″)	136	125	1	76	45	0	0
				total mg =	**2807**	**1374**	**156**	**1293**
Total Energy Choice = 1718 kcals				**%Cal =**	**1.47%**	**0.72%**	**0.08%**	**0.68%**

TABLE 19-7
Meal Times For 15% Plan That Gives 15% n-6 HUFA in Overall HUFA

Breakfast	Serving Size	grams	kcals	Servings	Short 6	Short 3	Long 6	Long 3
Mungo beans, mature seeds, boiled,	1 cup	180	95	0.5	22	302	0	0
Rice, white, long-grain, regular, cooked	1 cup	158	103	0.5	49	100	0	0
Mangos, raw	1 cup, sliced	165	107	1	23	61	0	0
Egg, whole, cooked, poached	1 large	50	75	1	572	17	71	21
Lunch	Serving Size	grams	kcals	Servings	Short 6	Short 3	Long 6	Long 3
Lettuce, cos or romaine, raw, shredded	0.5 cup	28	4	1	9	21	0	0
Lettuce, iceberg, raw, shredded	1 cup,	55	3	0.5	8	20	0	0
Spinach, raw	1 cup	30	3	0.5	3	17	0	0
Vinegar, cider	1 tbsp	15	2	1	0	0	0	0
Cheese, feta	1 oz	28	75	1	92	75	0	0
Squash, summer, zucchini, cooked,	1 cup, sliced	180	29	1	14	23	0	0
427 cold-pressed flaxseed oil	1	5	40	1	691	2558	0	0
Dinner	Serving Size	grams	kcals	Servings	Short 6	Short 3	Long 6	Long 3
Salmon, coho, wild, cooked, dry heat	0.5 fillet	178	247	1	100	190	39	1885
Beans, snap, green, cooked, boiled,	1 cup	125	44	1	70	111	0	0
Broccoli, cooked, boiled, drained	1 stalk,	280	157	2	213	722	0	0
Cauliflower, cooked, boiled, (1″ pieces)	0.5 cup	62	29	2	62	207	0	0
Squash, winter, hubbard, baked, cubes	1 cup	205	103	1	199	332	0	0
Cheese, fontina	1 oz	28	110	1	245	224	0	0
Rice, white, short-grain, cooked	1 cup	186	242	1	76	17	0	0
Wild rice, cooked	1 cup	164	166	1	195	156	0	0
Snacks	Serving Size	grams	kcals	Servings	Short 6	Short 3	Long 6	Long 3
Finfish, herring, Atlantic, pickled, boneless	1 oz	28	74	1	60	0	0	416
				total mg =	**2702**	**5063**	**110**	**2322**
Total Energy Choice = 1706 kcals				**%Cal =**	**1.43%**	**2.67%**	**0.06%**	**1.22%**

Readers of this book can now consider a wide range of food choices that will provide a wide range of relative risks for excessive n-6 eicosanoid actions. I hope the information in this book gives readers the confidence to choose their own nutritional path to travel with family and friends in the future.

Now, with the software system available to implement personal goals, I find that people want an answer to "What tissue composition would be "optimal" for me?" Answering that question is not easy because the steady gradient of CHD mortality in Fig. 19-5 has no definite place for claiming an optimal balance in tissue HUFA. Values in the lower left seem better than those in the upper right. The biomedical literature has no clear evidence of adverse health conditions with 25% HUFA as n-6 HUFA, in contrast to the much higher CHD mortality rate at 80 % n-6 HUFA in total HUFA. Knowledge about n-6 eicosanoid-mediated diseases described in earlier chapters of this book makes it unlikely that properly informed people would knowingly regard proportions above 60 percent n-6 in their tissue HUFA as either desirable or optimal. We have now arrived at a point in time when people are free to choose their own desired target value, and software will help them find foods to meet the desired goal for themselves and their families.

While there will always remain much that medical scientists do not know about specific disease mechanisms, there is now much that they do know. This small book includes some of the known facts to let readers make informed choices for themselves and their families. The goal of this second edition of *Fish, Omega-3 and Human Health* continues to be finding a fullness in life by balancing what we know with what we want. Insights and tools added to the book in 2005 may help readers take actions that did not occur very rapidly after the 1986 edition.

References

Krauss RM, Eckel RH, Howard B, et al. AHA Dietary Guidelines: revision 2000: a statement for healthcare professionals from the Nutrition Committee of the American Heart Association. *Circulation.*102:2284-2299, 2000.

Kris-Etherton PM, Harris WS, Appel LJ, for the Nutrition Committee. Fish consumption, fish oil, omega-3 fatty acids, and cardiovascular disease. *Circulation* 106:2747-2757, 2002.

Lands WEM. (2003) Primary prevention in cardiovascular disease: moving out of the shadows of the truth about death. *Nutr Metab Cardio Dis* 13:154-164, 2003.

Glossary

AcH (abbrev.), acetyl hydrolase is an enzyme that inactivates platelet activating factor (Chapter 5).

acetyl-CoA, is a common metabolic intermediate in converting the carbon and electrons of carbohydrates, fats and proteins into CO_2 and H_2O. The 2-carbon acetyl portion is attached to a complex derivative of the B vitamin, pantothenic acid.

acyl-CoA, is the form of pantothenic acid transfering 16- to 24-carbon fatty acids among their pathways of synthesis and oxidation.

adrenergic, refers to the signaling system acting with adrenaline and nor-adrenaline (or therapeutic agents that mimic these autacoids) and activating tissue and nerve receptors. Two different types of receptors, *alpha* and *beta*, mediate different signaling pathways in tissues.

allergic, defensive immune autacoid response(s) to materials from outside the body. The response(s) involve lymphocyte recognition of the material as 'non-self' and the formation of circulating antibodies and cytokines that trigger the self-healing defensive response when the foreign material is present (see also immune).

androgen, this class of hormones alters tissue responses of men and women. It produces gender-related aspects characteristic of males.

aneurysm, permanent distension of blood vessels that may cause rupture or leakage of blood into surrounding tissue and an impaired delivery of nutrients and oxygen to other regions. (For contrast, see *thrombosis*).

angina, sense of pain in different regions of the chest, neck and arm resulting from inadequate blood flow to the heart muscle

antioxidant, a material that diverts oxidative processes among tissue components.

apoptosis, cellular process of controlled self-destruction that creates less surrounding tissue damage than necrosis and allows tissues to develop new structures and functions.

arachidonic acid (AA), a polyunsaturated fatty acid containing 20 carbon atoms and 4 double bonds (20:4); one of several important highly unsaturated fatty acids (HUFA). This n-6 acid has the last double bond located six carbon atoms from the end carbon atom of the acid. It is abundant in meats.

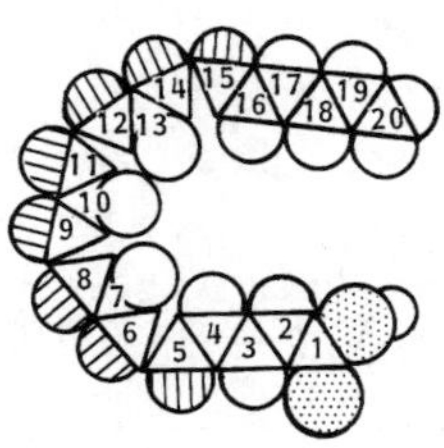

20:4*n*−6

arrhythmia, disturbance in the coordinated rhythmic contraction of the heart muscle.

arrhythmogenic, a condition or process that leads to (genesis) arrhythmia.

arthritis, chronic inflammatory destruction of joints and connective tissues.

asthma, complex set of reactions associated with a constriction of the airways to the lung; mediated perhaps by leukotrienes, especially following certain allergic events.

atherogenesis, the long series of events that over decades leads to (genesis) atherosclerosis.

atherosclerosis, inflammatory condition of blood vessels in which thickening of vessel wall narrows the space through which the blood flows, impairing delivery of nutrients and oxygen and increasing the risk of thrombosis.

atherosclerotic, about the condition of atherosclerosis.

autacoid, hormone-like compound that regulates transient "self-healing" (auto = self; akos = healing) adaptive responses of cells to stimuli.

autonomic, division of the nervous system that spontaneously (unconsciously) regulates and maintains normal body functions with a balance of two signaling systems, *sympathetic* (adrenergic) and *parasympathetic* (cholinergic).

B-cells, bone marrow-related white cells, also called *leukocytes* or *lymphocytes*, that participate in immune system interactions by forming and releasing specific antibodies (see Chapter 10).

biomarkers, molecules or events that can be measured reliably as indices of tissue status.

blood cells, cells normally circulating in the blood including red cells (that carry oxygen), white cells (that participate in immune inflammatory events), and platelets (that form thrombi).

bronchial asthma, see *asthma.*

cannabinoid, refers to a class of compounds that activate cannabinoid receptors in either self-healing or pharmacological tissue responses depending on the source of the compound.

cardiovascular, refers to the heart (cardio) and blood vessels (vascular) that constitute a system for distributing blood and the oxygen and nutrients that it carries to various tissues.

calcium (Ca), element that forms bones and also functions as an important regulator of cellular signaling and metabolic control.

carbon dioxide (CO_2), the end-product of oxidation of carbon compounds.

caspase, a family of destructive enzymes that cleave cellular proteins in association with programmed cell death or apoptosis.

cerebral artery disease, inflammatory vascular disease in the blood vessels to the brain; it involves processes similar to coronary heart disease.

CHD (abbrev.), coronary heart disease.

chemotactic, refers to the ability of a chemical to attract cells toward regions where the chemical occurs in higher concentrations.

cholesterol, a compound that is insoluble in water and that tends to accumulate in cell membranes when not being transported in the lipoproteins of the blood.

clinical signs, measurements agreed upon by expert committees for the International Classification of Disease (ICD) as indicating the presence of a particular disease.

clinical targets, molecular or physiological events thought to cause or mediate a disease process. Preventing or diminishing such targets is the goal of clinical intervention to reach a favorable healthy outcome.

coronary heart disease (CHD), progressive chronic impairment of blood flow to the heart that results from atherosclerosis in coronary blood vessels that supply the heart

coronary infarcts, loss of vital heart tissue usually following a prolonged loss of blood flow (ischemia).

coronary, related to larger blood vessels supplying nutrients and oxygen to the heart. (They are arranged like a crown.)

COX (abbrev.), cyclooxygenase, the enzymes that catalyze conversion of HUFA to prostaglandins.

CRP (abbrev), C-reactive protein is a biomarker of tissue oxidant stress which appears in plasma associated with inflammatory conditions and atherosclerosis

cytokine, an intercellular signaling protein that binds receptors on cell surfaces to trigger transient autacoid actions in immune and growth responses of cells.

cytosol, fluid contents of a cell.

CVD (abbrev.), cardiovascular disease.

DALY (abbrev.), Disability Adjusted Life Years, an epidemiological disease-specific measure of impaired health in a population.

delta 4, designating a chemical structure with a double bond starting at the 4th carbon, e.g 22:6n-3 has a delta-4 double bond.

depression, an abnormal loss of all interest and pleasure most of the day for at least two weeks with marked sadness and functional impairment. Separate related mood disorders are bipolar disorder and dysthymic disorder (linked to EFA in Chapter 3).

dermal, pertains to the skin.

desaturase, an enzyme that catalyzes the process of forming a double bond, called desaturation (discussed with elongation in Chapter 13).

diabetes, a metabolic disease characterized by elevated blood glucose values, inadequate insulin actions and imbalanced storing, mobilizing and metabolizing of fat (Chap.10).

DNA (abbrev.), deoxyribonucleic acid, the complex polymer that codes genetic information.

docosahexaenoic acid (DHA), a polyunsaturated fatty acid with 22 carbon atoms and 6 double bonds (22:6)—a member of the HUFA type of acid (see arachidonic acid). It has an n-3 structure and is very abundant in seafoods.

docosapentaenoic acid (DPA), refers to a polyunsaturated fatty acid with 22 carbon atoms and five double bonds (22:5)—a member of the HUFA type of acid (see arachidonic acid). The n-3 type is often abundant in seafoods.

double bond, a chemical structure with double the number of electrons shared between two carbon atoms; see *unsaturated.*

EAE (abbrev.), experimental allergic encephalitis.

EFA (abbrev.), essential fatty acids, vitamin-like nutrients with many vital functions (Chapter 3).

EGF (abbrev.), epidermal growth factor, one of several proteins that activate cellular receptors which trigger signal pathways causing extensive intracellular adaptations.

Eicosanoid, a term designating any of a large family of hormone-like compounds that contain 20 carbons, for which the most common precursor is the 20-carbon acid, arachidonate. The eicosanoids include two major types of biologically active agents: prostaglandins and leukotrienes that mediate self-healing autacoid responses.

eicosapentaenoic acid (EPA), a polyunsaturated fatty acid with 20 carbon atoms and 5 double bonds (20:5)—a member of the HUFA type of acid (see arachidonic acid). The common form has an n-3 structure, and is particularly abundant in seafoods.

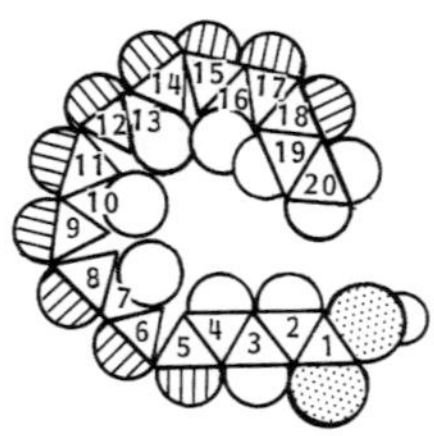

20:5*n*−3

ELISA (abbrev.), enzyme-linked immunospecific assay which allows quantitative measurement of small amounts of biological molecules using highly selective antibodies.

elongation, a multi-enzyme process of adding two carbons to a fatty acid, often associated with desaturation (Chapter 13).

embolism, a state of reduced blood flow due to blockage by abnormal material, usually a blood clot comprised of clotting proteins and platelets (see thrombosis).

en% (abbrev.), the percentage of total daily food calories that are in a particular type of item; e.g., 20 en% indicates 20% of the daily energy.

endocannabinoids, are autacoid signaling agents formed in tissues from essential fatty acids.

endothelial cell, a type of cell that forms a thin inner lining of blood vessels. These cells form the endothelium lining that is the largest organ of the body. It is in constant interaction with the blood and blood cells, and when stimulated, it produces the potent antithrombotic eicosanoid, prostacyclin, and the vasodilating autacoid, nitric oxide.

energy percent (en%), the percentage of total daily food calories that are in a particular type of item; e.g., 20 energy percent (20 en%) indicates 20% of the daily energy.

eskimo, a group of people (often called Inuits) who live in Arctic regions and whose traditional ethnic diet consists primarily of meats of maritime origins and other materials from the sea.

essential fatty acid (EFA), type of polyunsaturated fatty acid needed for normal health. It must be provided in the diet, since it cannot be formed in the body. Both n-6 and n-3 types of polyunsaturated fatty acid provide essential structures and functions. Recent data are indicating more functions (see Chapter 3) for which dietary supplies of EFA are needed.

expression, term for forming new molecules, especially in the context of translating genetic deoxyribonucleic acid (DNA) information into messenger ribonucleic acid (mRNA), which guides the synthesis of new proteins and alters cellular actions and functions.

fat, a storage and transport form of fatty acids combined with glycerol. Fats include butter, lard, margarine, vegetable oil, and fish oil.

fatty acid, an organic weak acid that usually contains a chain of an even number (e.g., 16 or 18) of carbon atoms. These chains give the physical character to fats that are commonly recognized: soft, greasy, oily, etc. Butter and margarine have many saturated fatty acids, whereas vegetable oil and fish oil have many unsaturated fatty acids. Short-chain fatty acids have 2-8 carbons and long-chain fatty acids may have 20 or 22 carbons.

folate, ionic form of folic acid, an important water-soluble vitamin that is vulnerable to oxidant stress. It works with vitamin B_{12} to help form and metabolize methyl groups.

fibrin, a protein (formed by cleaving fibrinogen), which holds blood components together in insoluble clots associated with thrombosis. Fibrin destruction or fibrinolysis breaks clots.

"free" fatty acids, fatty acids released from their usual ester linkage in tissue lipids are not water soluble and are more accurately called nonesterified fatty acids (NEFA) because they readily bind to proteins, ensuring that they are never "free".

gas chromatography, a method for separating, quantitatively analyzing the many different fatty acids that occur in mixtures in Nature (sample results from hundreds of people in Fig.17-1).

HDL (abbrev.), high density lipoproteins, a family of complex mixtures of proteins and lipids known to carry antioxidant enzymes and be positively related to good health.

hemorrhage, loss of blood from the blood vessels.

HMG-CoA (abbrev.), hydroxyl methylglutaryl-coenzyme A, is a metabolic intermediate that is formed from overabundant acetyl-CoA and leads to formation of isoprenoids and cholesterol

HRV (abbrev.), heart rate variability reflecting autonomic tone related to heart attacks and depression.

HUFA (abbrev.), refers to **20- and 22-carbon highly unsaturated fatty acids** with three or more double bonds.

hypolipidemic, condition of having lower than average amounts of lipid (fat) in the bloodstream.

ICAM (abbrev.), intercellular adhesion molecule, a protein at the outer surface of a cell that binds to receptors on adjacent cells and facilitates cooperative cellular interactions.

IDL (abbrev.), intermediate density lipoproteins, a family of complex mixtures of proteins and lipids resulting from progressive removal of fat by lipoprotein lipase action in the blood on circulating VLDL and LDL precursors.

immune, used in this text to refer to the defensive network of responses developed when a material is recognized (correctly or incorrectly) as "nonself" or alien to the system. The network includes signals between white cells (macrophages and lymphocytes) that lead to further amplified responses via the release of mediators of inflammatory responses. Thus different immune inflammatory events can involve different components of this network of signals.

induction, process of stimulating or activating gene expression to form messenger RNA.

infarction, a term for a region of dead tissue that is formed following continued lack of blood flow (ischemia).

inflammation, condition of localized immune cell response to stimuli that often involves redness, heat, pain, swelling, and loss of normal tissue function due to release of inflammatory mediators.

inflammatory, about inflammation.

interleukins (e.g., IL-6), a large family (more than a dozen) of cytokine proteins that provide intercellular communication by being released from one cell and binding to receptor on other cells; e.g., interleukin-1 (IL-1) is an inflammatory cytokine.

ischemia, a condition of reduced blood flow that can cause inadequate levels of oxygen and nutrients in a tissue and cause cell death if extended too long. Also spelled *ischaemia.*

ischemic heart disease, chronic impairment of blood flow to the heart muscle usually due to atherosclerosis. Also spelled *ischaemic.*

isoprostanes, a family of prostaglandin-like compounds formed during oxidant stress.

kinase, an enzyme that catalyzes placing a phosphate group on another molecule; glucokinase phosphorylates glucose and protein kinases phosphorylate proteins.

LDL (abbrev.), low-density lipoproteins, a family of complex mixtures of proteins and lipids resulting from progressive removal of fat by lipoprotein lipase action in the blood on VLDL precursors released earlier from the liver.

leukotriene, a class of polyunsaturated eicosanoids (LTA, LTB, LTC, LTD, and LTE) that is formed following the action of a lipoxygenase. These compounds have their double bonds rearranged to adjacent locations within the carbon chain and do not have the cyclic ring system that is present in prostaglandins.

linoleic acid, an 18-carbon fatty acid with two unsaturated (or double) bonds that are arranged with the last double bond six atoms from the end of the chain (making it an n-6 acid). It is the most common form of essential polyunsaturated fatty acid in our diet. The term, linoleate, refers to its derivatives.

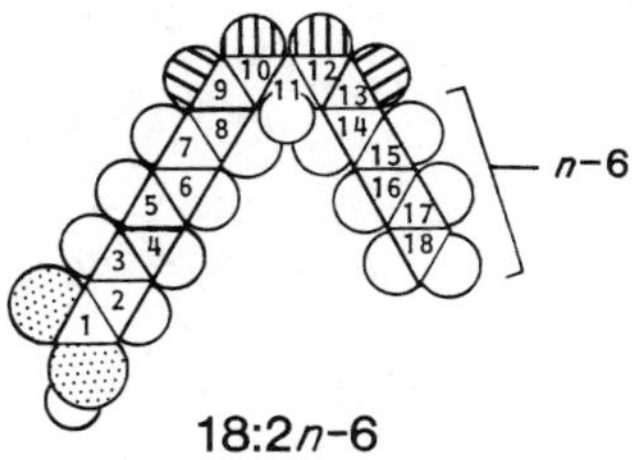

18:2*n*-6

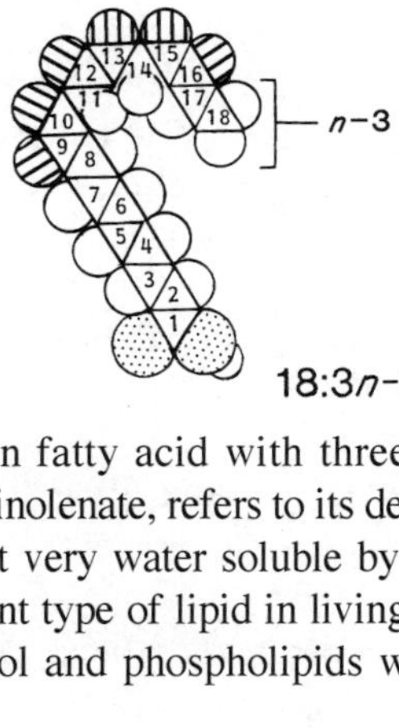

18:3*n*-3

linolenic acid, an 18-carbon fatty acid with three unsaturated bonds in an n-3 arrangement. The term, linolenate, refers to its derivatives.

lipid, a compound that is not very water soluble by virtue of its content of carbon atoms. The most abundant type of lipid in living tissues is fat, but other important forms are cholesterol and phospholipids which are present in cell membranes and lipoproteins.

lipoproteins, a complex of specific protein mixtures with lipids, including cholesterol. Low density lipoproteins are associated with increased atherosclerosis, whereas high density lipoproteins diminish atherogenic processes.

lipoxygenase, a type of oxidizing enzyme that catalyzes conversion of HUFA to leukotrienes.

macrophage, a white cell, or leukocyte, that can be activated to release inflammatory signaling molecules and promote inflammation.

MAPK (abbrev.), mitogen activated protein kinase, an enzyme in a signaling pathway from cell surface mitogen receptors which transmits the signal by phosphorylating specific sites on target proteins, modifying their continued action and altering cell physiology.

messenger, a term especially used to indicate special ribonucleic acid, messenger RNA (mRNA), that carries genetic code information and guides synthesis of new proteins.

monocytes, a white cell (leukocyte) that may engulf foreign materials and participate in immune inflammatory events.

multiple sclerosis, a disease of the nervous system that may result from an imbalanced immune regulation or an autoimmune disorder.

myocardial infarction, a condition of regional death of heart muscle usually due to impaired blood flow to the region.

n-3, "n minus three", a structural notation designating the location in a fatty acid of a double bond three carbons from the methyl terminus; i.e., the omega (or "nth" carbon) minus three position. Other structures include n-6, n-7 and n-9 arrangements.

neurohumoral, refers to a system of autacoid signaling involving nerves and the blood system

neutrophils, a white cell (leukocyte) that is the chief cell in the blood stream that engulfs foreign material and participates in inflammatory events.

NADH (abbrev.), reduced form of **nicotinamide adenine dinucleotide**,which carries electrons that can generate useful forms of energy during their transfer to oxygen. However, the alternate fate of reacting with NADH oxidase, produces reactive oxidant species that promote inflammatory and proliferative events.

NADPH (abbrev.), reduced form of **nicotinamide adenine dinucleotide phosphate**, which carries electrons that can generate useful forms of energy during their transfer to oxygen. However, the alternate fate of reacting with NADPH oxidase, produces reactive oxidant species that promote inflammatory and proliferative events.

NEFA (abbrev.), nonesterified fatty acids.

NFkappaB (abbrev.), nuclear factor kappa B, a very important activator of gene expression that carries signals to the nucleus from outer portions of the cell when triggered by signaling pathways.

NIDDM (abbrev.), noninsulin dependent diabetes mellitus.

nitric oxide (NO), this simple molecule of two atoms affects vascular dilation and tissue respiration.

NSAID (abbrev.), nonsteroidal anti-inflammatory drug, a family of therapeutic compounds that give benefits principally by inhibiting cycloxygenase and decreasing prostaglandin formation.

oleic acid, an 18-carbon unsaturated fatty acid of the n-9 type. It can be formed by our tissues and is abundant in olive oil.

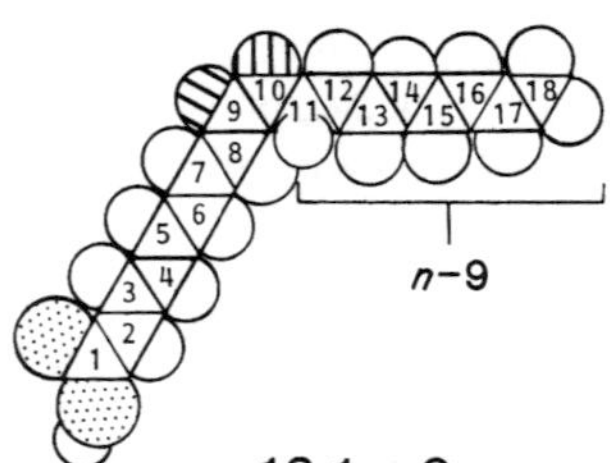

18:1n-9

oxidant, a molecule that accepts electrons from other molecules at different energy levels. Atmospheric oxygen is the ultimate oxidant for humans.

oxidase, an enzyme that catalyzes electron removal from a metabolite (i.e., oxidation).

p38, a phosphorylated protein of 38 kilodalton size, usually mitogen activated protein kinase (MAPK), which transmits the signal by phosphorylating specific sites on target proteins, modifying their continued action and altering cell physiology (see Chapter 5).

p42/44, phosphorylated proteins of 42 and 44 kilodalton size, usually extracellular receptor kinase (ERK), which transmit their signal by phosphorylating specific sites on target proteins, modifying their continued action and altering cell physiology (see Chapter 11).

parasympathetic, a major portion of the autonomic nervous system that complements the sympathetic system to maintain and regulate body functions without conscious attention.

PAF (abbrev.), platelet activating factor.

palmitoleic acid, a 16-carbon unsaturated fatty acid of the n-7 type that can be formed by our tissues.

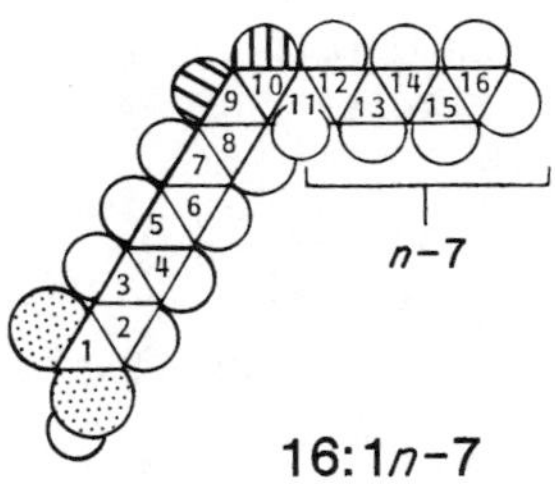

16:1n−7

PDAY (abbrev.), Pathobiological Determinants of Atherosclerosis in Youth, a large study of autopsy materials which showed evidence of the need for CHD primary prevention efforts to start before adolescence

PDGF (abbrev.), platelet derived growth factor, a cytokine that binds to cell receptors and triggers signaling pathways that alter cell functions

PGH (abbrev.), prostaglandin H, the intermediate formed from HUFA by cycloxygenase, which is then rearranged by various synthases to form PGD, PGE, PGF, PGI and thromboxane, TXA.

phagocytic, a cellular process of engulfing material to bring it inside the cell.

phosphatase, an enzyme that removes phosphate groups from molecules, reversing the action of kinases.

phospholipase, an enzyme that catalyzes cleavage of phospholipids.

phospholipid, a term for the complex water-insoluble compounds that contain fatty acids linked to glycerol and phosphate and are major components of cellular membranes.

PKC (abbrev.), protein kinase C is a phosphorylating enzyme that acts in signaling pathways to modify actions of other signaling proteins.

PLA (abbrev.), phospholipase A is an enzyme that releases fatty acids from phospholipids.

placebo, an untreated experimental component used to compare outcomes with treated components.

plasma, the fluid portion of blood in which the blood cells are suspended.

platelets, a specialized type of blood cell that adheres to blood vessel walls and can aggregate to form a plug or thrombus that stops blood flow.

polyunsaturated, description of a molecule containing two or more unsaturated (double bonds. The two main types are designated n-6 and n-3, and both types are essential nutrients. *Polyunsaturated fatty acids* can help lower the amounts of cholesterol and triglycerides in serum.

pre-β-lipoproteins, a type of lipoprotein in the blood that when present at elevated levels, is associated with risk of atherosclerosis.

postpartum, state of being immediately after birth of an infant.

postprandial, state of being immediately after a meal.

prostacyclin, a special type of prostaglandin that may be the most important antithrombotic eicosanoid. It is produced by endothelial cells of blood vessels.

prostaglandin, a type of compound derived from a polyunsaturated fatty acid by oxidation and rearrangement. Prostaglandins (PGD, PGE, PGF, PGG, PGH, PGI) contain a five-membered ring of carbon atoms and three or more oxygen atoms as shown in Chapter 14.

psoriasis, a chronic inflammatory disease of skin.

PTK (abbrev.), protein tyrosine kinase, an enzyme that phosphorylates specific tyrosine groups of target proteins, altering their interactions with other signaling proteins. The modification is reversed by protein tyrosine phosphatase (PTP) action.

PUFA (abbrev.), polyunsaturated fatty acid, fatty acids with two to six unsaturated groups (double bonds).

Ras, a nucleotide-binding protein important in signaling pathways linking the cell surface to the nucleus.

renal, refers to the kidney.

risk factor, a measurement that predicts (to some degree) the likelihood of developing a particular disease.

ROS (abbrev.), reactive oxidant species, molecules like hydrogen peroxide, superoxide and other peroxides that create oxidant stress conditions.

SAA (abbrev.), serum amyloid, a protein found in the blood and associated with neural health.

saturated, refers to carbon compounds in which all atomic connections are single bonds to either carbon or hydrogen and no carbons have double (unsaturated) bonds.

serum, the fluid portion of blood remaining after coagulation occurs that is similar but not identical to blood plasma (having altered the proteins during coagulation).

SHR (abbrev.), spontaneously hypertensive rats.

SLE (abbrev.), systemic lupus erythematosis, an immune disease with inflammatory aspects (Chapter 10).

sympathetic, a major portion of the autonomic nervous system that complements the parasympathetic system, coordinating tissue functions without conscious attention.

T-cells, thymus-related white cells, also called *leukocytes* or *lymphocytes*, that participate in immune system interactions as either T-helper (Th-1 or Th-2) or T-suppressor cells (see Chapter 10)

thrombocytes, platelets, the thrombus-forming cells of the bloodstream.

thrombosis, the formation of a blood clot of platelets and blood coagulation proteins within a blood vessel that restricts the flow of blood.

thrombotic, refers to thrombosis.

thromboxane, An eicosanoid derived from a prostaglandin intermediate. The active form, TXA, causes aggregation of platelets and contraction of muscles, but it rapidly degrades to inactive TXB.

tone, a condition balanced temporarily between rising and falling tendencies such as muscle tone, autonomic tone, neural tone or peroxide tone.

transcription, process of forming RNA from DNA prior to guiding protein synthesis.

triglycerides, a technical name for fat; the type of compound that has three fatty acids attached to glycerol.

TNF (abbrev.), alpha, tumor necrosis factor alpha, a major inflammatory cytokine

tyrosine kinase, refers to an enzyme transferring phosphate to a specific tyrosine in a protein.

unsaturated, refers to the portion of a carbon compound at which a double bond occurs between two carbons. That bond is regarded to be not fully saturated with hydrogen. The commercial conversion of polyunsaturated vegetable oils to the more saturated margarines is achithe cavity within a blood vessel through which blood flows.

About the Author

WILLIAM E. M. LANDS (Born: July 22, 1930, Chillicothe, Missouri) was Professor of Biochemistry at the University of Michigan (1955-1980) and the University of Illinois (1980-1991) where he studied the metabolism of fats, phospholipids, and prostaglandins. He authored over 250 papers and the book, *Fish and Human Health.* One of the world's 1000 most cited scientists in 1965-1978, he received numerous awards including the 1969 Glycerine Research Award, the 1979 Verhagen Lectureship at Rotterdam University, honorary membership in the Australian Rheumatism Association, the 1985 Pfizer Biomedical Research Award, the 1997 AOCS-Supelco Lipid Research Award and selection as a Fellow of the American Association for the Advancement of Science, the Society for Free Radical Biology and Medicine and the American Society for Nutritional Sciences. After retiring from university teaching, he directed the basic research program at the National Institute on Alcohol Abuse and Alcoholism (1990-1997) and served as Senior Scientific Advisor to the Director (1997-2002). He is now fully retired and serves on the board of directors of Omega Protein, Inc. He can be contacted at wemlands@att.net. Some of his research interests are in the reviews:

Lands, W.E.M. (1965) Lipid Metabolism. *Ann. Rev. Biochem. 34*, 313-346.

Lands, W.E.M. (1979) The Biosynthesis and Metabolism of Prostaglandins. *Ann. Rev. Physiol. 41*, 633-652.

Lands, W.E.M. (1991) Biosynthesis of Prostaglandins. *Annual Review of Nutrition 11*, 41-60.

Lands, W.E.M (1995) Cellular signals in alcohol-induced liver injury: A Review. *Alcoholism: Clin. & Exper. Resh, 19*: 928-938.

Lands, W.E.M (1998) A review of alcohol clearance in humans. *Alcohol 15*: 147-160.

Lands, W.E.M. (1999) Alcohol, slow wave sleep, and the somatotropic axis. *Alcohol 18*: 109-122.

Lands, WEM (2000) Stories about acyl chains. *Biochim. Biophys. Acta, 1483*: 1-15.

Lands, WEM (2002) Would it make a difference? *Inform* (two parts), 342-349; 418-422.

Lands, WEM. (2003) Functional foods in primary prevention or nutraceuticals in secondary prevention? *Current Topics in Nutraceutical Research 1(2)*: 113-120.

The shadows stretch
As we turn away
From the sun
To sleep—and dream
Of tomorrow.

Index

A

Acyl-CoA pathways
  biomarkers of EFA availability, 127–128
  catalysis of elongation and desaturation, 122
  competition among actions, 120–121
  conversion of foods, 121–122
  desaturase processes, 126–127
  described, 120
  impact of high dietary n-6 EFA, 125
  metabolic shifts due to competition, 123–125
  overeating consequences, 117–118, 125
  studies and data
    acyltransferase influences recognition, 130–132
    comparison of DPA and DHA, 132–133
    competition among actions, 129–130
    influences on gene expression, 133–134
  tissue acids changes after diet changes, 128–129
Alaskan natives. *See* Eskimos
Allergic responses, 13–14
Alpha-blockers, 65
American Heart Association, 32
Analgesics, 13
Antioxidants
  atherosclerosis and, 38–40
  oxidant stress inhibited by, 42
Antiplatelet Trial Collaboration, 52
Arachidonate
  conversion to eicosanoids, 47
  disease mechanism and, 13–15
  essentiality of, 21–22
Arrhythmias, 65
Arteriosclerosis, 18
Aspirin
  anti-inflammatory effect, 13
  coronary thrombosis and, 52–54
  inhibition of eicosanoids formation, 47
Asthma, 97–98
Atherosclerosis and serum lipids
  antioxidants and, 38–40
  atherosclerosis described, 31
  cause of atherosclerosis, 18
  cellular interactions involved, 34–35
  CHD lifetime risk development, 35–37
  diet-related inflammation and oxidative stress, 37–38
  inflammation markers as mediators, 42–43
  inflammatory process and EFA, 40–41
  lowering of lipids by dietary fish oils, 33–34
  mediation of cellular interactions by diet, 35
  oxidant stress inhibited by antioxidants, 42
  oxidative stress and inflammation, 41–42
Autacoids, 8, 16–17
Autoimmune disorders and hypertension, 78–80. *See also* immune system responses

B

Beta-blockers, 65

C

Cancer
  cellular DNA and, 105
  diet and, 108–109
  epidemiological comparisons, 108–109
  metastasis and eicosanoids, 106–108
  studies linking diet to, 109–110
Canola oil, 171

Cardiac output. *See* vascular spasm
Catecholamines, 76
Cell-mediated immunity, 83
Cereals, grains, and breads, 178
Cholesterol
anti-inflammatory effect of medications, 37–38
coronary disease and, 5–6
Coronary heart disease (CHD)
diet and, 5–6
ethnic differences in incidence, 9–11
factors involved in, 31–32
lifetime risk development, 35–37
Coronary thrombosis
aspirin and, 52–54
dietary connection studies and data, 55–58
dietary practices and, 50–52
fibrin formation and, 57–58
fish oil intake effects on platelet aggregation, 49–50
n-6 HUFA vs. HUFA intake in risk factors, 54–55
platelet function and eicosanoids, 47–49
COX-1/2/3, 109, 145–147
C-reactive protein (CRP), 42
Cyclooxygenase
blocking by aspirin, 52
different forms of, 145–147
link to cancer, 109
rate of action and prostaglandins, 143–144
requirement for hydroperoxide activator, 140–142
cytokines, 98

D

Dairy and egg products, 179
Danes
diabetes incidence and diet, 99
incidence of sickness and death, 3–4
DART trial, 53
Department of Agriculture, U.S. (USDA), 18, 178
DHA (docosahexaenoic acid), 43, 109
Diabetes, 99–101
Diet
alternative diets evaluation
decrease dietary linoleate/increase dietary linolenate, 188–189, 192
increase dietary n-3 HUFA, 189, 192
increase linoleate-based caloric intake, 186–187
lower n-6 acids intake, 187, 188, 192
recommendations, 189–190
asthma and, 97–98
average intake of fat per person, 172
biochemical links with disease, 115–118
cancer and, 108–110
connection to coronary thrombosis, 50–52, 55–58
coronary disease and, 5–6
diabetes and, 99–101
EFA and (*see* essential fatty acids)
fish oil and (*see* fish oil)
hydrogenation and oils, 172–173
imbalance in intake of n-6 to n-3, 24–25
individualized diet planning, web-based, 168
isolation and stability of, 182–184
lowering of lipids by dietary fish oils, 33–34
multiple sclerosis and, 96–97
n-3 EFA effects on, 33–34
need for primary prevention interventions, 191
nutritional factors role in disease, 6, 7, 9
overeating's impact on acyl-CoA esters, 117–118, 125
personal menu plans, 192, 193–199, 200
proportion of n-3 and n-6 HUFA in food pyramid categories, 178–181
prostaglandin formation following changes in, 152–153
questions to ask about food choices, 177
related inflammation and oxidative stress, 37–38
results of imbalances in n-6 and n-3 fats, 18
rheumatoid arthritis and, 90–93
sea vs. land-based, 3
sources of n-3 EFA, 171–172
stroke incidence related to, 71–73

systemic lupus erythematosis and, 94–95
worldwide diversity in food choices, 9
Disease
autacoids significance, 16–17
biochemical links with diet, 115–118
eicosanoids and, 5–6
ethnic differences in incidence, 9–11
factors involved in coronary disease, 31–32
focus on treating clinical signs, 17
health benefits from low n-6 eicosanoid signaling, 17
mechanism of, 13–15
mental disorders related to low n-3 EFA intake, 25–26
nutritional factors role in, 6, 7
PUFA relationship to, 14, 15–16
results of dietary imbalances in n-6 and n-3 fats, 18
risk factors for, 8
studies on disease incidence, 10–11
Docosahexaenoic acid (DHA), 43, 109

E

EAE (experimental allergic encephalomyelitis), 95
EFA. *See* essential fatty acids
Eicosanoids
cancer metastasis and, 106–108
disease and, 5–6
leukotrienes (*see* leukotrienes)
platelet function and, 47–49
prostaglandins (*see* prostaglandins)
significance of, 17
Eicosapentaenoic acid (EPA), 43
18:3n-3. *See* n-3 EFA
Endocannabinoids, 18–19
Eskimos
asthma incidence and diet, 98
diabetes incidence and diet, 99
incidence of sickness and death, 3–4
n-3 EFA intake, 49–50
salt intake and incidence of stroke, 71
studies on disease incidence, 10, 11
Essential fatty acids (EFA)
acyl-CoA pathways and, 127–128
brain development and, 26–27
dermal symptoms from deficit, 27
examples of content in foods, web-based, 178
imbalance in intake of n-6 to n-3, 24–25
n-6 activity, 21
n-6 dietary levels, 22–24
pituitary function and, 27–28
results of n-3 deficits, 25–26
risk factors for disease and, 8
vascular flammatory process and, 40–41
Experimental allergic encephalomyelitis (EAE), 95

F

Fish and seafood, 180
Fish oil
alternatives to, 176–177
chemical composition of n-3 HUFA in, 173
economics of, 174
intake effects on platelet aggregation, 49–50
isolation and stability of, 182–184
lowering of lipids by dietary, 33–34
pattern of PUFA in fish, 181–182
production of, 181
sources of, 171–172
sources of fatty acids in fish, 174, 175
world production, 173
Flaxseed oil, 171
Food pyramid, 178–181
Fruits, 179

G

GISSI-Prevenzione trial, 53
Greenland, 3, 10, 11

H

HDL (high density lipoprotein), 37
Heart attacks
coronary thrombosis (*see* coronary thrombosis)
factors involved, 31–32
incidence among maritime people, 3

Heart disease
atherosclerosis (*see* atherosclerosis and serum lipids)
factors involved, 31–32
Heparin, 72
High density lipoprotein (HDL), 37
Highly unsaturated fatty acid (HUFA), 23, 165–167. *See also* n-3 EFA
Histamine, 16–17
Homocysteine, 43
Humoral immunity, 83
Hypertension
autoimmune disorders and, 78–80
described, 75
dietary n-3 fatty acids impact on, 76–77
immune system markers and, 77–78
stroke and, 71, 73
studies and data, 78–80

I

Immune system responses
adaptive, 83–84
asthma, 97–98
autoimmune disorders and hypertension, 78–80
diabetes, 99–101
intervention targets, 84–86
mediators and modulators of, 87–89, 90
multiple sclerosis, 95–97
rheumatoid arthritis, 90–93
systemic lupus erythematosis, 93–95
T-helper and T-suppressor cells, 86–87, 98
Infarction, 31
Inflammatory disorders, 13–14
Ischemia, 31
Isoprostanes, 42–43

J

Japan
asthma incidence and diet, 98
death rates from specific diseases, 7
heart attack incidence, 3, 4
salt intake and incidence of stroke, 71

K

Keep It Managed (KIM), 178, 192

L

LDL (low density lipoprotein), 37
Leukotrienes
contribution to disease, 14–15
immune system mediation and, 87–89
lipoxygenase pathway, 155–157
lipoxygenase products, 157–158
mediation of cellular responses and, 35
Linoleic acid, 21, 22
Linseed oil, 171
Lipoxygenase
pathway, 155–157
products, 157–158
Low density lipoprotein (LDL), 37
LTB/LTC/LTD. *See* leukotrienes
Lyon Diet Heart Study, 53

M

Maritime populations, 3–4
Meat, fish, and legumes, 179–180
Menu plans, 192, 193–199, 200
Multiple sclerosis, 95–97

N

n-3 EFA. *See also* essential fatty acids; fish oil
autoimmune disorders and, 94–95
chemical composition in fish oils, 173
effects on diet, 33–34
hypertension impacted by, 76–77
platelet function and, 51
proportion in food pyramid categories, 178–181
research studies, 184
sources of, 171–172
sources of in fats and oils, 171–172
n-6 EFA
activity of, 21
acyl-CoA pathways and, 125

brain development and, 26–27
dietary levels, 22–24
health benefits from preventing excessive signaling of, 17
heart disease and, 9
immune system mediation and, 88–89
n-6 HUFA vs. HUFA intake in risk factors, 54–55
nutritional imbalances with n-3, 18
proportion in food pyramid categories, 178–181
Nitric oxide, 17
NSAIDS, 143
Nurses' Health Study, 71

O

Omega-3. *See* n-3 EFA

P

PAF acetylhydrolase, 37
Paraoxonase, 37
Pathobiological Determinants of Atherosclerosis in Youth (PDAY), 18, 35
PGE receptors, 148. *See also* prostaglandins
PGH, 139. *See also* prostaglandins
PGI, 63
Physicians' Health Study, 52
Pituitary function
cyclooxygenase activity and, 145
EFA intake and, 27–28
Polyunsaturated fatty acids (PUFA)
analysis of populations, 168–169
dietary balance questions, 163
dietary linoleate intake changes impact, 164–165
in fish oils, 175
HUFA proportions available in tissues, 165–167
pattern in fish, 181–182
in plant oils, 176–177
relationship to disease, 14, 15–16
sources available to fish, 174
Pork, turkey, and chicken, 180
Prostacyclin, 15, 48
Prostaglandins
cancer metastasis and, 106–108
contribution to disease, 13–14
cyclooxygenase requirement for hydroperoxide activator, 140–142
cyclooxygenases forms, 145–147
factors involved in autacoid actions of, 142–143
formation following diet changes, 152–153
immune system mediation and, 87–89
mediation of cellular responses and, 35
oxidative pathways, 139–140
platelet function and, 47
rate of cyclooxygenase action and, 143–144
receptors, 147–148
receptor specificities, 148
selectivity of biosynthesis, 140, 141
vascular spasm and, 63–65

R

Rainbow trout, 27
Rapeseed oil, 171
Red wine consumption and atherosclerosis, 39
Rheumatoid arthritis, 90–93

S

Salt intake and incidence of stroke, 71, 75
Serotonin, 17
Serum amyloid A (SAA), 42
Serum lipids. *See* atherosclerosis and serum lipids
Soybean oil, 171, 172
Strokes
factors involved, 31–32
incidence related to diet, 71
salt intake and, 71, 75
vascular causes, 71–72
Sunflower oil, 171
Systemic lupus erythematosis, 78, 93–95

T

T-helper and T-suppressor cells, 86–87, 98
Thrombosis, 31
Thrombosis Prevention Trial, 52
Thromboxane, 9, 15, 47, 48, 53
Type-2 diabetes, 100

U

United States, 7
USDA (Department of Agriculture, U.S.), 18, 178

V

Vascular spasm
  described, 31
  extreme heart rhythms, 65–66
  prostaglandin and, 63–65
  studies and data, 66–67
  sudden death and, 66
  vasoconstriction defined, 63
Vegetable oil, 172
Vegetables, 178–179
Vitamins, 16